Health-Promoting and Health-Compromising Behaviors Among Minority Adolescents

Edited by Dawn K. Wilson, James R. Rodrigue, and Wendell C. Taylor

American Psychological Association
Washington, DC

Published by
American Psychological Association
750 First Street, NE
Washington, DC 20002

Copies may be ordered from
American Psychological Association
Order Department
P.O. Box 92984
Washington, DC 20090-2984

In the UK and Europe, copies may be ordered from
American Psychological Association
3 Henrietta Street
Covent Garden, London
WC2E 8LU England

Typeset in Palatino by PRO-Image Corporation, Techna Type Div., York, PA

Printer: Data Reproductions Corp., Rochester Hills, MI
Cover Designer: Jennifer Pritchard, Baltimore, MD
Technical/Production Editor: Catherine R. Worth

Library of Congress Cataloging-in-Publication Data
Health-promoting and health-compromising behaviors among minority
    adolescents / edited by Dawn K. Wilson, James R. Rodrique,
    Wendell C. Taylor.
        p.   cm.
    Includes bibliographical references and index
    ISBN 1-55798-397-6 (acid-free paper)
        1. Minority tennagers—Health and hygiene—United States.
    2. Minority teenagers—Health risk assessment—United States.
    3. Health promotion—United States.   4. Health behavior in
    adolescence—United States.   I. Wilson, Dawn K.   II. Rodrigue,
    James R.   III. Taylor, Wendell C.
    RJ102.H438   1996
    613'.0433'08693—dc20   96-34967
                                                                        CIP

British Library Cataloguing-in-Publication Data
A CIP record is available from the British Library

Printed in the United States of America
First edition

To the optimal health and wellness of all children,
especially minority adolescents, who have unique health
concerns during this critical stage of development.

Contents

Contributors

Jose O. Arrom, Midwest Latino Health Research Training and Policy Center, The Jane Addams College of Social Work, University of Illinois at Chicago

Bettina M. Beech, Tulane University Medical Center

Gilbert J. Botvin, Institute for Prevention Research, Cornell University Medical College

Ronald L. Braithwaite, Rollins School of Public Health, Emory University

Michael J. Brondino, Family Services Research Center, Department of Psychiatry and Behavioral Sciences, Medical University of South Carolina

Cleopatra Howard Caldwell, Institute for Social Research, University of Michigan

Kristin Cole, Columbia University School of Social Work

Sharon S. Cummings, Center for Health Promotion Research and Development, School of Public Health, University of Texas–Houston Health Science Center

Phillippe B. Cunningham, Family Services Research Center, Department of Psychiatry and Behavioral Sciences, Medical University of South Carolina

Mary Ann Forgey, Fordham University School of Social Work

Lawrence Friedman, Division of Adolescent Medicine, Department of Pediatrics, School of Medicine, University of California—San Diego

Aida L. Giachello, Midwest Latino Health Research Training and Policy Center, The Jane Addams College of Social Work, University of Illinois at Chicago

Barbara J. Guthrie, School of Nursing, University of Michigan

W. Rodney Hammond, School of Professional Psychology, Wright State University, Ellis Human Development Institute

Helen P. Hazuda, Clinical Epidemiology Division, Department of Medicine, University of Texas–San Antonio Health Science Center

Scott W. Henggeler, Family Services Research Center, Department of Psychiatry and Behavioral Sciences, Medical University of South Carolina

Andrea G. Hunter, Department of Psychology, University of Michigan

James S. Jackson, Institute for Social Research, University of Michigan

Robert M. Kaplan, Department of Family and Preventive Medicine, Division of Health Care Sciences, School of Medicine, University of California—San Diego

Jenelle S. Krishnamoorthy, Department of Internal Medicine, Division of Clinical Pharmacology and Hypertension, Medical College of Virginia, Virginia Commonwealth University

JoAnne Kuo, Rollins School of Public Health, Emory University

Celia M. Lescano, Center for Pediatric Psychology Research, University of Florida Health Science Center

Ana Monterrosa, General Medicine Division, Department of Internal Medicine, University of Texas–San Antonio Health Science Center

Susan C. Nicholson, Department of Internal Medicine, Division of Clinical Pharmacology and Hypertension, Medical College of Virginia, Virginia Commonwealth University

Roberta L. Paikoff, Institute for Juvenile Research, Department of Psychiatry, University of Illinois, Chicago

Sheila H. Parfenoff, Institute for Juvenile Research, Department of Psychiatry, University of Illinois, Chicago

Susan G. Pickrel, Family Services Research Center, Department of Psychiatry and Behavioral Sciences, Medical University of South Carolina

Ken Resnicow, Rollins School of Public Health, Emory University

James R. Rodrigue, Center for Pediatric Psychology Research, University of Florida Health Science Center

Melisa D. Rowland, Family Services Research Center, Department of Psychiatry and Behavioral Sciences, Medical University of South Carolina

Lawrence M. Scheier, Institute for Prevention Research, Cornell University Medical Center

Steven Schinke, Columbia University School of Social Work

Sonja K. Schoenwald, Family Services Research Center, Department of Psychiatry and Behavioral Sciences, Medical University of South Carolina

Sherrill L. Sellers, Institute for Social Research, University of Michigan

Wendell C. Taylor, Center for Health Promotion Research and Development, School of Public Health, University of Texas–Houston Health Science Center

Kenneth P. Tercyak, Jr., Center for Pediatric Psychology Research, University of Florida Health Science Center

Dawn K. Wilson, Department of Internal Medicine, Division of Clinical Pharmacology and Hypertension, Medical College of Virginia, Virginia Commonwealth University

Betty R. Yung, Ellis Human Development Institute, School of Professional Psychology, Wright State University

Foreword

The Division of Health Psychology (Division 38) of the American Psychological Association presents the third volume in its series highlighting the application and practice of health psychology. One of the driving forces behind the establishment of the division was interest in health promotion and disease prevention and treatment through the application of principles and procedures that were emerging in the research arena. The vitality of health psychology depends on an active dialogue between its researchers and practitioners. One of the important goals of the series is to further expand this dialogue. Attempts to translate research findings into applications and interventions, to test and evaluate the efficacy of these interventions, and to denote important clinical experiences and research needs of the practice of health psychology are the focus of these volumes. Transfer of knowledge; feedback to researchers regarding needs, failures, and successes of clinical interventions; and facilitation and expansion of necessary dialogue between scientist and practitioner are the objectives.

Toward these aims, the volumes in this series are meant to function as vehicles for translating research into practice, with an analysis of issues related to the evaluation, prevention, and treatment of health behaviors and health problems. These goals are met by treating clinical or applied health psychology as broadly as possible, including community and public health assessment and intervention methods and problems of health care use. Issues are considered across a variety of settings, including hospitals, the practitioner's office, community clinics, work-site settings, schools, and managed care settings. Each volume provides direction in areas of need and populations to be served by health psychology intervention; critically examines issues and problems involved in clinical evaluation, prevention, and treatment of specific disorders; and illustrates the effectiveness of novel clinical approaches to diagnosis and treatment that may guide future research and innovation. Each volume focuses on a topic, such as this book's emphasis on health promotion in minorities, and synthesizes research on a range of topics to reinforce the theoretical and scientific rationale for the practice of health psychology and to identify critical issues in the prevention, assessment, and management of health problems.

Andrew Baum
Margaret Chesney

Preface

Many health behaviors are undoubtedly established early in life, yet more attention—by clinicians, scientists, and laypeople—is needed to better understand the development of these behaviors, especially among children and adolescents. While attending both regional and national conferences on child and adolescent health over the past decade, we have been struck by several important issues. First, it is commonly believed that a majority of adolescents experiment with high-risk behaviors but that the study of such behavior in adolescents will yield little understanding of subsequent health behaviors in adulthood. Also, we have heard many comments from colleagues suggesting that adolescents are resistant to interventions and, therefore, any attempt to modify behavior during this stage of the developmental life cycle will result in little gain. In fact, many professionals have commented that "riding out the storm of adolescence" until adulthood is the only solution to the problem, implying that high-risk behaviors will somehow change or improve once adolescents reach adulthood. In sharp contrast to these perceptions, research has clearly shown that many high-risk health behaviors such as sexual activity, tobacco use, and alcohol use begin during adolescence and continue throughout adulthood. Thus, in our view, adolescence is the ideal developmental period in which to intervene and establish health behavior patterns that will set the stage for adulthood.

The United States is unquestionably a diverse country, with many different cultures and varying attitudes toward health and behavior. African American, Hispanic, Asian, and Native American populations have all grown considerably in recent years, yet many health providers continue to view health behavior through ethnocentric lenses or stereotypical filters, without considering the diverse cultural and sociopolitical influences affecting the health of minorities. Indeed, minorities are at increased risk for numerous health problems. However, despite the fact that behaviors—such as poor diet, substance abuse, lack of exercise, and high-risk sexual activity—are at the root of most health problems, the professional community and public have been slow to develop health-promotion programs for U.S. minority youth.

In this book, we attempt to highlight the scope of the health problems facing children and adolescents in this country, with special consideration of minority adolescents. Our intent was to bring together researchers and clinicians who work directly with minority youth in the conceptualization, design, implementation, and evaluation of health-promotion programs. This provides the reader with useful clinical information and a review of which interventions are effective, and under what circumstances, for minority youth. Clinicians, researchers, and students from many disciplines (e.g., psychology, psychiatry, pediatrics, health services, social work, sociology, public health, nursing, and medicine) will find this book useful as they consider how to best influence the health behaviors of these populations.

We would especially like to thank a number of colleagues who have provided us and fellow contributors with helpful suggestions for improving the quality and focus of this volume: Lucile L. Adams-Campbell, Norman B. Anderson, John N. Austin, Tom Baranowski, Karl Bauman, Charles Bordvin, Lesley Foulkes-Jamison, Linda M. Freeman, Gary Geffken, Michael Harris, Jonathan D. Klein, Shiriki Kumanyika, Karol Kumpfer, Velma McBride Murry, Mario A. Orlandi, Lawrence A. Palinkas, Vera S. Paster, LaVome Robinson, James F. Sallis, Kathy Sanders-Phillips, Mareasa Isaacs Shockley, Robert F. St. Peter, and Eric Weston. We are also grateful to Andrew Baum, who was instrumental in helping us to produce this volume, and to Kerry A. Todd for her outstanding secretarial support. Finally, Dawn K. Wilson would especially like to thank her husband, Greg King, for his support and understanding throughout the process of developing this volume.

James R. Rodrigue
Dawn K. Wilson
Wendell C. Taylor

Introduction

Because of the increasingly alarming prevalence rate of disease among minority populations, primary prevention will become a top national priority by the Year 2000. The adolescent years are a critical transition period, and during this time, youth experiment with health-compromising and health-promoting behaviors. Effective programs that are culturally sensitive to minority adolescents are needed to encourage health-promoting behaviors. The purpose of this volume is to provide an overview of relevant health behaviors that are of primary concern to adolescents of diverse ethnic backgrounds. The ethnic groups that are addressed in this book primarily include African Americans, Hispanics (including Puerto Ricans and Mexican Americans), Asians (Pacific Islanders and Asian Americans), and Native Americans. Research on the health behavior of adolescents in these specific ethnic groups is lacking. In fact, many investigators have combined these unique ethnic groups with little consideration for their distinct linguistic and sociocultural heritages. With these issues in mind, this volume provides a basis for guiding, in particular, clinicians and health care professionals in their efforts to understand and develop innovative approaches for intervening in minority adolescent populations. There are three central themes in the book: (a) highlighting the similarities and differences across diverse ethnic groups of adolescents while keeping in mind that the heterogeneity between and within these populations is of utmost importance, (b) emphasizing innovative and culturally based approaches to prevention, and (c) highlighting the clinical applications and elements that will assist health care providers in facilitating health behavior change among minority adolescent populations.

The first part of the book provides a theoretical framework for understanding minority adolescent health behaviors. The two chapters in this part point to the importance of developmental, biological, and sociocultural perspectives of conceptualizing adolescent health and provide the foundation for the remaining chapters of the book. For the purposes of this volume, we define *adolescence* on the basis of standards developed by the Society for Research in Adolescence, which recognize three stages of adolescence: early adolescence (ages 10–14 years), middle adolescence (ages 15–17 years), and late adolescence (ages 18–20). These stages have important implications for understanding adolescent health-related behaviors. The first chapter in Part I highlights the need to consider maturational transitions from childhood through adolescence. In particular, minority adolescents may be at increased risk of engaging in health-compromising behaviors because of racial and socioeconomic circumstances. Chapter 2 also emphasizes the need to consider sociocultural and generational–historical perspectives on adolescent minority health. This chapter provides a comprehensive life-course perspective for understanding cultural issues in targeted populations. Together, these chapters provide a unique perspective for conceptualizing and developing sound behavioral interventions targeted at minority adolescent populations.

Clinicians and health care providers are particularly interested in understanding the unique health problems that minority adolescents face. Adolescence is a challenging time, in that young people begin to make the transition into adulthood and are confronted with complex issues including autonomy, intimacy, and decision making about health-related behaviors. Because this period is a critical time of transition, adolescents who experience difficulties in making this transition may engage in a number of health-compromising behaviors. The second part of the book comprises six chapters that provide an overview of health-risk behaviors and health-promoting behaviors that are of primary concern to minority adolescents. Health-compromising behaviors are reviewed which include drug abuse, violence, sexually transmitted diseases (HIV and AIDS), teenage pregnancy, and eating disorders. Increasing evidence suggests that minority adolescents are more likely to engage in behavioral patterns that may result in detrimental health consequences. The chapters in Part II provide an interesting perspective on how to positively restructure the context in which minority youth make health-related choices. Several chapters also advocate increasing health-promoting behaviors, such as physical activity and healthy dietary habits. These chapters highlight the need for conceptualizing the determinants and the complex interactions of the environment, individual, and genetic influences in designing appropriate interventions. Because female adolescents in particular face unique health concerns, this group is specifically addressed in one chapter. In addition, one chapter presents a review of health behaviors that are relevant to preventing chronic illness within specific minority groups. In summary, Part II provides the clinician with a basis for selecting appropriate health behaviors and developing effective treatment approaches that match the individual needs of ethnically diverse adolescent groups.

The third part of the book focuses on examining a wide range of clinical interventions with special relevance to minority adolescent health. The four chapters in this part examine interpersonal, family-based, school-based, and community-based interventions. Each of the interventions reviewed are based in theory and have been empirically tested. The theoretical perspectives addressed include social–cognitive theory, family systems theory, and socioecological principles. These intervention approaches are particularly relevant for clinicians and health care providers because they examine the application of interventions from a clinical and public health perspective. This is especially relevant given the increasing need to provide the clinician with better guidelines for implementing therapeutic skills that will be effective among adolescent minority groups. At the same time, from a public health perspective, it has become necessary to provide clear evidence for the appropriateness and efficacy of various treatments. In short, the chapters in Part III provide excellent guidelines for conducting minority-focused interventions that are applicable in diverse settings and across multiple health-related contexts.

The final part of the book explores future directions and special concerns for minority adolescents with respect to health care access and policy issues. For the clinician and health care provider, these issues are particularly pertinent for understanding barriers within the health care system that may restrict efforts to promote healthy lifestyle changes among minority youth. Minority adolescents are at particularly high risk for having limited access to the health care system and for having little or no health insurance coverage. Unfortunately, this group is often overlooked in terms of relative importance when health policy is developed because adolescents tend to have little or no immediate illness. The two chapters in Part IV do an excellent job of outlining pertinent issues with regard to access and health-related policy. Chapter 13 suggests that poverty may be particularly instrumental in restricting minority families from health care access and provides practical solutions for facilitating access among minority adolescent groups. Chapter 14 also provides an enlightening perspective of health care policy issues as they apply to minority adolescent populations, offering specific suggestions for altering health initiatives that are particularly relevant to minority adolescent populations. Overall, the chapters in Part IV give an excellent summary of the health policy issues that must be addressed with regard to the specific needs of minority adolescents.

In summary, this volume specifically examines the importance of advocating healthy lifestyles among minority adolescent populations, who are at increased risk for particular health problems. Adolescents who are disadvantaged because of financial and environmental constraints face increased odds of engaging in health-risk behaviors that may have profound effects on their long-term health status. Throughout the volume, innovative and culturally appropriate interventions for clinicians and health care providers are highlighted that may improve the quality of life and longevity of culturally diverse groups of adolescents.

Dawn K. Wilson
James R. Rodrigue
Wendell C. Taylor

I

Conceptual Framework for Understanding Minority Adolescent Health

INTRODUCTION

Conceptual Framework for Understanding Minority Adolescent Health

Part I of the book gives the conceptual foundation for understanding adolescent health behaviors. Adolescence is a dynamic developmental stage that may be strongly influenced by biological as well as sociocultural factors. This part consists of two chapters that highlight the developmental and maturational issues and the psychological, social, and cultural issues that will help clinicians and health care providers in their health-promotion efforts. Specifically, chapter 1 provides an overview of the physical, interpersonal, cognitive, and socioemotional issues brought about by puberty. Chapter 2 expands on this by providing a theoretical perspective for understanding the sociocultural and historical context that is an essential part of comprehending minority adolescent health behaviors.

In chapter 1, Parfenoff and Paikoff review the developmental and biological aspects of minority adolescents' maturational transitions from childhood through adolescence. The authors specifically consider race and sociocultural context (i.e., poverty) as key elements that affect whether adolescents will engage in health risk behaviors. Research has suggested that early maturational development may lead to increased sexual activity, especially among female minority adolescents. The importance of involving family, peers, and the community in health-promotion efforts is also emphasized. However, as youth enter later adolescence, such issues as the pursuit of adult responsibilities and the need for establishing independence from parents become more prominent. Thus, at this stage, intervention efforts should focus on the unique individual needs of adolescents, who are faced with complex choices.

3

In chapter 2, Jackson and Sellers give a psychological, social, and cultural perspective of minority adolescent health. These authors highlight the need to better examine the sociocultural and historical contexts in which adolescents are embedded. This chapter provides a conceptualization for the use of race, ethnicity, and culture in research on adolescent health from a life-course perspective. Such a perspective emphasizes the need to examine cultural strengths and structural barriers in designing health-promotion efforts for adolescents. In summary, the chapters in Part I emphasize the importance of conceptualizing minority adolescent health within an appropriate context and provide an excellent introduction for understanding why adolescents experiment with health-compromising and health-promoting behaviors. In addition, these theoretical perspectives help shape the pathway for developing effective interventions within minority adolescent populations.

Dawn K. Wilson

1

Developmental and Biological Perspectives on Minority Adolescent Health

Sheila H. Parfenoff and Roberta L. Paikoff

Minority adolescents in the United States are at high risk for numerous health problems, yet they are far less likely to have a regular source of medical care than either young children or adults (National Research Council, 1993). Most of these problems are related to patterns of behavior set in earlier developmental phases, which occur in response to environments; therefore, the salient causes of many of these problems are preventable (Millstein, Peterson, & Nightingale, 1993). How should efforts be designed so that they effectively

We gratefully acknowledge the support of the National Institute of Mental Health Office on AIDS (Grant 1R01 MH50423-02) and the William T. Grant Foundation Faculty Scholar Award (to Roberta L. Paikoff) during the completion of this chapter. We wish to thank Stephanie Williams for her assistance with the preparation of this manuscript.

work to prevent health problems in minority adolescents and additionally serve to promote health behaviors? Mainly, prevention efforts should be concerned with adolescent development such that particular health issues are addressed at the appropriate time (e.g., delay of early sexual debut before the age of exposure to sexual activity). In addition, prevention efforts are expected to be most effective when they are designed to be sensitive to cultural and ethnic issues (Earls, 1993). In this chapter, we focus on biological and contextual factors assumed to be central to the transitions into and out of adolescence, particularly for ethnic minority adolescents. We begin with a discussion of the transition into adolescence, focusing on the physical, interpersonal, cognitive, and socioemotional issues brought about by puberty. We then briefly explore some of the issues adolescents must confront when making the transition from adolescence into adulthood.

Biology and Developmental Psychology

Adolescence is a period of transition and change from childhood to adulthood. Adolescents experience physical change as they reach puberty and sexual maturity as well as changes in their cognitive abilities, social–emotional selves, and social contexts (Brooks-Gunn, 1989; Brooks-Gunn & Paikoff, 1992). These changes have numerous implications for the development of health behaviors that promote health or lead to health risk. Because adolescence is a period of transformation, it is a time of opportunity for encouraging health-promoting behaviors that will lead to a healthier adulthood.

The field of developmental psychology recognizes the importance of transitions as periods of preparation for the next stage of development (Montemayor, Adams, & Gullotta, 1990). These developmental transitions are challenging, and the individual's response to the challenge as well as the context in which he or she meets the challenge can lead to divergent developmental pathways (Peterson & Ebata, 1987). Adolescence is influenced by the resources and vulnerabilities acquired during childhood and the expectations one has for adulthood. In addition to examining such individual factors as resilience and vulnerability, a developmental psychological perspective also examines sociocultural influences on development that can lead to various trajectories or paths of health behavior, particularly as individuals can select contexts (Scarr & McCartney, 1983). Social, economic, and structural forces will likely influence the resources available to the adolescent. Therefore, opportunities for healthy development—physical health as well as psychological well-being—are influenced by ethnicity, minority status, gender, and poverty level (Crockett & Peterson, 1993).

The Transition Into Adolescence

Puberty. Puberty is a set of biological events that mark the beginning of reproductive maturity. These events include hormonal changes, pubic hair growth, genital development, breast and facial hair growth, and the growth spurt. Some of these events are purely physical (e.g., pubic hair growth), whereas others are both physical and social because they are visible to others (e.g., breast and facial hair growth). Many scholars believe that adolescence begins with the onset of puberty. However, although the sequence of biological events in puberty is similar across cultures, the timing of these events varies (Brooks-Gunn & Reiter, 1990). The physical and social nature of puberty and varying rates of timing for the events of puberty combine to produce a complex psychological process for the young adolescent. Many researchers have examined the effects of pubertal status and variation in timing of pubertal events in terms of the subsequent psychosocial and behavioral outcomes for adolescents (see Buchanan, Eccles, & Becker, 1992; Paikoff & Brooks-Gunn, 1991, for reviews). Overall, effects of puberty on psychosocial factors appear linked more frequently to pubertal timing than to pubertal status (Connolly, Paikoff, & Buchanan, in press).

Early developing females reach adult biological status before their male and female peers, putting them in a position of being different (not a comfortable state for young adolescents, who desire conformity). As a result, some evidence suggests, early maturing girls may experience unhappiness and lower self-esteem (Susman, Nottelmann, Inoff-Germain, Dorn, & Chrousos, 1987). Research has also indicated that because of their physical appearance, early maturing girls may interact with older boys and begin sexual activity earlier than other girls, putting them at greater risk for sexually transmitted diseases and pregnancy (Hayes & Hofferth, 1987; Stattin & Magnusson, 1990). Irwin and Millstein (1992) have suggested that early maturing girls with older peers may also expose themselves to other health risks, such as early substance use and motor vehicle accidents.

The effects of early maturation may be more problematic for urban minority adolescent girls who live in communities with drug problems. These girls are likely to be exposed to situations that require mature decision making regarding social pressure to engage in health-risk behaviors, such as early sexual activity and substance use. This process may operate for early maturing boys as well. Some research has pointed to risk for early development in boys as well as girls (Irwin, Millstein, Adler, & Turner, 1989; Westney, Jenkins, Butts, & Williams, 1984); however, early maturation for boys is less "off the time" with regard to the peer group than is the case for early maturing girls. More research is needed to examine the nature of experiences for urban minority girls and boys who mature early. This is particularly true given the well-known data regarding ethnic differences in pubertal timing (Brooks-Gunn & Reiter, 1990). For example, African American children hit all developmental milestones earlier than other children, which may in part account for reported differences in onset of sexual activity (Centers for Disease Control and Prevention [CDC], 1992).

Representing the opposite end of the spectrum of variation in pubertal development are late maturing boys. This group has not been studied as closely as early maturing girls; however, a psychosocial perspective does raise some interesting questions regarding health risks specific to such boys. For example, research has found that late maturing boys may be at a social disadvantage compared with other boys (Irwin & Millstein, 1986), perhaps because they do not yet have the physical attributes that are valued for males (i.e., muscular build and height). Researchers (e.g., Irwin & Millstein, 1986) have postulated that late maturing boys are more likely to take health risks as a form of gaining recognition. For example, to compensate for a lack of sexual development, such boys may engage in substance use and reckless behavior (e.g., unsafe driving).

In addition to puberty, many other changes occur during adolescence. Social relationships begin to change, advanced cognitive abilities develop, and self-definitional issues arise (i.e., identity and individuation). The physical changes of puberty and the psychosocial and cognitive changes are believed to influence one another and, thus, should be considered in conjunction with one another (Paikoff & Brooks-Gunn, 1991). We begin by discussing the changes that adolescence brings to social relationships.

Puberty and family relationships. The transition into adolescence is believed to be a time of realignment for the parent–child relationship, with parents and children renegotiating issues of autonomy and control (Holmbeck, Paikoff, & Brooks-Gunn, 1995). Findings from the literature do indicate some impact of puberty on the relationship between parents and their children. Specifically, with physical maturity, father–son relationships change such that there are increases in emotional distance (Steinberg, 1987), and fathers increase their assertiveness while sons decrease their assertiveness (Steinberg, 1981). Physically mature girls have also been shown to experience more conflict with parents during puberty, particularly with their mothers (Hill, 1988).

To date, much of the research in this area has been conducted with White, middle-class, two-parent families (Paikoff & Brooks-Gunn, 1991; Spencer & Dornbusch, 1990). However, with the increasing emphasis on understanding normative developmental processes in minority human development, this focus is likely to change. For example, in our study of African American preadolescents living in urban poverty (and largely in single-parent, female-headed families; Sagrestano, Parfenoff, Paikoff, & Holmbeck, 1995), we found effects of physical maturation and pubertal timing on boys' relationships with their mothers. However, we found no such effects for girls, although we did find other pubertal timing effects. Continued work with our sample (particularly at longitudinal follow-up, which will enable more extensive analyses of pubertal timing as well as status) and with others will further understanding of the degree to which normative developmental processes vary across cultures, social classes, and family structures.

In addition to parent–child relationships, sibling relationships may be important in understanding family processes during the transition to adolescence. Siblings are thought to have a more direct effect on each other than parents, and siblings serve as models for one another (Abramovitch, Corter, Pepler, & Stanhope, 1986; Bryant & DeMorris, 1992). Also, older siblings may serve as caretakers for younger siblings, with such caregiving arrangements likely to range from health-enhancing to less adaptive situations for both siblings, depending on family functioning. In our research with African American preadolescents and their families (Sagrestano et al., 1995), approximately 7% of the parents named older children as caregivers for younger children.

This research and the research of others may begin to examine possible psychological health effects that might occur for older siblings charged with caring for younger siblings, as well as effects on younger siblings and parents. Overall, research findings so far have provided evidence that sibling relationships are likely to affect health behaviors and, thus, should be considered in the development of intervention and health-promotion programs with adolescents.

Unfortunately, as mentioned above, the extensive research literature on parent–adolescent relationships and sibling relationships during adolescence has generally been limited to the study of majority-status adolescents (Spencer & Dornbusch, 1990). Therefore, very little is known about puberty and such relationships among minority adolescents (Paikoff & Brooks-Gunn, 1991). Because family interaction styles and family structure may vary by ethnicity, these relationships may also vary differently for minority adolescents during puberty (Harrison, Wilson, Pine, Chan, & Buriel, 1990; Spencer & Dornbusch, 1990; Tolson & Wilson, 1990).

When studying family interaction styles and structure for ethnic and minority groups, it is important for researchers to account for social influences and other contextually relevant variables (e.g., socioeconomic status and neighborhood safety). One must appreciate not only differences between ethnic and minority groups but also differences within these groups (e.g., Black African Americans vs. Black Caribbean Americans). There is much variability within ethnic and minority group families as well, and, again, socioeconomic status may adversely compound this variability (Garcia Coll, Meyer, & Brillon, 1995). For example, Garcia Coll et al. reported that poor families living in dangerous urban neighborhoods were likely to be more punitive in their parenting practices because of the fear of exposing their children to danger. Parenting practices, a kind of family interaction style, may subsequently have implications for the health behaviors and risks taken by adolescents, particularly in certain contexts (i.e., unsafe, poor neighborhoods). Perhaps parents who are punitive better manage to prevent their children from finding themselves in risky situations. But it is also possible that punitive parenting practices interfere with children's opportunities to learn the problem-solving skills that are necessary for them to function independent of their family. Thus, there is a need for normative information on families of different groups, to describe family interaction across different ethnic and minority groups as well as to address within-group differences.

In particular, research aimed at understanding or influencing health promotion among minority adolescents should examine parent–adolescent communication patterns around pubertal events, as this is a time of change in the adolescent and subsequently in the adolescent's relationship with his or her parents. Such research has been done with majority adolescents. Ruble and Brooks-Gunn (1982), examining the content of discussions regarding menarche between mothers and daughters, found that communication tends to center around practical concerns rather than feelings. Parents may be uneasy discussing pubertal change with their children, perhaps because pubertal changes are associated with sexual and reproductive maturity (Paikoff & Brooks-Gunn, 1991). But, because parents continue to play an important guiding role as their children enter adolescence, despite relationship changes at this time (Holmbeck et al., 1995), the nature of adolescent–parent communication around pubertal events has important implications for health risks (such as likelihood of early sexual intercourse) as well as for programs of health promotion (e.g., engaging parents in programs to delay early sexual intercourse and prevent high-risk sexual behavior). Minority adolescents are at greater risk for sexually transmitted diseases, including HIV and AIDS (CDC, 1995; Shafer et al., 1984); thus, it is of paramount importance that parent–adolescent communication among these youth be better understood.

In addition to family process, family structure (e.g., constellation of individuals residing in a household or participating in an extended kin network) is important. For minority adolescents, a focus on "traditional" two-parent families may be inappropriate given cultural and social resource considerations (Chase-Lansdale, Brooks-Gunn, & Paikoff, 1991; Harrison et al., 1990; Hogan, Hao, & Parish, 1990; Jarrett, 1994). Urban minority families are likely to vary widely in terms of family coresidential arrangements (Kellam, Branch, Agrawal, & Ensminger, 1975) and are overrepresented in the population of single-parent, female-headed families (Children's Defense Fund, 1991). A series of studies have found children living in mother-alone families to be at higher risk for health-compromising behavior (Garfinkel & McLanahan, 1990; Kellam et al., 1975). Extrafamilial supports and extended kin networks can ameliorate these risks (Jarrett, 1994); however, many families do not have adequate supports to meet parenting and child-care needs (Hogan et al., 1990).

In summary, family-based intervention programs have the potential to be important, albeit complex components of health promotion for minority adolescents. Health-promotion and intervention efforts for minority adolescents should include parents, recognizing the importance of the parent–adolescent relationship and appreciating that little is known about the nature of this relationship during the transition into adolescence. Furthermore, such efforts should explore ways of involving siblings and others who might exert less traditional family influences.

Peer relationships. Adolescents spend an increasing amount of time with peers as adolescence progresses (Savin-Williams & Berndt, 1990). Closeness or intimacy and sharing private thoughts with peers increases from mid-childhood through adolescence, exceeding closeness with parents, which remains relatively stable (Youniss & Smollar, 1985). The closeness occurs first with same-sex peers and does not reach cross-sex peer relationships until mid-adolescence (Sharabany, Gershoni, & Hofman, 1981). These changes in the importance and intensification of the peer relationship affect the level of influence that peers have over one another for health-risking behaviors (e.g., drug and alcohol use or early sexual activity). Peer influence depends on the existence of peer pressure and the susceptibility of the individual to such pressure. Peer pressure seems to be greatest for older adolescents (Brown, Clasen, & Eicher, 1986), and susceptibility to peer pressure is greatest for younger adolescents (Berndt, 1979).

Peer relationships are likely to be magnified in their importance for minority adolescents (Spencer & Dornbusch, 1990). In particular, among immigrant youth, peers give emotional support and guidance through the similarity of their experiences with acculturation. They provide a feeling of brotherhood or sisterhood within a new culture, which can protect against feelings of isolation. Alternatively, dependence on peers may be detrimental in some cases, because peers may view some behaviors negatively if they reflect goals of the majority population (e.g., success in school; Fordham & Ogbu, 1986). It is likely that for minority adolescents, as for other youth, friendship choices influence the degree to which they find themselves in situations where health is compromised. Thus, understanding the relationship between friendship choices and other social relationships (such as those with family) is critical to health-promotion efforts for minority youth.

Adolescent cognition. As young people enter adolescence, they acquire cognitive abilities that can be both helpful and problematic for health promotion. Many adolescents develop the ability to reason abstractly, to think hypothetically, to use abstract concepts, and to apply formal logic. Health-promotion intervention efforts for adolescents need to consider the potential variability in thinking among preadolescents and young adolescents. The idea of "intelligence" was initially conceptualized as unimodal and emphasizing a particular form of cognitive processes; however, more recent theoretical and empirical writings have emphasized the importance of diverse types of intelligence in promoting health and preventing risk (Furby & Beyth-Marom, 1990; Keating, 1990). To understand the effects of cognitive abilities and styles on minority adolescent health promotion, researchers need to understand the naturalistic contexts in which cognition influences behavior (Weitzman, Paikoff, & Brooks-Gunn, 1995). Unfortunately, little work has been done to map out these areas of inquiry in either majority or minority youth (Keating, 1990).

Changing cognitive abilities can enable some adolescents to reason that engaging in risky or harmful health behavior today can affect their health tomorrow. They can reflect on their behavior and consider its long-term consequences—an advantage for health-promotion efforts—or they may use the same abilities to rationalize against making behavioral changes or engaging in risk behaviors as effects of particular behaviors that may be long-term and probabilistic—a deterrent to health promotion. Additionally, research (Keating, 1990) has shown that adolescents have strong misconceptions about the world. These misconceptions often do not change, even when contrasting evidence is presented (Linn, 1983), posing problems for interventions centered around health education.

Decision-making abilities are also critical to helping adolescents choose health-promoting behaviors. As adolescents grow increasingly independent, they are likely to face situations where they must make decisions regarding drug and alcohol use, sexual activity, risk of injury, and so on. The question is, are they capable of making wise decisions in situations that may be risky to their health? Young adolescents can generate options, examine situations from a number of perspectives, anticipate the consequences of their decisions, and evaluate the credibility of information sources (Furby & Beyth-Marom, 1990; Mann, Harmoni, & Power, 1989). However, they are less skilled at making decisions than are older adolescents and adults. In addition, it is difficult for both adolescents and adults to use higher cognitive-reasoning abilities in situations that require spontaneous thought and are emotionally arousing (Hamburg, 1986).

For minority adolescents, socialization and cognitive development come together to form unique demands of cognitive and social flexibility in the context of discontinuity. Biculturalism—that is, functioning in both the ethnic and nonethnic communities—requires greater cognitive and social flexibility, resulting in a synthesis of both cultures as well as a separateness (Harrison et al., 1990; LaFramboise, Coleman, & Gerton, 1993). Bilingual children, for example, show greater flexibility in the use of language as a tool of thought. Research has found that problem-solving tasks are affected by cognitive flexibility: In particular, African American children perform better on tasks that are presented in a varied format as opposed to an unvaried format (Boykin, 1979). In addition, minority adolescents must contend with the discontinuities between their ethnic community and the majority culture. The problems of discontinuity are particularly pronounced when the adolescent goes from the home environment to the school environment. Research has shown that the stress of discontinuity (i.e., difficulties in learning) can be adjusted when the context of the learning environment is consistent with students' ethnic background (Boykin, 1979; Holliday, 1985).

Adolescent social–emotional issues. In Western conceptualizations of adolescence, young people are involved in a process of understanding the self, known as identity development. That is, they are beginning to understand what they will do in their adult lives, what job or career they will pursue, what their political and religious beliefs are, and with whom they wish to associate (Erikson, 1959; Marcia, 1966). The search for identity is constrained by opportunities and experiences available in the environment. Minority adolescents probably experience restricted opportunities in their identity search because of discrimination. Research has shown that minorities experience such barriers to identity formation as conflicting values with the broader society, exposure to stereotyping and prejudice, and a lack of adult role models with positive ethnic identities (Spencer & Markstrom-Adams, 1990). In their review, Spencer and Markstrom-Adams found that minority adolescents tend to "foreclose" on their identities; that is, they do not go through a period of questioning, but simply identify with their parents and take on their beliefs and lifestyles. Socially and emotionally, an inability to break away from parents and carve out a separate identity may make some young people vulnerable to health risks (e.g., for mental health problems such as anxiety or depression or for nonuse of health services). For example, Asian American parents have a reputation for expecting academic excellence from their children, but such achievement may not be possible for all Asian American adolescents; such discontinuities may result in mental health problems for developing adolescents. Additionally, much of the research on minority adolescents' identity exploration is confounded by socioeconomic status and ethnicity. Socioeconomic status may also account for high rates of foreclosure among these adolescents, because parents with low socioeconomic status generally have lower education levels and fewer resources and, thus, opportunities for their children are restricted. Such families frequently live in poverty, restricting opportunities to adopt health-promoting behaviors, such as regular use of health care services. Although theory describes the importance of exploring one's identity during adolescence (Erikson, 1959), it may be that exploration may not be desirable when the young person is recognized and rewarded for their identification with the community (Spencer & Markstrom-Adams, 1990).

In summary, there are numerous biological and developmental characteristics of the young adolescent that have important implications for health behavior. For example, puberty—particularly its timing—has implications for the experience of adolescence; that is, the timing of puberty may "set the tone" for the individual's adolescence. As previously described, early pubertal timing for girls can lead to a greater likelihood of exposure to various health risks. In this sense, the timing of puberty can set a trajectory that will influence the adolescent's health behavior for later development and quality of life. In addition, negotiation of the transition into adulthood may be influenced by the health risks experienced in adolescence. The period of developmental transition from adolescence into adulthood may also be the time to change health behaviors as a result of experiences during adolescence.

The Transition Into Adulthood

Studies of the transition from adolescence into adulthood have been rare and less sophisticated than studies of the transition from childhood to adolescence. The reason for this is likely to be the great range and breadth of change involved in the early adolescent years, where growth is greater than any other period of development with the exception of infancy. However, developmental research on late adolescence has indicated that social–emotional and contextual changes as well as continued refinement of cognitive abilities occur during this period. As a result, events that occur in early adolescence can have very different meaning than if they were to occur in late adolescence. For example, engaging in first sexual intercourse at age 13 has different health implications than engaging in first intercourse at age 19. To fully appreciate the long-term consequences of health behaviors, it is important to distinguish between the developmental periods of early and late adolescence (Sherrod, Haggerty, & Featherman, 1993).

In late adolescence and during the transition into adulthood, the young person experiences issues surrounding the pursuit of adult responsibilities and goals. Because this is a time of growth and change, it is also a time for opportunity. In particular, this can mean that young people take this time as a chance to move away from risky health behaviors and to start anew (Aseltine & Gore, 1993). On the other hand, some health-related behaviors may have consequences that cannot be avoided later in life (e.g., sexually transmitted disease or unintended pregnancy). Therefore, the transition to adulthood needs to be viewed in two ways. The first is as a time to change from unhealthy behavior to health-promoting behavior, given the developmental advantages brought about by entry into adulthood (primary prevention). The second perspective is of the transition as a time to address coping with past health mistakes, such that the quality of life can be improved and other unhealthy behaviors can be avoided (secondary prevention).

Unfortunately, researchers have seldom examined differences in paths to adulthood among members of minority groups. In addition, in some minority populations, it is difficult to find adult work other than parenting. Does parenting then become an adaptive step into adulthood for some young adults who have little or no other opportunities? Considering the trade-offs between employment, education, and parenting in late adolescence for urban minority youth is tremendously complex because of the need for reconciling "mainstream" societal goals with the restricted opportunities that many of these young people face. Although teenage and young adult parenting does appear to negatively influence short-term adaptation for many adolescents, long-term studies have reported tremendous heterogeneity of outcomes for teenage mothers (Furstenberg, Brooks-Gunn, & Morgan,

1987), suggesting much room for secondary prevention efforts to ameliorate individual and social costs of teenage pregnancies.

These contextual issues of the transition to adulthood for minority adolescents and young adults have important implications for setting up health-promotion programs that fit the diverse paths taken by individuals at this stage in the life span. Unlike earlier periods of development, this period is not as easily characterized, particularly given the lack of research on minority individuals' transitions into adulthood. It is necessary for program developers to appreciate the importance of individual paths at this time of development in relationship to the choices available to those from minority groups. We now turn to a brief discussion of major issues in adolescent minority health and the implications of developmental, biological, and epidemiological data for the design, implementation, and evaluation of health-promotion programs for minority youth.

Prevention of Health Problems: Prevention and Health-Promotion Programs

As we have described, adolescents experience change in the areas of physical maturation, cognitive development, and social–emotional development. Change occurs in the social contexts of the family, peer relationships, school, and the neighborhood and community. These areas of change have many implications for the prevention of health risks and for promoting healthy behaviors. In the development and implementation of prevention and health-promotion programs, health professionals should consider three issues: First, who should be involved in prevention and health-promotion efforts so as to effectively reach minority adolescents? Second, what sort of delivery of the prevention and health-promotion message should be used so that, in terms of developmental issues, adolescents will best respond? Finally, one should appreciate the complete picture of the life of a minority adolescent, including possible constraints for adequately promoting health in the targeted population. We address each of these issues in turn.

Many health-risk-taking behaviors begin in early adolescence. For example, alcohol or cigarette use tends to begin at this period of development. This may set up a developmental trajectory in which substance abuse precedes the use of other substances or the onset of sexual behavior (Irwin & Millstein, 1992; Irwin et al., 1989); such a trajectory may differ as a function of ethnicity and social class (see Paikoff, 1995, for a discussion of early sexual behavior as a gateway to other health-compromising risk behaviors for urban, African American youth). Ideally, prevention and health-promotion efforts should begin in late childhood, before the transition to adolescence begins. At this stage, one is more likely to "catch" the older child before he or she becomes involved in health-risk behaviors and, thus, to help establish health-promoting behaviors rather than health-risk behaviors.

Theory and research have indicated that adolescents at risk for early substance use are heavily influenced by families, peers, and community (for a review, see Petraitis, Flay, & Miller, 1995). Parents and friends can serve as role models to young people who, at this stage, are quite dependent on such groups of people for guidance and other social–emotional needs. Emotional attachments to peers who are involved in substance use is believed to be caused, in part, by weak attachments to family and community. As a result of these weak attachments, young adolescents feel that they have little to lose by attachment to deviant peers. Similar findings are associated with early sexual intercourse, in which exposure to peers who have engaged in sexual activity, along with a poor family relationship, is believed to leave a young adolescent at risk for early intercourse (Parfenoff, Paikoff, Brooks-Gunn, Holmbeck, & Jarrett, 1995). Therefore, prevention and health-promotion efforts need to involve all of the players (i.e., family, friends, and community) important to the social–emotional development of the older child. Benefits would be derived from involving family, peers, and community by strengthening attachments to these groups, instilling close relationships both at home and in the community, and presenting role models that can help to deter children from early health-risk behaviors. For example, churches and other community organizations as well as teachers can present urban minority youth with a variety of role models that may be otherwise unavailable in communities with high rates of joblessness (Jarrett, 1994).

For minority youth, family, peers, and community play a different role in terms of the nature of emotional attachments. As previously explained, minority youth must negotiate their attachment to their ethnic group with their interaction with the larger culture, which perhaps makes these relationships even more important to prevention and health promotion. That is, it may be imperative that a dialogue regarding health behavior be started and cultivated with parents who may be perceived as out of the mainstream by their children. For example, different levels of acculturation are thought to be a potential source of conflict between older and younger generations in Hispanic families. Puerto Rican families have reported particularly severe conflict when daughters have sought more freedom (Allison & Takei, 1993). Alternatively, research has found that African American mothers are more likely to be involved in a family planning clinic visit with their daughters (under age 20) than are White mothers (Nathanson & Becker, 1986). African Americans may acknowledge and discuss certain health risks, although parental knowledge and teaching of these health risks has not been explicitly examined.

Authoritative parenting is associated with higher self-reliance and lower psychological distress among adolescents across ethnic, socio-economic, and family structure (i.e., intact versus nonintact) groups (Steinberg, Mounts, Lamborn, & Dornbusch, 1991). However, characterizing parents who are minorities against constructs tested in research with parents in the majority culture obviously does not necessarily generalize to the very poor and is perhaps not a good fit. In general, prevention and health-promotion efforts with minority adolescents should examine the importance of parenting practices and the influence of community on the health behaviors of minority youth. Where positive parenting relationships are not possible, it is important to link youth with some supportive role model from the community.

Older adolescents should also be distinguished as a group with unique developmental prevention and health-promotion needs. As described earlier, they are a much different group from early adolescents, with different social–emotional concerns (i.e., desire for adult roles and consideration of work goals), more life experience, greater need for independence, and enhanced cognitive abilities. Additionally, with this age group, changing previous health-risk behaviors may need to be the focus of health-promotion efforts along with prevention of other health-risk behaviors. For older adolescents, one should consider the diversity of paths taken into adulthood, and health-promotion efforts should focus on individual needs as a result of these diverse paths. For example, some adolescents entering adulthood may have already laid out an adult path by having children. As a result, prevention and health-promotion efforts should revolve around teaching late adolescents to set an example of health behavior for their children as well as to manage parenting stressors while attempting to continue to pursue their own developmental needs (e.g., education and work goals). In this way, programs can establish positive health behaviors in both parents and children and possibly prevent poor emotional health among mothers (e.g., depression).

Also at issue in the development of prevention and health-promotion programs is how to convey the importance of adapting healthy behaviors to minority adolescents. First, delivery of programs in the schools is likely to be optimal for young adolescents, who spend most of their time in this setting. The school often serves as a center to the community as well. Peer acceptance of a program is probably essential because of the importance of peers to adolescents in general and to minority adolescents in particular. However, those schools with a large minority group are in a better position to address the unique health issues of that group without segregating the minority from the majority group, which may or may not be encouraging for participation in such programs. Second, school personnel can model healthy behaviors in ways intrinsic to their school curriculum and schedule. For instance, schools can issue a no-smoking policy, provide nutritional school lunches, emphasize physical education programs and the importance of regular exercise, and provide opportunities to learn conflict management and resolution in an effort to reduce or avoid violent behavior. Finally, school-based health centers allow easy access for the provision of health and counseling services or for referrals within the community to adolescents who may not otherwise have adequate access to these services. For older adolescents and young adults, the probability of high-school dropout reduces the appropriateness and effectiveness of school programs, because those believed most at risk are often no longer in school. Further exploratory research is necessary to better understand these issues and provide optimal mechanisms to reach these youth.

Because adolescents are concerned with such issues as achieving independence from parents and establishing an identity for themselves, they are likely to appreciate a perspective of health-promoting behavior as an opportunity to exercise their need to address these issues. Adolescents would benefit from knowledge of possible consequences to health and the presentation of decision-making skills in the context of personal choice and control, thus enhancing the need to exercise autonomy and define their identities. Programs should also attempt to minimize health-risk behaviors often associated with adolescents and their need for independence. For those minority groups that are susceptible to health-risk behavior because of high risks in their communities, the message of prevention and health promotion needs to focus on balancing the need to be independent with avoiding dangerous situations within the community. For minority adolescents who generally do not question parental choices and lifestyles, programs may need to explore possible problems to development of autonomy and exploration of identity as putting the adolescent at risk for poor mental health (e.g., depression or anxiety).

The delivery of prevention and health-promotion programs should also take into consideration the need to make programs contextual. That is, programs should attempt to be similar to the home environment whenever possible, to reduce any discontinuity experienced between the majority culture associated with the program and the minority culture. This will likely facilitate learning and memory of health-related information as well as help encourage adolescents to apply what they learn. Participation of members of the minority culture in program design would enhance the appreciation of contextual issues to be addressed.

Finally, health professionals should appreciate the complete picture of the life of a minority adolescent, including possible constraints for adequately promoting health among these youth. Contextual issues such as the experience of discontinuity between cultures, incidence of poverty among those of minority status, and opportunities available within the majority culture are interrelated with such developmental factors as a growing need for independence from parents, the need to define adult goals, and prospects for the quality of life in adulthood. This interrelatedness of context and development is also affected by the timing of events, such that developmental trajectories are set up to either enhance healthy lifestyles or to leave adolescents at a health deficit. The timing of puberty, for example, can set up a trajectory that puts young adolescents at risk to become parents—a responsibility that they are not financially, emotionally, or educationally ready to assume. The developmental needs of the adolescent, coupled with the contextual issues associated with minority status in the United States, leave adolescent parents at risk for living in poverty and subsequently experiencing poor access to adequate health care. Program efforts need to be alert to the importance of understanding the whole life experience of the minority adolescent. In this way, health professionals can identify those at risk (e.g., those entering puberty early) and develop programs that address appropriate contextual and developmental factors.

Conclusion

The purpose of prevention and health promotion with adolescents is to promote and maintain positive growth and healthy behaviors while helping youth to avoid health-risk behaviors that might interfere with later quality of life. For minority adolescents, prevention and health promotion must focus on social context. Social context—the interaction with family, peers, and community within the minority culture—is the construct that raises many of the important questions and issues regarding health for minority adolescents. Because adolescents are likely to be striving for independence, they interact more between social contexts (e.g., family and peers, minority and majority culture), and they experience unique risks to health and opportunities for health promotion. Again, for the minority adolescent, these risks and opportunities are different than those of the majority status adolescent. As health professionals, we must encourage program development that is sensitive to the issues and needs of being a minority adolescent in the United States as well as to biological and developmental needs. The likely result will be programs that are carefully tailored to specific groups (i.e., age, ethnicity, race, and community) and that better target risks to health while enhancing preexisting health-promoting behaviors.

REFERENCES

Abramovitch, R., Corter, C., Pepler, D. J., & Stanhope, L. (1986). Sibling and peer interaction: A final follow-up and a comparison. *Child Development*, 57, 217–229.

Allison, K. W., & Takei, Y. (1993). Diversity: The cultural contexts of adolescents and their families. In R. M. Lerner (Ed.), *Early adolescence: Perspectives on research, policy, and intervention* (pp. 51–69). Hillsdale, NJ: Erlbaum.

Aseltine, R. H., & Gore, S. (1993). Mental health and social adaptation following the transition from high school. *Journal of Research on Adolescence, 3,* 247–270.

Berndt, T. (1979). Developmental changes in conformity to peers and parents. *Developmental Psychology, 15,* 608–616.

Boykin, A. W. (1979). Psychological behavioral verve: Some theoretical explorations and empirical manifestations. In A. W. Boykin, A. J. Franklin, & J. F. Yates (Eds.), *Research directions of Black psychologists* (pp. 351–367). Newbury Park, CA: Sage.

Brooks-Gunn, J. (1989). Pubertal processes and the early adolescent transition. In W. Damon (Ed.), *Child development today and tomorrow* (pp. 155–176). San Francisco, CA: Jossey-Bass.

Brooks-Gunn, J., & Paikoff, R. L. (1992). Changes in self-feelings during the transition towards adolescence. In H. R. McGurk (Ed.), *Childhood social development: Contemporary perspectives* (pp. 63–97). Hillsdale, NJ: Erlbaum.

Brooks-Gunn, J., & Reiter, E. O. (1990). The role of pubertal processes. In S. Feldman & G. Elliott (Eds.), *At the threshold: The developing adolescent* (pp. 16–53). Cambridge, MA: Harvard University Press.

Brown, B., Clasen, D., & Eicher, S. (1986). Perceptions of peer pressure, peer conformity, dispositions, and self-reported behavior among adolescents. *Developmental Psychology, 22,* 521–530.

Bryant, B. K., & DeMorris, K. A. (1992). Beyond parent-child relationships: Potential links between family environments and peer relations. In R. D. Parke & G. W. Ladd (Eds.), *Family-peer relationships: Modes of linkage* (pp. 159–189). Hillsdale, NJ: Erlbaum.

Buchanan, C. H., Eccles, J. S., & Becker, J. B. (1992). Are adolescents the victims of raging hormones? Evidence for activational effects of hormones on moods and behavior at adolescence. *Psychological Bulletin, 111,* 62–107.

Centers for Disease Control and Prevention. (1992). Selected behaviors that increase risk for HIV infection among high school students. *Morbidity and Mortality Weekly Report, 41*(14), 231–240.

Centers for Disease Control and Prevention. (1995). *HIV/AIDS surveillance report* (Vol. 6). Atlanta, GA: Author.

Chase-Lansdale, L. P., Brooks-Gunn, J., & Paikoff, R. L. (1991). Research and programs for adolescent mothers: Missing links and future promises. *Family Relations, 40,* 396–404.

Children's Defense Fund. (1991). *The adolescent and young adult fact book.* Washington, DC: Author.

Connolly, S. D., Paikoff, R. L., & Buchanan, C. M. (in press). Puberty: The interplay of biological and psychosocial processes in adolescence. In G. Adams, R. Montemayor, & T. Gullota (Eds.), *Psychosocial development in adolescence: Vol. 8. Advances in adolescent development.* Newbury Park, CA: Sage.

Crockett, L. J., & Peterson, A. C. (1993). Adolescent development: Health risks and opportunities for health promotion. In S. G. Millstein, A.C. Peterson, & E. O. Nightingale (Eds.), *Promoting the health of adolescents: New direc-*

tions for the twenty-first century (pp. 13–37). New York: Oxford University Press.

Earls, F. (1993). Health promotion for minority adolescents: Cultural considerations. In S. G. Millstein, A. C. Peterson, & E. O. Nightingale (Eds.), *Promoting the health of adolescents: New directions for the twenty-first century* (pp. 58–72). New York: Oxford University Press.

Erikson, E. (1959). *Identity and the life cycle.* New York: Norton.

Fordham, C., & Ogbu, J. (1986). Black students' school success: Coping with the burden of "acting White." *Urban Review, 18,* 176–206.

Furby, L., & Beyth-Marom, R. (1990). Risk-taking in adolescence: A decision-making perspective. Washington, DC: Carnegie Council on Adolescent Development.

Furstenberg, F. F., Brooks-Gunn, J., & Morgan, S. P. (1987). *Adolescent mothers in later life.* Cambridge, England: Cambridge University Press.

Garcia Coll, C. T., Meyer, E. C., & Brillon, L. (1995). Ethnic and minority parenting. In M. H. Bornstein (Ed.), *Handbook of parenting: Vol. 2. Biology and ecology of parenting* (pp. 189–209). Hillsdale, NJ: Erlbaum.

Garfinkel, I., & McLanahan, S. (1990). The effects of the child support provisions of the Family Support Act of 1988 on child well-being. *Population Research and Policy Review, 9,* 205–234.

Hamburg, B. (1986). Subsets of adolescent mothers: Developmental, biomedical, and psychosocial issues. In J. B. Lancaster & B. A. Hamburg (Eds.), *School-age pregnancy and parenthood: Biosocial dimensions* (pp. 115–145). New York: Aldine de Gruyter.

Harrison, A. O., Wilson, M. N., Pine, C. J., Chan, S. Q., & Buriel, R. (1990). Family ecologies of ethnic minority children. *Child Development, 61,* 347–362.

Hayes, C. D., & Hofferth, S. L. (1987). *Risking the future: Adolescent sexuality, pregnancy, and childbearing* (Vol. 2). Washington, DC: National Academy Press.

Hill, J. P. (1988). Adapting to menarche: Familial control and conflict. In M. Gunnar & W. A. Collins (Eds.), *Minnesota symposia on child development* (Vol. 21, pp. 43–77). Hillsdale, NJ: Erlbaum.

Hogan, D. P., Hao, L. X., & Parish, W. L. (1990). Race, kin networks, and assistance to mother-headed families. *Social Forces, 68,* 787–812.

Holliday, B. G. (1985). Developmental imperative of social ecologies: Lessons learned from Black children. In H. P. McAdoo & J. L. McAdoo (Eds.), *Black children* (pp. 53–71). Beverly Hills, CA: Sage.

Holmbeck, G. N., Paikoff, R. L., & Brooks-Gunn, J. (1995). Parenting adolescents. In M. H. Bornstein (Ed.), *Handbook of parenting: Vol. 1. Children and parenting* (pp. 91–118). Hillsdale, NJ: Erlbaum.

Irwin, C. E., Jr., & Millstein, S. G. (1986). Biopsychosocial correlates of risk-taking behaviors during adolescence: Can the physician intervene? *Journal of Adolescent Health Care, 7*(Suppl. 6), 82S–96S.

Irwin, C. E., Jr., & Millstein, S. G. (1992). Risk-taking behaviors and biopsychosocial development during adolescence. In E. J. Susman, L. V. Feagans,

& W. J. Ray (Eds.), *Emotion, cognition, health, and development in children and adolescents* (pp. 75–102). Hillsdale, NJ: Erlbaum.

Irwin, C. E., Jr., Millstein, S. G., Adler, N. E., & Turner, R. (1989). Pubertal timing and adolescent risk-taking: Are they correlated? [Abstract]. *Pediatric Research, 25,* 8.

Jarrett, R. L. (1994). Living poor: Family life among single-parent, African-American women. *Social Problems, 41,* 30–49.

Keating, D. P. (1990). Adolescent thinking. In S. S. Feldman & G. R. Elliott (Eds.), *At the threshold: The developing adolescent* (pp. 54–89). Cambridge, MA: Harvard University Press.

Kellam, S. G. , Branch, J. D., Agrawal, K. C., & Ensminger, M. E. (1975). *Mental health and going to school: The Woodlawn program of assessment, early intervention, and evaluation.* Chicago: University of Chicago Press.

LaFramboise, T., Coleman, H. L. K., & Gerton, J. (1993). Psychological impact of biculturalism: Evidence and theory. *Psychological Bulletin, 114,* 395–412.

Linn, M. C. (1983). Content, context, and process in reasoning during adolescence: Selecting a model. *Journal of Early Adolescence, 3,* 63–82.

Mann, L., Harmoni, R., & Power, C. N. (1989). Adolescent decision making: The development of competence. *Journal of Adolescence, 12,* 265–278.

Marcia, J. (1966). Development and validation of ego identity status. *Journal of Personality and Social Psychology, 3,* 551–558.

Millstein, S. G., Peterson, A. C., & Nightingale, E. O. (1993). *Promoting the health of adolescents.* New York: Oxford University Press.

Montemayor, R., Adams, G., & Gullotta, T. (1990). *Advances in adolescent development: Vol. 2. From childhood to adolescence: A transitional period?* Newbury Park, CA: Sage.

Nathanson, C. A., & Becker, M. H. (1986). Family and peer influence on obtaining a method of contraception. *Journal of Marriage and Family, 48,* 513–525.

National Research Council. (1993). *Losing generations: Adolescents in high risk settings.* Washington, DC: National Academy of Sciences.

Paikoff, R. L. (1995). Early heterosexual debut: Sexual possibility situations during the transition to adolescence. *American Journal of Orthopsychiatry, 65,* 389–401.

Paikoff, R. L., & Brooks-Gunn, J. (1991). Do parent–child relationships change during puberty? *Psychological Bulletin, 110,* 47–66.

Parfenoff, S. H., Paikoff, R. L., Brooks-Gunn, J., Holmbeck, G. N., & Jarrett, R. L. (1995). *Early sexual behavior and the risk for HIV/AIDS in early adolescence: The contribution of family and contextual factors.* Manuscript submitted for publication.

Peterson, A. C., & Ebata, A. (1987). Developmental transitions and adolescent problem behavior: Implications for prevention and intervention. In K. Hurrelmann, F. X. Kaufman, & F. Losel (Eds.), *Social intervention: Potential and constraints* (pp. 167–184). New York: Walter de Gruyter.

Petraitis, J., Flay, B. R., & Miller, T. Q. (1995). Reviewing theories of adolescent substance use: Organizing pieces in the puzzle. *Psychological Bulletin, 117,* 67–86.

Ruble, D. N., & Brooks-Gunn, J. (1982). The experience of menarche. *Child Development, 53,* 1557–1566.

Sagrestano, L. M., Parfenoff, S. H., Paikoff, R. L., & Holmbeck, G. N. (1995). *Conflict and pubertal development in low income urban African American adolescents: Links to experiences in sexual possibility situations.* Manuscript in preparation.

Savin-Williams, R. C., & Berndt, T. J. (1990). Friendship and peer relations. In S. S. Feldman & G. R. Elliott (Eds.), *At the threshold: The developing adolescent* (pp. 277–307). Cambridge, MA: Harvard University Press.

Scarr, S., & McCartney, K. (1983). How people make their own environments: A theory of genotype–environment effects. *Child Development, 54,* 424–435.

Shafer, M. A., Blain, B., Beck, A., Dole, P., Irwin, C. E., Sweet, R., & Schlacter, S. (1984). Chlamydia trachometis: Important relationships to race, contraceptive use, lower genital tract infection, and papanicolaou smears. *Journal of Pediatrics, 104,* 141–146.

Sharabany, R., Gershoni, R., & Hofman, J. (1981). Girlfriend, boyfriend: Age and sex differences in intimate friendship. *Developmental Psychology, 17,* 800–808.

Sherrod, L. R., Haggerty, R. J., & Featherman, D. L. (1993). Introduction: Late adolescence and the transition to adulthood. *Journal of Research on Adolescence, 3,* 217–226.

Spencer, M. B., & Dornbusch, S. M. (1990). Challenges in studying minority youth. In S. S. Feldman & G. R. Elliott (Eds.), *At the threshold: The developing adolescent* (pp. 123–146). Cambridge, MA: Harvard University Press.

Spencer, M. B., & Markstrom-Adams, C. (1990). Identity processes among racial and ethnic minority children in America. *Child Development, 61,* 290–310.

Stattin, H., & Magnusson, D. (1990). *Pubertal maturation in female development.* Hillsdale, NJ: Erlbaum.

Steinberg, L. D. (1981). Transformation in family relations at puberty. *Developmental Psychology, 17,* 833–840.

Steinberg, L. D. (1987). The impact of puberty on family relations: Effects of pubertal status and pubertal timing. *Developmental Psychology, 23,* 451–460.

Steinberg, L. D., Mounts, N. S., Lamborn, S. D., & Dornbusch, S. M. (1991). Authoritative parenting and adolescent adjustment across varied ecological niches. *Journal of Research on Adolescence, 1,* 19–36.

Susman, E. J., Nottelmann, E. D., Inoff-Germain, G., Dorn, L. D., & Chrousos, G. P. (1987). Hormonal influences on aspects of psychological development during adolescence. *Journal of Adolescent Health Care, 8,* 492–504.

Tolson, T. F. J., & Wilson, M. N. (1990). The impact of two-and-three generational Black family structure on perceived family climate. *Child Development, 61,* 416–428.

Weitzman, P. F., Paikoff, R. L., & Brooks-Gunn, J. (1995). *Mastering the possibilities: An exploratory look at how pre- and young adolescents define and approach decisions.* Manuscript submitted for publication.

Westney, Q. E., Jenkins, R. R., Butts, J. D., & Williams, I. (1984). Sexual development and behavior in Black adolescents. *Adolescence, 19,* 558–568.

Youniss, J., & Smollar, J. (1985). *Adolescents' relations with mothers, fathers, and friends.* Chicago: University of Chicago Press.

2

Psychological, Social, and Cultural Perspectives on Minority Health in Adolescence: A Life-Course Framework

James S. Jackson and Sherrill L. Sellers

R esearch on the health of adolescents of color encompasses a wide variety of topics and areas. In comparison, and somewhat paradoxically, theoretical approaches are rather narrow. For the most part, work on adolescent health has been "problem focused," centering on issues of substance abuse, teen pregnancy, and violence. To our way of thinking, these problems are too often divorced from the sociocultural and historical context in which adolescents are embedded. In this chapter, we focus on a conceptual framework for understanding the health of adolescents of color in the United States. We suggest that to understand physical and psychological health status in adolescence, to implement policies and research agendas, and to develop effective health-promotion programs among adolescents of color, researchers must conceptualize health-related factors and outcomes at multiple levels across the life course (J. S. Jackson & Sellers, in press).

We have three interrelated aims in this chapter. Our first aim is to briefly outline the contours of a life-course framework of race and ethnic influences on physical and psychological health in adolescence. We argue for the importance of historical and cohort factors that may specifically influence the life trajectories of ethnic and racial minority populations (Cobb, 1992; Dragastin & Elder, 1975). Given the considerable variation in definitions and uses of the concepts of race, ethnicity, and culture in the research, our second aim is to identify promising definitions and conceptualizations of these concepts as they relate to adolescent health. Our third aim is to specify two areas of sociohistorical context that may be of particular importance to examination of the health of adolescents of color: structural lag and birth cohort. Although M. W. Riley and Riley (1994) have focused their attention on the latter years of the life course, we believe that the concepts related to structural lag may be even more important for the often volatile and rapidly changing periods of childhood and adolescence (Dragastin & Elder, 1975; Hill, 1993).

There is growing recognition of the importance of ethnic background among all groups for understanding a wide array of psychological and social health conditions. We focus our discussion on groups of color, because their relative deprivation in comparison with White ethnic groups differentially shapes the nature of their human development and life-course experiences (Barresi, 1987; J. S. Jackson & Sellers, in press; Sokolovsky, 1985; Stanford & DuBois, 1993). The approach we take has particular relevance for racially defined and oppressed groups, and we draw much of the background for this chapter from our work on health and mental health among Americans of African descent (Gibson & Jackson, 1991; J. S. Jackson, Chatters, & Taylor, 1993; J. S. Jackson & Kalavar, 1994). Because the findings among African Americans may not always generalize to other cultural, racial, and ethnic groups (Barresi, 1987) and because there are differences in the life-span experiences of African, native Hispanic, Asian, and other American racial and ethnic groups (Harper, 1990; J. S. Jackson et al., 1996), we recognize that we are constrained by the limits of available data. Unfortunately, comparable research findings in the field of human development, particularly relating to adolescence, are rarely available across all racial ethnic groups (J. S. Jackson & Sellers, in press). However, we believe our approach may also be useful for examining the health behaviors of and prevention or intervention strategies for other ethnic or cultural groups. We discuss this aspect of our approach in the chapter summary.

Finally, we assume that there are important scientific, ethical, and practical considerations that must be addressed in reinventing the conceptualizations of health needs, access to health care, and health delivery in ethnic and racial minority communities more generally (J. S. Jackson, 1992; Klein, Slap, Elster, & Schonberg, 1992). It is now almost axiomatic that current models of health status, health promotion, and health services do not adequately take the structural, social, and cultural context of ethnic and racial minority adolescents into consideration when thinking about health promotion and health interventions (Earls, 1993; Spencer & Dornbusch, 1993). Most of the scientific and professional models that have been used to orient and provide service, health promotion, and health intervention are not equally applicable for all groups and individuals. This cultural heterogeneity must be included in models of health behaviors and health interventions if they are to be accurate and effective (J. S. Jackson, 1992; Klein et al., 1992).

Racial, Ethnic, and Cultural Categorization

Culture

How the concepts of culture, race, and ethnic group are defined and categorized is vitally important in models of human life-course development (J. S. Jackson, 1993; Wilkinson & King, 1987). It is essential to know more about the conditions under which race, ethnicity, sociocultural, and socioeconomic factors may serve as important resources in the coping processes and adaptation of ethnic groups of color to their relatively disadvantaged circumstances (Dressler, 1985, 1991; Small, 1994; Wilkinson & King, 1987). Development of more encompassing models of adolescent development and health may be best accomplished by understanding the ways in which ethnicity, culture, and race contribute to human developmental processes at every point in the life-course (Cobb, 1992; J. S. Jackson, 1989; Keith, 1990). Yet these categories—race, ethnicity, and culture—are conceptualized, defined, and operationalized in a variety of ways. Researchers may use these categorizations in post hoc analyses to explain away unexpected find-

ings or, worse, may "control for" these categorizations without artic-
ulating the possible differences in trajectories. More precisely, adolescents of color may "look like" their White, non-Hispanic counterparts
along a number of dimensions. However, the processes by which they
arrive at these endpoints may vary (Sellers & Hunter, 1996). Race and
ethnic issues are of central importance in understanding health status
and health behaviors. The failure of current health models to adequately encompass these issues in the lives of minority groups of
color, especially in adolescence, has contributed to the lack of success
in implementing delivery of health-promotion interventions and services in ethnic and racial communities (Airhihenbuwa, 1993; Earls,
1993).

Culture has been defined in many different ways (Jackson, Antonucci, & Gibson, 1990a). We use Swidler's (1986) definition of culture
as a symbolic vehicle of meaning, including beliefs, ritual practices,
art forms and ceremonies, and such informal practices as language,
gossip, stories, and rituals of daily life. At the basis of this definition
is the role of culture in providing strategies of action, continuity in
the ordering of these actions through time, and a template for con-
structing action. This perspective provides a useful backdrop for development of health-promotion and illness-prevention programs for
adolescents of color. Two examples are particularly powerful, both in
the area of substance abuse prevention. For African American adolescents, the family (defined intergenerationally) may be an important
base for prevention efforts. Millstein (1993) speculated that extended
family members may provide additional resources for African American adolescents, such that these family members are viewed as significant sources of assistance with a substance use problem. A second
example relates to Hispanic adolescents. Schinke, Botvin, and Orlandi
(1991) found that alcohol use among female Mexican American adolescents increases with acculturation. This suggests that prevention
efforts for such girls may need to focus on balancing the tensions
between wider society's acceptance of moderate drinking and the
Mexican cultural norm of abstinence for women.

Ethnicity

The concept of ethnicity is defined within a larger societal context.
Just as with other concepts in the social sciences, several distinctly

different definitions of ethnicity exist. Yinger (1985) suggested the following definition of an ethnic group:

> a segment of larger society whose members are thought, by themselves and/or others, to have a common origin and to share important segments of a common culture and who, in addition, participate in shared activities in which the common origin and culture are significant ingredients. Some mixture of language, religion, race and ancestral homeland with its related culture is the defining element. No one by itself [sic] demarcates an ethnic group. (p. 159)

In the United States, the recent arrival of Haitian immigrants as well as immigrants from other Caribbean nations and from African countries highlights the historical fact of the diversity among African Americans. This diversity may be best captured in ethnic rather than racial terms. Current theories of ethnicity assume that the development and persistence of ethnicity—the crystallization of solidarity and identification—depend on structural conditions in society (J. S. Jackson et al., 1996; Nielsen, 1985). In contrast, older, pluralist notions of ethnicity held that shared cultural heritage was the major basis for ascriptive group identity. Several researchers have taken a self-identifying approach to the definition of ethnicity (e.g., Roberts, 1987; Sokolovsky, 1989). This view emphasizes the dynamic interactions among cultural traits, socialized patterns of social behavior, and environmental influences. Barth (1969) defined ethnicity in a minimalist manner, in which the group must identify and be identified by others as a distinct category of people. His definition, as Nielsen (1985) suggested, was presumably made on the basis of racial or cultural markers, such as language, religion, or customs. Closely linked to definitions of ethnicity is the term *minority group*, proposed by Wirth (1945), which adds dimensions of inequality and discrimination.

Race

We are tempted to conclude that the term *race* should be discarded. However, the reality of research and social policy suggests the futility of such an idea. Instead, we suggest that the concept of race requires considerable rethinking. Specifically, race should be defined within the larger cultural context. Yinger (1985) suggested that "there is now widespread if not universal agreement that racial differences derive social significance from cultural diversity" (p. 159). Cooper (1984, 1991) and others (e.g., Williams & Collins, 1995) have asserted that the concept of race has no scientific meaning and that social definitions of race and ethnicity should be viewed solely as clues for searching out environmental causes of observed differences between groups (Small, 1994). Research in behavioral medicine, for example, has revealed that cultural and lifestyle differences among racial groups play an independent role in accounting for behavioral and health outcomes (Cooper, 1984, 1991; Dressler, 1985, 1991; Driedger & Chappell, 1988; J. S. Jackson, 1993; Williams & Collins, 1995).

The tendency of most researchers to address race and ethnicity as demographic characteristics rather than as distinct, predisposing cultural and social environment orientations (J. S. Jackson, 1993) has precluded the types of research and analyses that examine the contributory role of sociocultural factors to health behaviors within racial and ethnic groups (James, 1984; Myers, 1984). The appropriateness and validity of current socioeconomic status and other sociocultural measures (e.g., occupation, coping resources, and lifestyle factors) have been questioned by James (1984), Myers (1984), and others (J. J. Jackson, 1988; J. S. Jackson, 1993) when making comparisons across race and ethnic groups (Markides, Liang, & Jackson, 1990; Williams & Collins, 1995). Ethnic group members are often portrayed in the scientific literature in a simplistic and undifferentiated manner. An underlying assumption has been that there is extensive homogeneity in values, motives, social and psychological statuses, and behaviors among members of these populations (J. S. Jackson, 1991; Jaynes & Williams, 1989). Although categorical treatment can and often does produce extensive group uniformity in attitudes and behaviors, it is equally true that much heterogeneity exists within the same ethnic groups (J. S. Jackson, 1991, 1993).

Significant improvements in the life circumstances of ethnic and racial groups, particularly in health, have occurred over the past 40 to 50 years (National Coalition of Hispanic Health and Human Service Organizations [NCHHHSO], 1994; J. S. Jackson, 1991; Siegel, 1993). Recent literature (e.g., Farley & Allen, 1987; Jaynes & Williams, 1989; NCHHHSO, 1994), however, continues to document the negative life conditions of many ethnic groups of color in the United States. Although the exact causal relationships are not known (Williams, 1990; Williams & Collins, 1995), it is clear that such factors as poverty, poor health care, poor health behaviors, and exposure to environmental toxins are predisposing factors for high morbidity and mortality across the entire life span of ethnic people of color (Dressler, 1991; Haan & Kaplan, 1985; Hamburg, Elliott, & Parron, 1982).

Life-course considerations are key components in an approach to understanding racial and ethnic influences on individuals. Different ethnic and racial groups have divergent life experiences (Driedger & Chappell, 1988). These different experiences will have profound influences, both positive and negative, on individual, family, and group well-being at all stages of the life course, ultimately influencing adjustments to major life transitions (e.g., schooling, work life, marriage, loss of spouse, retirement, and disability). We conceptually consider race (and to some extent, ethnicity as well) as a social construct that represents numerous social, psychological, and, possibly, biological variables (Wilkinson & King, 1987). More information is needed about how these factors contribute to individual and group coping and adaptive mechanisms in alleviating the distinct socioeconomic and psychological disadvantages over the life-course (Stanford, 1990; Stanford & DuBois, 1993).

Finally, we emphasize the need to separate the constructs of minority group, race, ethnicity, and culture (Holzberg, 1982; J. S. Jackson et al., 1996; Small, 1994). We suggest that ethnicity and culture be viewed as mutable and changeable over the life-course for different cohorts, with continuity over time and generations (Holzberg, 1982; J. S. Jackson et al., 1990a). Race (an externally imposed social construction), ethnicity (a self- and other-imposed group construction), and cultural distinctiveness (the peculiar patterning of artifacts, beliefs, and values across generations) all have to be conceptualized as more than stratification variables. Instead they should be conceptualized as potential individual and group resources, providing psychological, social, and personal identity as well as group connections for ethnic group members (J. S. Jackson et al., 1996).

Ethnicity, national origin, and culture all play important roles in human development and life-course-related processes. It is apparent that other social group memberships also contribute significantly to individuals' developmental processes, for example, gender (Verbrugge, 1989) and socioeconomic status (J. S. Jackson, 1993; Williams & Collins, 1995). Many of these factors operate in parallel or interact with race and ethnicity to influence changes over a person's life-course (Jackson, Antonucci, & Gibson, 1990b). These influences are often subtle. For example, the health problems, issues, and concerns of adolescents of color may reflect their minority status. That is, compared with their White counterparts, adolescents of color may be more strongly affected by discrimination and struggles with self- or group identity. In an examination of adolescents' perspectives on health, Millstein (1993) reported a series of findings which suggest that adolescents of color *feel* their vulnerable status. She wrote that, "compared to white adolescents, black adolescents rate their health as poor, think more about their health, are more concerned about future illness and believe they are more susceptible to specific diseases, such as cancer" (p. 103). She also noted that, compared with their White counterparts, African American and Hispanic adolescents feel more vulnerable to such negative health outcomes as cancer, pregnancy, HIV, and AIDS. Although few of the studies Millstein reviewed controlled for social economic status, these findings are nonetheless suggestive.

Demographic Composition Among Adolescent Groups of Color

According to Hoberman (1992), the 1990 U.S. Census documented 35 million persons between the ages of 10 and 19. At the time, then, adolescents represented 15% of the U.S. population. At present, groups of color constitute 21% of the total American population; however, 40% of public school children are minorities (Feldman & Elliot, 1993). Although definitions of adolescence vary greatly (Feldman & Elliot, 1993; Hill, 1993), it has been estimated that by the Year 2000 approximately 31% of U.S. adolescents will belong to an ethnic minority group (Hill, 1993). However, these overall statistics mask vast heterogeneity among the groups of color.

African Americans constitute about 12% of the total U.S. population. Nearly 50% of the African American population is under 18 years of age (Bennett, 1995; Hoberman, 1992). As a result of growth among other groups, African American adolescents will increasingly constitute a shrinking proportion of the minority adolescent population (Jaynes & Williams, 1989). It is estimated that 43% of all African American adolescents live in poverty, and some estimates have indicated that, by the Year 2000, as many as 80% of all African American children will live a significant portion of their lives in a poverty-level household (Jaynes & Williams, 1989).

Hispanic adolescents have a different pattern. Exemplifying the issue of intragroup heterogeneity, the term *Hispanic* masks large differences among several major groups. For example, Cubans constitute a smaller proportion (6%) of the Hispanic population than do Puerto Ricans (14%), and the former group has significantly fewer adolescent-age individuals. Alternatively, Mexican-descent Hispanics constitute nearly two thirds (60%) of the total population of Hispanics, but not the same proportion of adolescents. Significant differences exist in the material advantages of these different Hispanic groups and in their social–historical backgrounds, political affiliations, and orientations. It is projected that by the Year 2000, the Hispanic population will increase by 42% and represent nearly 12% of the total U.S. population, which is nearly an 80% increase from their current 7% of the total population. Approximately 42% of the Hispanic population is made up of individuals under 18 years of age, and like African Americans, 40% of these reside in poverty-level households (Dryfoos, 1990).

Similarly, the category of Asian and Pacific Islanders encompasses broad differences in backgrounds and national origins, including 30 distinct groups. This group is also experiencing large increases among its respective populations, second only to Hispanics. Similar to Hispanics, the proportions of those in various age subpopulations vary greatly. These large differences in the proportions of populations are fueled by past immigration policies and the nature and makeup of current and projected rates of immigration and fertility. Approximately 33% of Asian Americans are under the age of 18; foreign-born adolescents represent 50% of this total (Hoberman, 1992).

The proportion of Native American, Alaska Natives, and Aleuts has, in general, also shown recent changes. Native Americans are the smallest of the ethnic minority groups (1%), but their numbers have doubled since 1970; adolescents make up 25% of this population. Nearly 50% of Native American adolescents live in poverty-level or near-poverty-level households; only 24% live on reservations, whereas the vast number reside in large urban areas. Similar to Americans of African, Hispanic, and Asian descent, Native Americans are individuals who differ widely in language, lifestyle, worldviews, and socioeconomic resources and belong to many different nations.

For the most part, groups of color are marked by vast heterogeneity in their respective adolescent populations. Even within groups, vast differences in poverty rates, single-parent households, and school dropout rates prevail. Some groups are especially disadvantaged (e.g.,

African Americans, Puerto Ricans, Cambodians, and Native Americans), whereas other groups are relatively well-off (e.g., Chinese, Japanese, and Cubans). However, given the growth and age distribution of these groups in many parts of the country, especially central cities, minority youth constitute the largest proportions of adolescents, the largest proportions of public school enrollees, and disproportionate numbers of school dropouts (Hoberman, 1992).

Emerging demographic changes in the United States that are shifting the composition of the general and elderly populations will have important implications for the process of adolescence. Overall, adolescents will represent a shrinking proportion of the total population (Bennett, 1995; Siegel, 1993). Due to these demographic transitions policy makers, researchers, and program planners are revising and reconsidering household structure, divorce, child rearing, parental relationships, and processes of development (Hill, 1993).

Physical and Mental Health Status of Minority Adolescents

Although the same quality data are not available on all groups, epidemiological studies consistently describe the health risks to adolescents of color (NCHHSO, 1994). For the most part, many have viewed the period of adolescence as relatively healthy. However, recent evidence (Klein et al., 1992) has pointed to serious physical and mental disorders among youth, conditions that may be exacerbated by ethnic and minority status. On the basis of a Congressional Office of Technology report, Klein et al. (1992) determined that 5%–10% of all U.S. adolescents have chronic diseases or disabilities, such as asthma, heart disease, vision impairment, or hearing loss, with approximately half having daily activity limitations. This report also estimated that 20%–50% of adolescents have a wide array of other less serious, but no less debilitating problems, including acne, dysmenorrhea, or gynecomastia. Public health problems abound, including homicide, suicide, pregnancy, sexually transmitted diseases, and substance abuse. Unintentional injuries and violence cause 76% of the deaths among adolescents and contribute to most of their disability. These problems are exaggerated among minority adolescents and youth. Among minority adolescents, poverty, homicide, HIV risks, substance abuse, violence, and gang involvement all show elevated rates (Klein et al., 1992).

The problems of ethnic and minority adolescents may begin at birth. Children of many groups of color are born with a nonzero probability of being in poverty during a significant portion of their life-course (Bennett, 1995). For example, some researchers (e.g., Jaynes & Williams, 1989) have estimated that upward of 80% of African American children born over the next decade will spend the bulk of their childhoods in poverty. It is reasonable to suggest that there is considerable potential for negative outcomes for children born in such circumstances. Possible consequences include poor early health care, exposure to toxic environments, problematic material resources, and potentially problematic socialization, all of which point to increased poor psychological and physical health outcomes. Compared with their White counterparts, African American children are 3 times more likely to live in poverty, to die of abuse, and to be classified as learning disabled and 4 times more likely to be murdered before their first birthday (Hale, 1992).

Childhood experiences of a large proportion of children of color may not be sufficient preparation for the rigors of adolescence. Among preadolescent boys and girls, lack of educational opportunities, material resources, and poor early health care are already beginning to take a toll. Educational opportunities for children of color may be limited by shrinking property taxes, resulting in fewer new books, limited extracurricular activities, and scant technological innovations. Furthermore, parents may lack the material resources to provide developmentally important but expensive luxuries, such as computers, summer enrichment camps, and extensive after-school programming. These factors provide the foundation for underachievement and school dropout. Additionally, diets insufficient in basic nutrients and high in fat and starches may be laying the groundwork for later hypertension, heart disease, and cardiovascular problems.

In terms of their educational, social, and psychological preparation, vast numbers of children of color may be inadequately prepared for adolescence. Environmental stressors such as racism and systemic barriers to mobility may further challenge adolescents' developmental tasks. In addition, children and adolescents spend a great deal of time watching television. Much of the media's focus is on crime and violence, and this focus is often racialized, in that the "bad guy" is disproportionately portrayed by a person of color. The environmental messages for youth of color are clear: (a) Violence is an acceptable means of achieving a goal and (b) other, more socially acceptable means of accomplishment may not be available to them. Combined with hormonal and physical changes, the lack of psychological resources and perceived material means to success may take their toll early in the lives of many adolescents of color. Opportunities for often lucrative criminal activity, school dropout, early family development, and drug use and abuse compound these early experiences, making health-compromising behaviors explicable, if no less acceptable (J. S. Jackson & Sellers, in press).

A Life-Course Approach

A central premise of a life-course perspective is that already-born cohorts of ethnic and racial groups have been and are being exposed to conditions that will profoundly influence their social–psychological and health status as they reach adolescence and adulthood (Baltes, 1987; Elder, 1987). There is a growing consensus among health practitioners about the need for resource-based, life-span models of culture and ethnicity that transcend traditional notions of culture and assimilation. For example, findings from research on cultural differences in illness expression, personality differences, patterns of family and friend interaction, and coping and adaptation all point to the existence of distinct and measurable ethnic, cultural, and racial dimensions that influence (and are influenced by) biological, social, and psychological developmental processes (J. S. Jackson et al., 1990b, 1993). We contend that the life-course framework can contribute to theoretical models that help explain the influence of cultural and ethnic factors in human development at all points in the life-course, but especially in adolescence (Dragastin & Elder, 1975). We suggest that health status and conditions among adolescents cannot be divorced from considerations of social, environmental, and psychological conditions of conception and gestation, prenatal care, birth, infancy, childhood, and early pre-adolescent development (Airhihenbuwa, 1993; Millstein & Litt, 1990). We therefore believe that an intergenerational framework is needed—one that examines the larger family network and the manner in which parental and other familial influences provide the context, resources, and socialization filter for the larger environmental, physical, and social worlds of minority youth (see J. S. Jackson & Sellers, in press, for a more complete development of this model). Recent theorizing about the process of adolescent development views it as a period of development involving a negotiated transition into a wider social world, rather than as a dramatic shift or the unquestioning adoption of parental values and lifestyles (Hill, 1993; Millstein, 1993). This more recent evolving view of adolescence is much more consonant with a contextualized, structurally embedded view of adolescence, emphasizing multifactorial and interactive social, cognitive, emotional, and biological influences (Hoberman, 1992). Such an interactive view, we feel, provides a more accurate descriptive account of transitions among adolescents of color in the United States (Hill, 1993).

Period and Cohort Influences

Our aim is to outline a life-course approach within which the nature of the economic, social, and psychological lives of African Americans and other Americans of color might be comprehended, explained, and understood in the context of historical and current structural disadvantage and blocked-mobility opportunities (J. S. Jackson, 1991; J. S. Jackson & Kalavar, 1994). Central to this effort is addressing the question of how structural disadvantages in the environment are translated at different points in individual and group life-courses into physical, social, and psychological aspects of group and self. How these different birth cohorts, historical and current environmental events, and individual differences in developmental and aging processes interact forms the overall context of the model that is needed. The overarching framework of this model is one that contextualizes specific individual and group experiences by birth cohort, period events, and individual development and aging processes.

Although several authors have indicated the necessity of considering life-course models (e.g., Barresi, 1987; Soldo & Manton, 1985) and history, cohort, and period effects in the nature of ethnic and racial group status, few have actually collected the type of data or conducted the analyses that would shed any light on these processes. We have reviewed the material on health, mortality, morbidity, and risk factors, and it appears that examination of the health status of adolescents of color has been conducted in a relative vacuum. As Klein et al. (1992)

noted, this is because suitable conceptual models of minority health status and quality trend data on sizable representative samples of these groups are lacking.

The differential cohort experiences of groups of color undoubtedly play a major role in the nature of their health experiences over the lifecourse in terms of the quality of health care from birth, exposure to risk factors, and the presence of exogenous environmental factors. Confounding these cohort experiences for large numbers of recent immigrants are factors related to acculturation. Another contributing factor is the stressor role of prejudice and discrimination, even though it may differ in form and intensity as a function of birth cohort, ethnic group, period of life, and age (Baker, 1987; Cooper, Steinhauer, Schatzkin, & Miller, 1981; Dressler, 1991).

Structural Lag and Opportunities for Adolescents of Color

We believe the health-status and health-promotion needs of adolescents of color cannot be understood outside of a systems, life-course perspective—one that considers the intersections of the economic, social, political, historical, and cultural realms in which these youth reside (Earls, 1993). At the same time, it has been long recognized that adolescence brings a peculiar set of life tasks as individuals make the developmental transition from childhood to adulthood (e.g., Havighurst, 1972). The interrelationship of the former, largely structural perspectives with the latter, largely psychological developmental focus of individual transition have rarely been linked in integrated models.

M. W. Riley and colleagues (J. W. Riley & Riley, 1994; M. W. Riley 1994a, 1994b; M. W. Riley & Riley, 1994) have proposed that cohort succession and structural lag must be considered in models of human development and, especially, of aging. Their main argument is that as people age, they encounter changing role opportunities and circumstances in society. This interplay between individual lives and role opportunities can never be in synchrony; the two elements must always be asynchronous (i.e., one or the other lags behind). Thus, there will always be structural lags.

The notion of structural lag highlights the problems of allocating such things as health care, education, work, and leisure time over the life-course. For example, the rapid technological advances in medicine and related scientific fields may quickly outstrip the training of physicians, requiring extensive re-education and training. Similarly, adolescents of color whose racial socialization was consistent with the racial climate (and structure) of their parents' may be ill-prepared for the shifting racial climate of later times (Cose, 1993).

One of the issues only briefly touched on in Riley's work on structural lag and age integration (e.g., M. W. Riley, 1994a, 1994b; M. W. Riley & Riley, 1994) is the role of the family as an important mediator in the relationship between individual and social structure. For many ethnic and racial minorities in the United States, and, in fact, many countries around the world, human development and age integration is accomplished not so much by individuals having direct relationships to complex social structures but, instead, through family systems that provide productive relationships and connections across the life span. Some of these functions are formal, such as the transitions to leadership positions in complex tribal and family economic systems with age. Many more of these role functions are informal, however, involving important work within the family as counselors, helpers for the youngest and most dependent, or sources of informal work contributing to the economic and social well-being of the family. This has certainly been true among Americans of African, Hispanic, and Asian descent.

Now, because of some structural changes (e.g., a shift from a manufacturing to service economy), these formal and informal familial arrangements are in danger. These changes threaten to remove one important buffer and facilitator in the lives of many ethnic and racial groups in America, a buffer that has shielded them—especially children and adolescents—from such changes but that also has protected them against the continuing pernicious effects of discrimination and racism (which, especially in its institutional forms, transcends the types of structural changes that have occurred). In fact, the continuing oppression of racism and discrimination interact with structural changes, making them more difficult to cope with (e.g., the continuing systematic barriers to quality education and training that exist for racial and ethnic minorities). Although prediction of future events and structural circumstances is hazardous, it is clear that structural change will continue to be asynchronous with the course of individual lives. Thus, we must develop flexible structures and processes for changes in opportunities and norms that are responsive to structural lags and the course of individual lives.

Summary

In considering a life-course perspective on adolescent health, it is important for one to consider the entire life span. In this chapter, we have suggested that to develop effective health-promotion programs, policies, and research agendas, practitioners must conceptualize and assess the health outcomes of racial and ethnic groups at multiple levels and across the life-course. One central implication of this framework is the need to design programs that address the health of these groups comprehensively, over the life-course, and as members of racialized groups embedded in a particular sociohistorical context. Put simply, our work and emerging conceptualization suggests that health outcomes are a complex interaction of individual, group, and structural factors, all of which must be considered simultaneously if the disparities in health outcomes among adolescents of differing backgrounds are to be lessened.

Given the structural changes that we discussed earlier (e.g., M. W. Riley, 1994b), with each succeeding generation, increasing numbers of adolescents of color may actually be less prepared materially and psychologically to cope with new political, economic, and social realities in succeeding historical periods. For example, some adolescent research has suggested that poorer health outcomes are associated with increased acculturation among newer immigrants of color (Vega, Kolody, Kwang, & Noble, 1993). The seeming intractability of teen pregnancy among African American and Latino youth, the inexorable rise in poverty, and deteriorating family structures all point to the increasing problems of structural lag in adolescence. Designing and implementing cost-effective health-promoting interventions and ensuring good health behaviors and health status among adolescent groups of color are becoming increasingly more complicated and difficult. We do not mean to imply that improving the quality of health status and health behaviors of this population is impossible. However, it is difficult and will become increasingly more so in the decades to come. If practitioners are to provide effective health interventions among adolescents of color, then systemic life-course, culturally appropriate models are needed to address adolescents' health-status, health-promotion, and health-service needs. Now would be a good time for the design and implementation of such models.

REFERENCES

Airhihenbuwa, C. (1993). Health promotion and disease prevention strategies for African Americans: A conceptual model. In R. Braithwaite & S. Taylor (Eds.), *Health issues in the Black community* (pp. 267–280). San Francisco: Jossey-Bass.

Baker, F. M. (1987). The Afro-American life cycle: Success, failure, and mental health. *Journal of the National Medical Association, 7*, 625–633.

Baltes, P. B. (1987). Theoretical propositions of life-span developmental psychology: On the dynamics between growth and decline. *Developmental Psychology, 23*, 611–626.

Barresi, C. M. (1987). Ethnic aging and the life course. In D. E. Gelfand & C. M. Barresi (Eds.), *Ethnic dimensions of aging* (pp. 18–34). New York: Springer.

Barth, F. (1969). *Ethnic groups and boundaries: The social organization of culture and indifference.* London: Allen and Unwin.

Bennett, C. E. (1995). *The Black population in the United States: March 1994 and 1993.* (U.S. Bureau of the Census, P20–480). Washington, DC: U.S. Government Printing Office.

Cobb, N. (1992). Foundations of adolescent development: A life-span perspective on adolescence. In Nancy J. Cobb (Ed.), *Adolescence: Continuity, change, and diversity* (pp. 27–39). Mountain View, CA: Maryfield.

Cooper, R. (1984). A note on the biological concept of race and its application in epidemiological research. *American Heart Journal, 108*, 715–723.

Cooper, R. (1991). Celebrate diversity—or should we? *Ethnicity and Disease, 1*, 3–7.

Cooper, R., Steinhauer, M., Schatzkin, A., & Miller, A. (1981). Improved mortality among U.S. Blacks, 1968–1978: The role of antiracist struggle. *International Journal of Health Services, 11*, 511–522.

Cose, E. (1993). *The rage of a privileged class.* New York: Harper Collins.

Dragastin, S. E., & Elder, G. H., Jr. (Eds.). (1975). *Adolescence in the life cycle.* Washington, DC: Hemisphere.

Dressler, W. W. (1985). Extended family relationships, social support, and mental health in a Southern Black community. *Journal of Health and Social Behavior, 26*, 39–48.

Dressler, W. W. (1991). Social class, skin color, and arterial blood pressure in two societies. *Ethnicity and Disease, 1*, 60–77.

Driedger, L., & Chappell, N. (1988). *Aging and ethnicity: Toward an interface.* Toronto, Ontario, Canada: Butterworths.

Dryfoos, J. G. (1990). *Adolescents at risk: Prevalence and prevention.* New York: Oxford University Press.

Earls, F. (1993). Health promotion for minority adolescents: Cultural Considerations. In S. G. Millstein, E. O. Nightingale, & A. C. Petersen (Eds.), *Promoting the health of adolescents: New directions for the twenty-first century* (pp. 58–72). New York: Oxford University Press.

Elder, G. (1987). Families and lives: Some developments in life-course studies. *Journal of Family History, 12,* 179–199.

Farley, R., & Allen, W. (1987). *The color line and the quality of life in America.* Newbury Park, CA: Sage.

Feldman, S., & Elliot, G. (1993). Progress and promise of research on adolescence. In S. Feldman & G. Elliot (Eds.), *At the threshold: The developing adolescent* (pp. 479–505). Cambridge, MA: Harvard University Press.

Gibson, R. C., & Jackson, J. S. (1991). The Black oldest old: Health, functioning, and informal support. In R. M. Suzman, D. P. Willis, & K. G. Manton (Eds.), *The oldest old* (pp. 506–515). New York: Oxford University Press.

Haan, M. N., & Kaplan, G. A. (1985). The contribution of socioeconomic position to minority health. In *Report of the Secretary's Task Force on Black and Minority Health: Crosscutting issues in minority health, 2.* Washington, DC: U.S. Government Printing Office.

Hale, C. (1992). A demographic profile of African Americans. In R. Braithwaite & S. Taylor (Eds.), *Health issues in the Black community* (pp. 6–20). San Francisco: Jossey-Bass.

Hamburg, D. A., Elliott, G. R., & Parron, D. L. (1982). *Health and behavior: Frontiers of research in the biobehavioral sciences.* Washington, DC: National Academy Press.

Harper, M. S. (1990). *Minority aging: Essential curricula content for selected health and allied health professions* (DHHS Pub. No. HRS P-DV090-4). Washington, DC: U.S. Government Printing Office.

Havighurst, R. J. (1972). *Developmental tasks and education* (3rd ed.). New York: D. McKay.

Hill, P. (1993). Recent advances in selected aspects of adolescent development. *Journal of Child Psychiatric Development, 34,* 69–99.

Hoberman, H. M. (1992). Ethnic minority status and adolescent mental health services utilization. *The Journal of Health Administration, 19,* 246–267.

Holzberg, C. (1982). Ethnicity and aging: Anthropological perspectives on more than just the minority elderly. *The Gerontologist, 32,* 249–257.

Hunter, A. G., & Sellers, S. L. (1996). *Feminist attitudes among African American men and women.* Unpublished manuscript.

Jackson, J. J. (1988). Social determinants of the health and aging Black populations in the United States. In J. S. Jackson (Ed.), *The Black American elderly: Research on physical and psychosocial health* (pp. 69–98). New York: Springer.

Jackson, J. S. (1989). Race, ethnicity, and psychological theory and research. [Review]. *Journal of Gerontology: Psychological Sciences, 44,* 1–2.

Jackson, J. S. (Ed.). (1991). *Life in Black America*. Newbury Park, CA: Sage.

Jackson, J. S. (1992). Conducting health behavior research in ethnic and minority communities. In D. M. Becker, D. R. Hill, J. S. Jackson, D. M. Levine, F. A. Stillman, & S. M. Weiss (Eds.), *Health behavior research in minority populations: Access, design and implementation* (NIMH Pub. No. 92-9269; pp. 13–22). Washington, DC: U.S. Government Printing Office.

Jackson, J. S. (1993). Racial influences on adult development and aging. In R. Kastenbaum (Ed.), *The encyclopedia of adult development* (pp. 18–26). Phoenix, AZ: Oryx Press.

Jackson, J. S., Antonucci, T. C., & Gibson, R. C. (1990a). Cultural, racial, and ethnic minority influences on aging. In J. E. Birren & K. W. Schaie (Eds.), *Handbook of the psychology of aging* (3rd ed., pp. 103–123). San Diego, CA: Academic Press.

Jackson, J. S., Antonucci, T. C., & Gibson, R. C. (1990b). Social relations, productive activities, and coping with stress in late life. In M. A. P. Stephens, J. H. Crowther, S. E. Hobfoll, & D. L. Tennenbaum (Eds.), *Stress and coping in later life families* (pp. 193–212). Washington, DC: Hemisphere.

Jackson, J. S., Brown, T., Williams, D. W., Torres, M., Sellers, S., & Brown, K. (1996). Perceptions and experiences of racism and the physical and mental health status of African Americans: A thirteen-year national panel study. *Journal of Ethnicity and Disease, 6*(1,2), 132–147.

Jackson, J. S., Chatters, L. M., & Taylor, R. J. (1993). Status and functioning of future cohorts of African-American elderly: Conclusions and speculations. In J. S. Jackson, L. M. Chatters, & R. J. Taylor, *Aging in Black America* (pp. 301–323). Newbury Park, CA: Sage.

Jackson, J. S., & Kalavar, J. (1994). Equity and distributive justice across age cohorts: A life-course family perspective. In L. Cohen (Ed.), *Justice across generations: What does it mean?* (pp. 175–183). Washington, DC: American Association of Retired Persons.

Jackson, J. S., & Sellers, S. L. (in press). A multi-dimensional life-course perspective. In P. M. Kato & T. Mann (Eds.), *Health psychology of special populations: Issues of age, gender, and ethnicity.* New York: Plenum.

James, S. A. (1984). Coronary heart disease in Black Americans: Suggestions for research on psychosocial factors. *American Heart Journal, 108,* 833–838.

Jaynes, G. D., & Williams, R. K., Jr. (Eds.). (1989). *A common destiny: Blacks and American society.* Washington, DC: National Academy Press.

Keith, J. (1990). Age in social and cultural context. In R. Binstock & L. George (Eds.), *Handbook of aging and the social sciences* (3rd ed., pp. 91–111). San Diego, CA: Academic Press.

Klein, J. D., Slap, G. B., Elster, A. B., & Schonberg, S. K. (1992). Access to health care for adolescents: A position paper of the Society for Adolescent Medicine. *Journal of Adolescent Health, 13,* 162–170.

Markides, K. S., Liang, J., & Jackson, J. S. (1990). Race, ethnicity, and aging: Conceptual and methodological issues. In L. K. George & R. H. Binstock (Eds.), *Handbook of aging and the social sciences* (3rd ed., pp. 112–129). San Diego, CA: Academic Press.

Millstein, S. (1993). A view of health from the adolescent's perspective. In S. G. Millstein, A. C. Petersen, & E. O. Nightingale (Eds.), *Promoting the health of adolescents: New directions for the twenty-first century* (pp. 97–145). New York: Oxford University Press.

Millstein, S., & Litt, I. (1990). Adolescent health. In S. Feldman & G. Elliot (Eds.), *At the threshold: The developing adolescent* (pp. 431–456). Cambridge, MA: Harvard University Press.

Myers, H. F. (1984). Summary of workshop, III: Working group on socioeconomic and sociocultural influences. *American Heart Journal, 108,* 706–710.

National Coalition of Hispanic Health and Human Service Organizations. (1994). *Growing up Hispanic: National chart book* (Vol. 2). Washington, DC: Author.

Nielsen, F. (1985). Toward a theory of ethnic solidarity in modern societies. *American Sociological Review, 50,* 133–149.

Riley, J. W., & Riley, M. W. (1994, June). Beyond productive aging: Changing lives and social structure. *Aging International,* 15–19.

Riley, M. W. (1994a). Aging and society: Past, present, and future. *The Gerontologist, 34,* 436–446.

Riley, M. W. (1994b). Changing lives and changing social structures: Common concerns of social science and public health. *American Journal of Public Health, 84,* 1214–1217.

Riley, M. W., & Riley, J. W., Jr. (1994). Age integration and the lives of older people. *The Gerontologist, 34,* 110–115.

Roberts, R. (1987, December). *Depression among Black and Hispanic Americans.* Paper presented at the National Institute of Mental Health Workshop on Depression and Suicide in Minorities, Bethesda, MD.

Schinke, S. P., Botvin, G. J., & Orlandi, M. A. (1991). *Substance abuse in children and adolescents: Evaluation and intervention.* Newbury Park, CA: Sage.

Siegel, J. S. (1993). *A generation of change.* Newbury Park, CA: Sage.

Small, S. (1994). *Racialized barriers: The Black experience in the United States and England in the 1980s.* London: Routledge.

Sokolovsky, J. (1985). Ethnicity, culture and aging: Do differences really make a difference? *The Journal of Applied Gerontology, 4,* 6–17.

Sokolovsky, J. (Ed.).(1989). *The cultural context of aging.* New York: Bergin & Garvey.

Soldo, B., & Manton, K. (1985). Dynamics of health changes in the oldest old: New perspectives and evidence. *Milbank Memorial Fund Quarterly, 63,* 206–285.

Spencer, M., & Dornbusch, S. (1993). Challenges in studying minority youth. In S. Feldman & G. Elliot (Eds.), *At the threshold: The developing adolescent* (pp. 123–146). Cambridge, MA: Harvard University Press.

Stanford, E. P. (1990). Diverse Black aged. In Z. Harel, E. A. McKinney, & M. Williams (Eds.), *Black aged: Understanding diversity and service needs* (pp. 99–117). Newbury Park, CA: Sage.

Stanford, E. P., & DuBois, B. C. (1993). Gender and ethnicity patterns. In J. E. Birren, R. B. Sloane, & G. D. Cohen (Eds.), *Handbook of mental health and aging* (2nd ed., pp. 99–117). San Diego, CA: Academic Press.

Swidler, A. (1986). Culture in action: Symbols and strategies. *American Sociological Review, 51,* 273–286.

Vega, W. A., Kolody, B., Kwang, J., & Noble, A. (1993). Prevalence and magnitude of perinatal substance exposures in California. *New England Journal of Medicine, 329,* 850–854.

Verbrugge, L. M. (1989). The twain meet: Empirical explanations of sex differences in health and mortality. *Journal of Health and Social Behavior, 30,* 282–304.

Wilkinson, D. T., & King, G. (1987). Conceptual and methodological issues in the use of race as a variable: Policy implications. *The Millbank Quarterly, 65,* 56–71.

Williams, D. R. (1990). Socioeconomic differentials in health: A review and redirection. *Social Psychology Quarterly, 53,* 81–99.

Williams, D. R., & Collins, C. (1995). U.S. socioeconomic and racial differences in health: Patterns and explanations. *Annual Review of Sociology, 21,* 349–386.

Wirth, L. (1945). *The science of man in the world crisis.* New York: Columbia University Press.

Yinger, J. (1985). Ethnicity. *Annual Review of Sociology, 11,* 151–180.

II

Health-Compromising and Health-Promoting Behaviors in Minority Adolescent Populations

INTRODUCTION

Health-Compromising and Health-Promoting Behaviors in Minority Adolescent Populations

Part II specifically focuses on examining health-damaging and health-promoting behaviors among culturally diverse groups of adolescents. Because adolescence is a unique developmental stage in which adolescents experiment with health-compromising and health-promoting behaviors, the chapters in this part of the book take a special look at these behavioral patterns. Six chapters address a wide range of health behaviors, including drug abuse; sexually transmitted diseases (STDs); physical activity; diet; and special health concerns of female adolescents, such as eating disorders, teenage pregnancy, and STDs. This part also includes a chapter that takes a unique look at health behaviors that may be important for preventing the development of chronic illness among "at-risk" minority populations. With the clinician in mind, each chapter also highlights the treatment implications for developing effective programs for diverse groups of minority adolescents.

Drug addiction has serious consequences for any adolescent while also posing serious threats to future health. In chapter 3, Botvin and Scheier take a special look at the issue of drug abuse and violence among minority adolescents. The authors provide an excellent overview of the incidence rates of drug use across ethnic groups and summarize effective school-based approaches from several different theoretical perspectives. In chapter 4, Rodrigue, Tercyak, and Lescano emphasize the seriousness of the prevalence of STDs, such as HIV and AIDS, among minority adolescents. These authors provide an overview of important issues that may be key to developing effective prevention programs for STD's and HIV among adolescent minorities. In chapter 5, Taylor, Beech, and Cummings review the current trends in

53

physical activity levels, determinants, and interventions among minority adolescents. They point to the need for further research in these areas and specifically request that health care professionals capitalize on their unique opportunities to intervene in minority adolescent populations. Wilson, Nicholson, and Krishnamoorthy, in chapter 6, emphasize the important role that diet may have in preventing the incidence of morbidity and mortality among minority adolescents. These authors provide a framework for understanding the significance of environmental, individual, and genetic influences on developing dietary interventions for specific minority adolescent populations. In the next chapter, Guthrie, Caldwell, and Hunter provide a review of the antecedents and correlates of several health problems currently affecting minority female adolescents. They outline social, cultural, and psychological contextual factors that may have significant impact on future health-promotion efforts targeted at this population. Finally, in chapter 8, Hazuda and Monterrosa present prevalence rates of chronic illnesses among specific minority groups. In particular, this chapter reviews health behaviors that are relevant in preventing chronic illness.

In summary, Part II provides an overview of a variety of health risk and health-promoting behaviors. As a whole, these chapters describe an important profile of health-related behaviors. This profile can serve as a basis for guiding clinicians in their efforts to improve minority adolescent health.

Wendell C. Taylor
Dawn K. Wilson

3

Preventing Drug Abuse and Violence

Gilbert J. Botvin and Lawrence M. Scheier

Drug abuse and violence are two of the most serious public health problems in the United States. Etiological studies have shown strikingly similar causes for these problems. Although drug abuse and violence prevention efforts have evolved independently, there is a surprising degree of overlap in the objectives and methods of many approaches. Moreover, empirical data and theoretical formulations suggest that an array of adolescent problem behaviors (including drug abuse and violence) are interrelated, raising the possibility that multiple problem behaviors may be prevented by a common intervention strategy. Although racial and ethnic differences have been observed with respect to drug abuse and violence, there appear to be considerable similarities across populations in the risk factors associated with these problems. However, available evidence concerning the etiology and prevention of drug abuse and violence in racial and ethnic minority populations is limited.

This chapter is not intended to be a comprehensive review of the existing literature. Rather, it was designed to summarize what is known about effective school-based approaches to drug abuse prevention and to discuss the kind of prevention model that might have dual applicability to drug abuse and violence. We begin with a summary of the prevalence and current trends in drug use and violence, discuss the relationship between drug abuse and violence with respect to etiology, and then suggest a general developmental model for drug abuse and violence that integrates several theoretical perspectives. We describe school-based approaches to drug abuse prevention along with evaluation data concerning their effectiveness—for youth in general and with respect to minority populations in particular. Although most of the existing literature consists of studies conducted with predominantly White populations, this literature provides an important point of departure for identifying approaches that might also be effective with racial and ethnic minority adolescents. Where empirical evidence exists, we discuss racial and ethnic differences in prevalence rates and etiology as well as research concerning the effectiveness of preventive interventions targeting minority youth.

Prevalence and Current Trends in Drug Use

Recent national survey data (Johnston, O'Malley, & Bachman, 1994) have shown a sharp rise in marijuana use among eighth, tenth, and twelfth graders as well as an increase for all three grade levels in the use of cigarettes, stimulants, LSD, and inhalants. This reversal of the decade-long downward trend in drug use underscores the importance of developing more effective strategies to prevent drug abuse. Among high school seniors, 31% had used illicit drugs in the past year, and 42.9% had done so during their lifetime. Specific drug use data were as follows: The annual prevalence rates were 26% for marijuana, 7% for inhalants, 6.8% for LSD, and 8.4% for stimulants. The lifetime rates for these respective drugs were 35.3%, 17.4%, 10.3%, and 15.1%. For alcohol use, the annual rate was 76% and the lifetime rate was 87%. Although annual rates for smoking were not provided, the lifetime rate was 61.9%, and the 30-day rate was 29.9%.

Since 1991, when racial and ethnic differences were included in the national estimates for secondary school students, Black youth have reported the lowest prevalence estimates for all drugs mentioned in the survey, whereas Hispanic youth have reported the highest lifetime, annual, and recent 30-day prevalences. A different picture emerges, however, from the National Household Survey (National Institute on Drug Abuse [NIDA], 1991), which lumps together a broader age range inclusive of individuals from 12 through 17 years of age (thus, high school seniors are included along with eighth graders). In this survey, which relied on face-to-face interviews, prevalence estimates for marijuana use in the past year were largely the same for Blacks (10.4%), Whites (10.3%), and Hispanics (9.4%). Recent data from the 1993 NIDA survey showed that annual illicit drug use among Hispanics had soared from 13.3% to 17.6% and usage was at the highest level among the three largest racial groups. Whites were second at 13.5%, followed by Blacks (11.0%), for any illicit drug use in the past year (NIDA, 1993).

Given disproportionately higher rates of drug-related problems among minority populations relative to Whites, it might reasonably be expected that rates of drug use would be correspondingly higher. The fact that a number of national, state, and local surveys have found that the prevalence of drug use is either the same or lower for ethnic minority youth than for White youth has led to considerable speculation. Attempts to account for lower than expected rates of drug use found in several surveys for different racial and ethnic groups (particularly for Black youth) have considered a range of possible explanations. Some of the explanations considered include differential truthfulness, larger than average within-group gender differences, differential school dropout rates leading to underrepresentation of drug users in school-based minority drug surveys, delayed initiation, and differences in discretionary income. However, empirical examination of these hypotheses using national survey data from the Monitoring the Future Study (Wallace, Bachman, O'Malley, & Johnston, 1995) has generally failed to adequately explain disparities between observed and expected prevalence rates for drug use among minority youth.

Role of Racial and Ethnic Factors

In addition to exploring racial variation in patterns of drug use, several researchers have begun to examine the specific ways in which ethnic and cultural factors contribute to different etiologies among White, Hispanic, and Black youth. Unfortunately, no clear consensus has emerged from these studies. For example, Dembo, Blount, Schmei-dler, and Burgos (1986) reported nonsignificant associations among perceived environmental risk (e.g., status given to gangs and drug availability), ethnicity, and drug use. In contrast, Barnes and Welte (1986) reported that Black and Hispanic youth had higher prevalence for alcohol-related social problems than did Whites, despite higher rates of drinking among Whites. They also noted that, on the basis of select analyses of students reporting high levels of illicit drug-related social problems, minority youth reported almost double the number of alcohol-related problems compared with White youth.

Newcomb and colleagues (Maddahian, Newcomb, & Bentler, 1988; Newcomb, Maddahian, Skager, & Bentler, 1987) reported that ethnic group membership was an essential factor in determining risk status and that it contributed independently to adolescent drug use. They also noted ethnic differences in the number of psychosocial risk factors and their relationships to drug use. Blacks were at the lowest risk for each of the individual risk factors studied (e.g., self-esteem, psycho-pathology, and low grades) and had the lowest scores on a summed unit-weighted risk index compared with White, Asian, and Hispanic youth. However, Black youth at greatest risk (seven-plus risk factors) were 100% more likely to be smoking cigarettes, and among Black youth there was also a significant positive association between being characterized as a heavy (daily) user of tobacco, alcohol, or marijuana and the number of risk factors. Thus, despite their comparatively lower rates of risk both for drug use and in terms of number of risk factors, a small proportion of Black drug-using youth appear to be at heightened risk (see also Maddahian, Newcomb, & Bentler, 1985).

Additional studies have also highlighted ethnic differences in cor-relative patterns between risk and drug use. Coombs, Paulson, and Richardson (1991) reported different predictors for licit and illicit drug use among Hispanic and White youth. Parental objection to selection of friends was significantly and negatively related to tobacco and al-cohol use for Hispanic youth but not for Whites. Gender, on the other hand, was an important predictor for White but not for Hispanic youth. Among Hispanics, a youth's attitude toward parental objection to friends was a significant predictor of marijuana use, whereas only perceived friends' use of marijuana entered into the equation for White youth. Other studies have corroborated the finding of differ-ential etiologies for Black and Hispanic youth. Flannery, Vazsonyi, Torquati, and Fridrich (1994), for example, reported that perceived friends' use of alcohol, a measure of aggression, school adjustment, and peer pressure predicted male Hispanic drug use, whereas friends' alcohol use, peer pressure, and aggression predicted drug use for White boys. The model for White girls included grades and parent–child relations in addition to the variables mentioned for boys; the model for Hispanic girls included only school adjustment as a significant predictor of drug use.

Prevalence and Current Trends in Violence

Related to drug abuse is the problem of violence, which has ascended to the very top of the U.S. national agenda in recent years and has become a public heath problem of significant magnitude. According to national data, over 20,000 deaths and 2.2 million nonfatal injuries occur each year as a result of interpersonal violence (Centers for Disease Control and Prevention [CDC], 1985). Although national sources of data (such as the Uniform Crime Reporting Program and the National Crime Survey) exist, it is generally acknowledged that the data on nonfatal injuries from assaultive violence are underreported and may actually be 2 to 3 times higher than national crime data indicate (Hammond & Yung, 1993). National trend data suggest that although the proportion of young people committing serious violent crimes (e.g., aggravated assaults, forcible rapes, and homicides) is about the same as in 1980, the frequency of violence against today's youth and its lethality have increased significantly (Federal Bureau of Investigation, 1992). Violence is the second leading cause of injury-related death in the United States, and homicide risk increases dramatically during adolescence (Rodriguez, 1990). In New York City, homicide is the leading cause of death for adolescents ages 15 to 19 years (New York City Department of Health, 1993). The results of a national survey conducted in 1991 indicated that 26% of high school students had carried a weapon at least once in the past month (Kann et al., 1993).

Ethnic minority youth are at particularly high risk for violence. As Hammond and Yung (1993) noted in their excellent review article, inner-city Blacks, Hispanics, and Native Americans are at greater risk for assaultive violence than Whites. Black youth are at 4 times greater risk for homicide than White youth of the same age; followed by Hispanics, at 3 to 4 times greater risk than Whites; and Native Americans, who are at twice the risk. Although murder rates are typically higher among males than females, the magnitude of risk for Black males and females relative to White males and females is equally great. Similar patterns of risk exist for assaultive violence not resulting in death. Ethnic differences also have been noted with respect to the sources of violence. Blacks have family-friend-acquaintance homicide rates that are 6 times higher than Whites. Hispanics have the highest homicide rates by gang-related violence. Asian Americans are less likely to experience violence from someone they know, but have the highest rates of violence from strangers.

Relationship Between Drug Abuse and Violence

Data from several sources suggest a strong interrelationship between drug abuse and violence (e.g., Elliott, Huizinga, & Menard, 1989; Kingery, Pruitt, & Hurley, 1992). It is not only that drug abuse is a predictor of later involvement in assaultive violence but that homicides and other types of assaultive violence occur while individuals are under the influence of alcohol (Dawkins & Dawkins, 1983) or illicit drugs or are involved in drug-related criminal activity (Tardiff & Gross, 1986). Suicidal behaviors, another form of violence, have also been found to be related to aggression and substance use among high school students (Garrison, McKeown, Valois, & Vincent, 1993). Despite these associations, the relationship between drug use and violence is complex and poorly understood. Several longitudinal studies (Kandel, Simcha-Fagan, & Davies, 1986; White, Pandina, & LaGrange, 1987) found little evidence that drug use either necessarily precedes or follows violence, only that they tend to co-occur in some individuals and are associated in frequency and severity. Neither is a necessary or sufficient condition for the other, but existing evidence suggests that both may have similar etiologies.

Etiological Factors

A common set of demographic, environmental, inter- and intrapersonal factors appear to be involved in the etiology of drug abuse and violence. According to review articles (e.g., Elliott, 1994; Hammond & Yung, 1993), a number of risk factors are associated with assaultive violence. Demographic factors include poverty, ethnic minority group membership, gender (i.e., being male), age, and living in the inner city. Family factors include weak family bonding; ineffective monitoring and supervision; exposure to and reinforcement of violence in the home; poor impulse control and problem-solving skills of caretakers; and the acquisition of expectations, attitudes, beliefs, and emotional responses that support or tolerate the use of violence. Media influences include the modeling of violent behavior as an appropriate response to a variety of situations as well as the desensitization to violence that comes from seeing an estimated 180,000 murders, rapes, armed robberies, and assaults during the 15,000 hours of cumulative viewing that have been spent watching TV during childhood and early adolescence (Comstock & Strasburger, 1990). Such dispositional or temperamental factors as antisocial personality, attention deficit disorder, or poor impulse control have also been implicated. Other psychosocial factors include commitment to conventional norms and values; expectations, attitudes, and beliefs about sources of violence; perceived threats and misattributions of others' intentions; normative beliefs about the appropriateness of violence as a problem-solving strategy; and difficulty coping with anger and frustration. In addition, lack of personal competence and independence, low self-efficacy, poor problem-solving skills, poor social skills, and difficulty in coping with stress and anger can be contributing factors. Related to this is the use of alcohol and drugs, poor academic performance, and involvement with a delinquent peer group (e.g., gang membership) in which violence is modeled and reinforced. According to Elliott (1994), violence is often used to achieve desired goals, such as power and status, or as a method of resolving conflict; for many it is viewed as the most effective means of achieving these goals. Many of these same factors have been associated with drug use (Botvin & Botvin, 1992; Hawkins, Catalano, & Miller, 1992).

Etiological Mechanisms

Similar etiological mechanisms also appear to accentuate or mitigate vulnerability for drug abuse and violence. Cognitive–mediational and social interaction models of aggression in children and young adolescents support the view that deficits in social problem solving and poor cognitive strategies foster the development of deviant and antisocial behaviors (Dodge, 1980, 1986). A conceptual basis for these models is that functional deficits in social information processing lead to inappropriate and often negative attributions, appraisals, and expectations regarding peer-instigated behavior (Lochman, 1987). A growing literature has also documented that aggressive youth are characteristically low in self-esteem, feel rejected by the larger (normative) peer group, and suffer from poor academic performance. On the basis of a number of empirical studies of aggressive and antisocial male children and adolescents, Coie, Lochman, Terry, and Hyman (1992) concluded that the combination of social withdrawal and peer rejection contributed largely to "channeling rejected, aggressive boys into deviant peer groups that in turn influence their members toward increased antisocial behavior" (p. 783). These associations serve to bolster self-esteem and promote social interactions circumscribed by behavioral standards and normative beliefs that favor aggressive responses (Lochman, 1992). Longitudinal studies of antisocial behavior (e.g., Patterson, 1986) have suggested that deficits in familial social interactions precede the development of inadequate social and cognitive skills in children. Deficiencies in these skills foster school problems, feelings of rejection from peers and family, and learned behavioral contingencies (coercive processes) that produce delinquent and antisocial behavior. According to Patterson's model, the combination of poor parenting practices, inappropriate parental discipline, and a lack of parental monitoring establishes a hostile and negative environment for a child. These conditions are often exacerbated by social and economic disadvantage, language barriers, and poor acculturation.

Figure 1 provides an overview of an aggression and violence model that incorporates elements of social–interactional and social–cognitive perspectives. Ideally, the behavioral transformations consistent with these views unfold developmentally from early childhood through early adolescence. The area designated as "parallel developmental contingencies" represents the more common risk-engendering psychological processes hypothesized to foster violence and drug abuse behavior. A variety of factors influence whether a youth will be prone to violence, drug abuse, or some combination of both, including (a) individual differences in vulnerability, (b) activation of protective mechanisms (e.g., low family tolerance of deviance), (c) exposure (e.g., when a specific risk factor operates along the developmental continuum), and (d) the intensification or amelioration of prior risk processes (e.g., dysfunctional family functioning that perseveres throughout childhood). For example, early family dysfunction and poor parental monitoring can lead to early stage delinquency, social strain, and poor social skills. Left unabated, these problems can accentuate

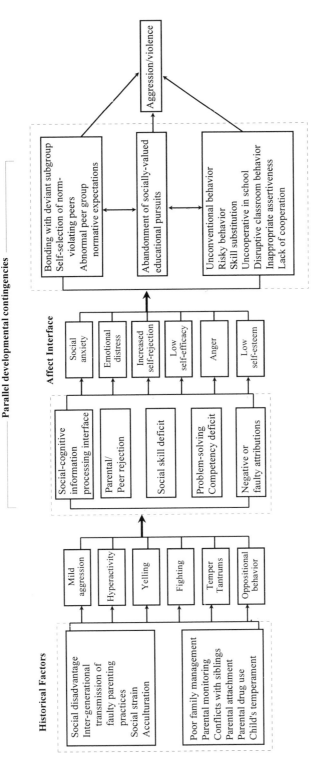

Figure 1. A hypothetical domain model depicting parallel developmental contingencies for aggression and violence.

peer rejection by prosocial groups and foster the need for deviant subgroup bonding. This type of bonding facilitates the adoption of inappropriate behavioral standards for aggression as well as drug use, which is more easily accessible and reinforced (Coie et al., 1992).

Most contemporary theories of adolescent drug abuse underscore similar risk mechanisms that lead to drug abuse (e.g., see Newcomb & Bentler, 1988). Although emphasizing somewhat different risk factors, different points of developmental inflection, or different causal relations, models of drug abuse and antisocial behavior share a common thread in the primacy of social and personal competence. Although previous explanatory models of violence and drug abuse have stressed the causal nature of these processes, many of the risk processes can be conceptualized as recursive or reciprocal pathways that reflect behavioral maintenance or exacerbation. Moreover, the earlier model as presented in Figure 1 is not intended to convey a sense of equilibrium or equipotentiality among the postulated causal processes. Numerous factors impinge differentially on the hypothesized relations, including duration of risk, intensity, amplification, buffering, or inoculation, to name just a few, all of which modulate the effects of risk over time.

Theoretical Considerations

A Problem Behavior Perspective

Theoretical formulations and empirical data point to relationships among multiple problem behaviors. Thus, the relationship between drug abuse and violence may merely be part of a larger constellation of interrelated behaviors that also includes truancy, delinquency, and precocious or unprotected sexual activity. Problem behavior theory (Jessor & Jessor, 1977) conceptualizes these behaviors as part of an overall syndrome of functionally similar behaviors with a common etiology. Empirical support for a problem behavior syndrome or general deviance latent construct can be found in Jessor's own work (e.g., Donovan & Jessor, 1985; Donovan, Jessor, & Costa, 1988) as well as the work of others (e.g., Farrell, Danish, & Howard, 1992; McGee & Newcomb, 1992). Coie et al. (1993) has extended and articulated the notion of a cluster of related behaviors with a common etiology or set of risk factors as a basic prevention principle in the mental health field.

The significance of these conceptualizations and the supporting empirical data is that once a common set of predictors or risk factors is identified and an effective intervention is developed, it may be possible to prevent several different problems or disorders with a single prevention approach.

General Developmental Risk Mechanisms for Violence and Drug Abuse

Figure 2 shows a general developmental risk mechanism with common pathways and developmental contingencies for aggression or violence and drug abuse. Elements from several prominent theories of drug abuse (e.g., self-derogation, social influence, and peer cluster) and antisocial behavior are included to represent a broad mixture of risk processes. Given the utility of many of the putative risk–protective factors for predicting a wide variety of outcomes (i.e., problem behaviors), a superordinate construct of "general deviance' is modeled as the criterion (e.g., Donovan & Jessor, 1985; McGee & Newcomb, 1992). Variations on this model can be contrasted statistically with structural equation modeling (SEM) techniques. The figure designates key areas for developmental change and individual growth. In effect, the model captures etiologic-specific risk processes as well as key intervention points. The figure suggests that the effects of early family processes, personality, social, and cognitive factors on the behavioral outcomes are sequentially processed through a series of social–cognitive filters that culminates with the decision to engage in aggressive behavior or drug use.

According to Dodge and others (Dodge, 1980; Dodge, Price, Bachorowski, & Newman, 1990), deficient processing at any point along this continuum leads to deviant and antisocial behavior. Thus, we hypothesize that youth characterized as impulsive, risk taking, lacking in diligence, having poor self-reinforcement skills, and having low self-esteem engage in drug use primarily for the positive social benefits (e.g., it makes them look cool, helps them obtain friends, and elevates peer status). The immediate and proximal motivational reasons are captured under "social influences" and allude to the acquisition of deviant and antisocial behavioral standards. This approach may best characterize early stage drug abuse, but the model is also applicable to early stage delinquency (e.g., bullying and fighting). For instance, we would hypothesize that impulsive, poor self-monitoring

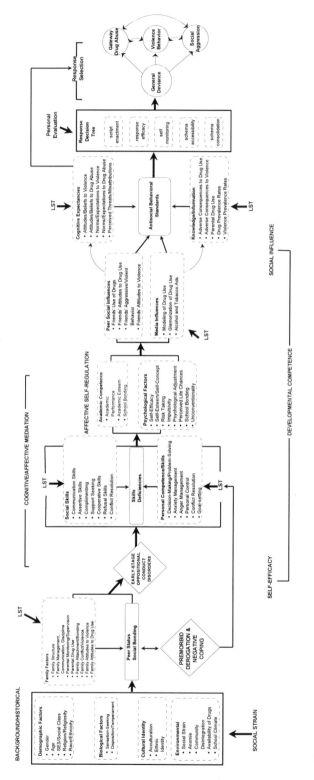

Figure 2. A common developmental pathway for violence-related and drug abuse behavior. Large, bold-headed arrows designate key areas for developmental change and individual growth. Risk processes are designated by diamonds, aggregate risk factors are enclosed by stippled lines, and hypothesized psychological filters are designated by large bold-faced boxes.

youth with low self-efficacy (low internal control) would have difficulty forming lasting ties with peers, school, or social institutions (i.e.,
clubs). For these youth, exacerbated drug use leads to violent behavior
(i.e., fighting, property destruction, and extreme forms of antisocial
behavior, including self-destruction). Although both drug use and violent behavior are considered under a single rubric of general deviance, risk processes specific to each construct may be examined using
SEM techniques (McGee & Newcomb, 1992).

Consistent with social strain and developmental models of aggression, our model hypothesizes that violence-prone or drug-abusing
youth have crafted a set of expectancies and values that originated in
childhood family interactive sequences and that these expectations regarding self and others have survived intact through their early adolescent years. The lack of preparation to address the high levels of
conventionality and emphasis on skill acquisition and development in
competitive environments such as in school stimulates a process by
which these youth disengage from learning and begin to drift toward
supportive, although highly deviant, peer groups that promote a new
set of working standards (Snyder, Dishion, & Patterson, 1986). These
standards usually include physical fighting as a vehicle to gain peer
approval, drug use to obtain peer acceptance, and unconventional and
high-risk behaviors to maintain peer status. A sequence of this nature
promotes heightened delinquency (truancy, vandalism, and crime).

It is important to note that, in its initial stages, drug abuse is not a
sufficient condition for violent behavior but instead accentuates certain vulnerabilities and risk-potentiating conditions. Thus, for many
youth, violent behavior is "caused" by a risk mechanism that also
includes long-term drug abuse. For instance, youth with low esteem
who lack personal competence and social skills are likely to bond with
other deviant friends to gain recognition and diminish their negative
derogation. Early stages of delinquency include fighting and aggression to maintain peer status, which contribute to the development of
behavioral standards. This activity enhances adolescents' expectancies
for violence or drug use (e.g., "drugs help me gain peer approval"),
which are consolidated through reinforcement and instrumental learning. However, continued drug use enmeshes these youth in a perpet-
ual cycle of deviance (or activities that promote deviant behavior). As
a second stage, our model hypothesizes that continued deviance in
the presence of drug use will lead to violence (e.g., fighting with teachers, parents, and associating with nondeviant school peers).

Intervention Approaches

Approaches to Drug Abuse Prevention

Reviews of the prevention research literature (Botvin & Botvin, 1992; Hansen, 1992) and meta-analytic studies (Bangert-Drowns, 1988; Bruvold & Rundall, 1988) have indicated that drug abuse prevention programs using information dissemination, affective education, and alternatives approaches are ineffective. Studies testing these approaches have not been able to produce reductions in drug use behavior. The most promising approaches, according to available evidence, are those that target the psychosocial factors implicated in the initiation of drug abuse (Bangert-Drowns, 1988; Botvin & Botvin, 1992; Bruvold & Rundall, 1988). All of these approaches have been designed to be implemented with junior high school students in classroom settings and to provide students with the information and skills necessary for resisting social influences to use drugs. Some also teach an array of personal and social skills to decrease potential motivations for using drugs.

Resisting Social Influences

The most widely researched psychosocial approach to drug abuse prevention relies on a prevention model that derives from social psychology. The underlying conceptualization of this model and its many variations is that adolescent cigarette smoking, for example, is the result of social influences (persuasive messages) from peers and the media in the form of offers to smoke cigarettes, advertising appeals, and exposure to smokers who may serve as role models.

The prevention approaches based on this model have typically contained two or more of the following components: psychological inoculation, correcting normative expectations, and resistance skills training (Evans et al., 1978; Flynn et al., 1992; Ross, Greene, & House, 1977). Early research with approaches based on this model emphasized psychological inoculation and modifying normative expectations. More recent approaches have tested variations on this model that emphasize resistance skills training. Some approaches have added other components, such as having students make a public commitment to not use drugs.

Evaluation Results

Researchers have conducted a number of studies evaluating the effectiveness of social influence approaches to drug abuse prevention over the past decade and a half. Results of both small- and large-scale studies have documented the effectiveness of these approaches (e.g., Arkin, Roemhild, Johnson, Luepker, & Murray, 1981; Luepker, Johnson, Murray, & Pechacek, 1983; Pentz et al., 1989; Perry, Killen, Slinkard, & McAlister, 1983; Snow, Tebes, Arthur, & Tapasak, 1992; Sussman, Dent, Stacy, & Sun, 1993; Telch, Killen, McAlister, Perry, & Maccoby, 1982). Most of these studies have focused on smoking prevention, with some researchers reporting results in terms of smoking onset (preventing the transition from nonsmoking to smoking), others reporting results in terms of overall smoking prevalence, and still others reporting results with respect to an index measure or scale of smoking involvement.

Several follow-up studies (e.g., Luepker et al., 1983; MacKinnon et al., 1991; McAlister, Puska, Koskela, Pallonen, & Maccoby, 1980; Pentz et al., 1989; Sussman et al., 1993; Telch et al., 1982) have reported positive behavior effects lasting for up to 3 years. However, data from several longer-term follow-ups (Bell, Ellickson, & Harrison, 1993; Ellickson, Bell, & McGuigan, 1993; Flay et al., 1989; Murray, Davis-Hearn, Goldman, Pirie, & Luepker, 1988) have shown these effects to gradually decay over time, suggesting the need for ongoing intervention or booster sessions. Because little is known about the nature and timing of booster interventions, additional research is needed. Also, because relatively little research has been conducted with substances other than tobacco, data concerning the durability of prevention effects on other substances are not yet available.

Teaching Resistance Skills and General Life Skills

The second major approach to drug abuse prevention emerging during the past decade and a half integrates the teaching of skills for resisting social influences to use drugs with the development of general personal and social skills. In our research at Cornell University, we have tested a prevention approach called Life Skills Training (LST) that is based on this prevention model. As indicated in Figure 2, the LST approach is designed to affect a number of the factors believed to play important roles in the etiology of drug abuse and violence. The LST prevention program can best be conceptualized as consisting of two general-skills-training components to enhance overall personal competence and a problem-specific component relating to drug abuse prevention. The program consists of 15 class periods, each roughly 45 min long. We have summarized the three components and the intervention methods and materials elsewhere (e.g., Botvin & Tortu, 1988; see also chap. 11, this volume).

Over the past 15 years, a series of evaluation studies (summarized by Botvin & Botvin [1992]) have been conducted to test the effectiveness of drug abuse prevention approaches based on the LST model. These studies have been conducted in a logical sequence intended to facilitate the development of a prevention approach that is effective with different problem behaviors when implemented by different types of providers and with different populations. The focus of the early LST research was on cigarette smoking and involved predominantly White middle-class populations. Later research extended this work to other problem behaviors, including the use of alcohol, marijuana, and, most recently, illicit drugs other than marijuana. These studies have shown that the LST approach can reduce drug use among junior high school students (compared with untreated control participants) by up to 87%. Long-term follow-up data collected at the end of high school have provided empirical support for the durability of these effects on drug use as well as their potential for preventing more serious levels of drug involvement (Botvin, Baker, Dusenbury, Botvin, & Diaz, 1995). In addition, this research has increasingly been focused on the utility of the LST approach with inner-city minority populations.

Prevention Among Racial and Ethnic Minority Youth

A gap in the drug abuse prevention field that has only recently begun to be addressed concerns the lack of high-quality research with minority populations. In developing preventive interventions for minority populations, researchers have followed two strategies. One strategy, based on the assumption that the etiology of drug abuse is different for different populations, involves the development of interventions designed to be population-specific. The other strategy, which is based on the assumption that the etiology of drug abuse is more similar than different across populations, involves developing interventions to be generalizable to a broad range of individuals from different populations. Research with the LST program has followed the second course; that is, where warranted, modifications have been made to maximize generalizability, cultural sensitivity, relevance, and acceptability across varied populations. Although there are only limited data concerning the etiology of drug abuse among minority populations, existing evidence does suggest that there is substantial overlap in the factors promoting and maintaining drug use and abuse among different racial and ethnic populations (e.g., see Bettes, Dusenbury, Kerner, James-Ortiz, & Botvin, 1990; Botvin, Epstein, Schinke, & Diaz, 1994; Botvin, Goldberg, Baker, Dusenbury, & Botvin, 1992; Dusenbury et al., 1992; Epstein, Botvin, Diaz, & Schinke, 1994). A second reason for pursuing this course is that most urban schools contain individuals from multiple racial and ethnic groups. For both logistical and political reasons, even if differences did exist across populations to warrant different interventions, it would be extremely difficult to implement separate interventions for different racial and ethnic groups in the school setting.

Although some Asians have been included in the studies conducted with the LST program, the major racial and ethnic groups involved in the most recent research studies with minority populations comprise Black and Hispanic youth. As was the case with earlier research among White middle-class youth, the initial focus of this research was on cigarette smoking, followed by a focus on other gateway substances. Research testing the generalizability of the LST prevention approach to inner-city minority youth has progressed through the following sequence: (a) exploratory and qualitative research, consisting of focus-group testing and key-informant interviews; (b) expert review of intervention methods and materials; (c) consumer-based review of intervention materials and methods; (d) small-scale pilot studies; and (e) large-scale randomized field trials. Modifications have been made as necessary throughout the process of development and testing. None of the changes deriving from the etiological literature concerning minority youth or the first three research phases outlined above involved the underlying prevention strategy. Rather, these changes related to the appropriateness of the reading level of intervention materials; the inclusion of appropriate graphics (e.g., illustrations or pictures of minority youth); and language, role-play scenarios, and examples appropriate to the target population.

Hispanic youth. In the first study testing the effectiveness of the LST approach with a minority population, Botvin, Dusenbury, Baker, James-Ortiz, and Kerner (1989) examined a sample of 471 seventh graders (46% male) attending eight public schools in the New York metropolitan area. The sample consisted predominantly of lower income Hispanic students (74%) as well as a small percentage of Black students (11%) and White (4%) students. Schools were randomly assigned to conditions. The authors found significant differences between the experimental and the control group, controlling for pretest smoking status, gender, social risk for becoming a smoker, and acculturation. They also found intervention effects for knowledge concerning the immediate consequences of smoking, smoking prevalence, the social acceptability of smoking, decision making, normative expectations concerning adult smoking, and normative expectations concerning peer smoking.

Data from a subsequent large-scale randomized trial (Botvin, Dusenbury, et al., 1992) demonstrated significant program effects when the LST program was implemented with predominately Hispanic urban minority students. This study involved 3,501 students from 47 public and parochial schools in the greater New York City area. Intervention materials were modified (on the basis of results from our pilot study and input from consultants, teachers, and students) to increase their relevance to Hispanic youth as well as to ensure a high degree of cultural sensitivity. Schools were randomly assigned to experimental and control conditions. Using school means as the unit of analysis, we found significant reductions in cigarette smoking for the adolescents who received the LST program in comparison with control participants at the end of the seventh grade. Follow-up data demonstrated the continued presence of prevention effects through the end of the tenth grade.

Black youth. Before testing the LST approach on Black youth, we once again subjected the intervention materials and methods to an extensive review to determine their cultural appropriateness for the target population. We then conducted a small-scale study with nine urban junior high schools in northern New Jersey (Botvin, Batson, et al., 1989). The pretest involved 608 seventh-grade students; of these, 221 were in the treatment group, and 387 made up the control group. The sample was 87% Black, 10% Hispanic, and 1% White; 2% were of some other ethnicity. Schools were randomly assigned to treatment and control conditions within each of the three participating communities. Students in the treatment schools received the LST program, whereas students in the control schools received the smoking education curriculum normally provided by their school. Throughout the prevention program, we collected both classroom observation data and teacher feedback. Results indicated that there were significantly fewer posttest smokers in the treatment group than in the control group, on the basis of self-reported smoking status in the past month. Significant treatment effects were also found for knowledge of smoking consequences, normative expectations regarding adult smoking prevalence, and normative expectations regarding peer smoking prevalence. A large-scale prevention trial (Botvin & Cardwell, 1992) involving predominantly Black youth from 46 inner-city schools in northern New Jersey provided additional empirical support for the effectiveness of this prevention approach with this population. We randomly assigned 46 schools to treatment ($n = 21$) or control conditions ($n = 25$). In the treatment condition, all eligible classes in participating schools received the LST intervention; in the control condition, all classes received the health (smoking) education normally provided to its students. The sample used in the final analysis included 97% minorities and 3% Whites. Of the total sample, 78% were Black, 13% were Hispanic, 1% were Native American, 1% were Asian, and 3% classified themselves as "other." Initial posttest results showed significantly less smoking for students in the treatment group, who received the intervention in the seventh grade and booster sessions in the fall of the eighth grade, in comparison with both the nonbooster treatment condition and the control condition. At the final follow-up, students who had received booster sessions and the original intervention smoked significantly less than the controls.

Tailoring interventions to the target population. In a recently completed study, Botvin, Schinke, Epstein, and Diaz (1994) tested the relative effectiveness of a broad-spectrum prevention approach (LST) previously found to be effective with White, Black, and Hispanic youth and a prevention approach specifically tailored to Black and Hispanic youth. Both prevention approaches were similar in that they taught students a combination of generic life skills and skills specific to resisting offers to use drugs. However, the tailored, or culturally focused, approach was designed to embed the skills-training material in myths and legends derived from Black and Hispanic cultures. Six junior high schools containing predominantly (95%) minority students were assigned to one of three conditions: (a) to receive the LST program, (b) to receive the culturally focused prevention approach, or (c) to serve as an information-only control group. The sample was 48% Black, 37% Hispanic, 5% White, 3% Asian, and 8% other. Students were pretested and posttested during the seventh grade. Results indicated that students in both skills-training prevention conditions had lower intentions to drink beer or wine relative to the information-only control participants, and the students in the LST condition had lower intentions to drink hard liquor and use illicit drugs. Both skills-training conditions also affected several mediating variables in a direction consistent with nondrug use. According to these results, both prevention approaches were equally effective, producing significant reductions in behavioral intentions to drink and use illicit drugs and suggesting that a generic drug abuse prevention approach with high generalizability may be as effective as one tailored to individual ethnic populations. These data also provide support for the hypothesis that a single drug abuse prevention strategy can be used effectively with multiethnic populations.

Two-year follow-up data ($N = 456$), collected at the end of the ninth grade for participants in Botvin, Schinke, et al.'s (1994) study showed significant prevention effects for both prevention approaches (Botvin, Schinke, Epstein, Diaz, & Botvin, 1995). Students in both skills-training prevention conditions drank alcohol less often, became drunk less often, drank less alcohol per drinking occasion, and had lower intentions to use alcohol in the future relative to the control participants. However, these data also showed that the culturally focused intervention produced significantly stronger effects on these variables than did the generic LST approach. The findings of this follow-up are particularly interesting because, while suggesting that it may be possible to develop a preventive intervention that is effective for a relatively broad range of students, they show that tailoring interventions to specific populations can increase effectiveness among inner-city minority populations.

Extending the LST Model to Aggression and Violence Prevention

Studies testing interventions for decreasing peer rejection and aggression (Coie & Koeppl, 1990) and aggressive, oppositional, and conduct disorder behavior (Kazdin, 1987) have included generic skills-training components similar to those in the LST approach to drug abuse prevention, along with some additional, problem-specific material. These interventions have typically emphasized teaching social skills, problem solving, and anger management by using cognitive–behavioral techniques. Both short- and longer-term effects have been produced with respect to the skills targeted as well as to self-esteem, social status with peers, and aggression. Some of these studies (e.g., Hammond & Yung, 1991; Lochman, Coie, Underwood, & Terry, 1993) have been conducted with inner-city minority youth. This literature and literature showing relationships among multiple problem behaviors suggest that modifying the current LST model to include material specific to aggression and violence may result in a prevention approach that is effective with both drug abuse and violence. In the sections that follow, we describe a version of the LST approach to preventing drug abuse that Botvin and his colleagues at Cornell's Institute for Prevention Research are currently developing to extend to aggression and violence prevention with inner-city minority youth. The adaptation includes both a school and a parent intervention, each of which we describe below. We are testing both interventions in a 5-year investigation funded by the National Institute on Drug Abuse.

School-Based Intervention

Although much of the material in the generic skills-training components has relevance for violence prevention as well as drug abuse prevention, some additional generic skills would also need to be included to further strengthen the intervention and render it appropriate as a violence prevention approach. Likewise, additional new material specific to the problem of violence is needed to render the LST model appropriate as a combined drug abuse and violence prevention approach. A combined drug abuse–violence prevention LST model would consist of training provided in seventeen 45-min class periods, which would be augmented by in-class video material and a parent intervention consisting of take-home videos and written material.

Personal skills component. This component is designed to affect an array of personal self-management skills. The personal skills component includes material that contributes to the following goals:

1. Fostering the development of decision making and problem solving (e.g., identifying problem situations, defining goals, generating alternative solutions, and considering consequences);
2. Teaching skills for identifying, analyzing, interpreting, and resisting media influences;
3. Providing self-control skills for coping with anxiety (e.g., relaxation training) and anger and frustration (inhibiting impulsive reactions, reframing, and using self-statements); and
4. Providing the basic principles of personal behavior change and self-improvement (e.g., goal setting, self-monitoring, and self-reinforcement).

Most of this material consists of generic self-management skills important to both drug abuse and violence prevention, except for the self-control skills that deal with anger and frustration management, which is more specific to violence prevention.

Social skills component. This component is designed to affect several important social skills and enhance general social competence. The social skills component contains material designed to help students overcome shyness and improve general interpersonal skills. Emphasis is on communication skills, general social skills (e.g., initiating social interactions, conversational skills, and complimenting others), skills related to boy–girl relationships, and both verbal and nonverbal assertive skills. This component is the same as that included in the drug abuse prevention LST model.

Drug-abuse-specific component. This component is designed to affect students' knowledge and attitudes concerning drug use, normative expectations, and skills for resisting drug use influences from the media and peers. The material contained in this component is similar to that of many psychosocial drug abuse prevention programs (e.g., Evans, Hansen, & Mittlemark, 1977; Hurd et al., 1980; McAlister, Perry, & Maccoby, 1979; Pentz, Dwyer et al., 1989). It concerns short- and long-term consequences of drug use; knowledge about the actual levels of drug use among both adults and adolescents, to correct normative expectations about drug use; information about the declining social acceptability of cigarette smoking and other drug use; information and class exercises demonstrating the immediate physiological effects of cigarette smoking; information about media pressures to smoke, drink, or use drugs; knowledge of techniques used by cigarette and alcoholic beverage advertisers to promote the use of these drugs, as well as skills for resisting them; and techniques for resisting direct peer pressure to smoke, drink, or use drugs.

Violence-specific component. The violence-specific component is designed to affect knowledge and attitudes concerning violence and aggression, normative expectations, and skills for resisting pro-violence influences from media and peers. This component helps students examine information concerning violence prevalence rates; sources of violence; the appropriateness and efficacy of using aggression and violence as a way of dealing with problems or conflicts; common situations leading to violence and how to avoid them; identifying hostile misattributions and distorted perceptions, and how to modify them; strategies for "saving face," maintaining status, and resolving conflict situations; and skills for identifying and resisting pro-violence influences from media and peers.

Parent Intervention

Notwithstanding the evidence supporting the effectiveness of school-based approaches to drug abuse prevention and their promise for preventing violence, considerable research has pointed to the need for interventions that target the family (e.g., Brook, Brook, Gordon, Whiteman, & Cohen, 1990). Kazdin (1993) and others have argued for the inclusion of family intervention components in prevention efforts targeting mental health. In a recent review, Kumpfer and Alvarado (1995) summarized the research conducted with family interventions targeting delinquency and drug abuse and highlighted the potential of including skills-based family intervention components in drug abuse and violence prevention programs.

A considerable literature exists that supports the potential of interventions targeting the family or parents for preventing drug abuse and violence in children (e.g., Kumpfer & Alvarado, 1995). Important focuses of family and parent interventions include parental monitoring and discipline, communication skills, drug abuse and violence prevention skills, and knowledge. For maximal effectiveness, parent interventions should be designed to complement and reinforce interventions being conducted in school settings. Because it may be difficult to involve more than a few parents in formal interventions (i.e., as this would require meetings), parent interventions should be easy to use, interesting, capable of being standardized, use a delivery channel that is widely available, and capitalize on the power of television.

Parent videotape. The parent videotape we used was designed to encourage parental monitoring and supervision of children, establishment of antidrug and antiviolence messages, effective communication, being a good (nonviolent and non-drug-using) role model, and practicing drug abuse and violence prevention skills with children. To promote synergy between the school and parent interventions, we included an introduction to the school-based prevention program for parents and a demonstration of the skills their children were learning in school.

Written materials. Another important part of a parent intervention is to supply a written manual for parents that provides information on both the causes and the consequences of drug use and violence, as well as on early warning signs for drug involvement and aggressive or violent behavior. We include the parents' manual to reinforce and more fully explain the skills covered in the videotape. Newsletters can also be distributed to parents to provide current information on drug abuse and violence prevention as well as information on their children's school-based intervention. Although the primary purpose of the written material is to convey information, a secondary purpose is to increase awareness of the problems of drug abuse and violence and to increase participation and support for the school-based intervention.

Homework assignments. Program leaders can also give students participating in the school-based intervention handouts and homework assignments that are designed to be completed with the parent or caregiver. Topics may include establishing family rules; goal setting, decision making, and problem solving; and practicing drug and violence prevention skills.

Parent workshops. Parents or caregivers of students involved in the drug abuse and violence prevention program can also be invited to attend a workshop. The workshop should be conducted on multiple occasions to increase the opportunity for all adults to attend. To increase the potential for parental involvement, program administrators should schedule these workshops at times that are convenient for parents (generally, early mornings, evenings, and weekends). The workshop agenda should consist of a videotape screening, a presentation on the causes and consequences of drug use and violence, and demonstrations and discussions of techniques that parents can use to help protect their children from drugs and violence. Workshop recruitment can be done through homework activities, mailed invitations, and parent–teacher conferences.

Conclusions and Implications for Practitioners

Drug abuse and violence are two of the most important public health problems facing the United States. After nearly a decade of decline, drug use among adolescents is once again on the increase. Violence has assumed new proportions as guns have proliferated and the lethality of violence among youth has increased dramatically. New urgency now exists for developing more innovative and effective solutions to two old problems.

Examination of the etiologies of drug abuse and aggression and violence has suggested considerable overlap in terms of risk factors and developmental mechanisms. Moreover, theoretical formulations and empirical work in several allied areas suggest a common problem behavior syndrome or general deviance syndrome. The implication for prevention practitioners is that theoretically and empirically related problems such as drug abuse and violence may be similar enough to be prevented by using the same intervention techniques.

Our own research with the LST prevention approach has demonstrated that such training can consistently produce substantial reductions in adolescent drug use. Longitudinal research has shown that preventive gains obtained with this approach can be maintained with booster sessions in subsequent years. Over a 15-year period, studies involving nearly 6,000 students from 56 schools have shown that the LST approach can reduce tobacco, alcohol, and marijuana use among adolescents. Preventive effects have also been found with respect to more severe levels of drug involvement, such as heavy cigarette smoking, immoderate drinking, and the use of multiple substances and illicit drugs. Overall, research with LST demonstrates the importance of using (a) an intervention model grounded in theory and empirical research concerning the etiology of drug abuse, (b) proven skills-training techniques, (c) an adequate intervention dosage, (d) a multi-year intervention that includes booster sessions, and (e) quality control to ensure adequate implementation fidelity.

Extending the LST model to include material related specifically to the problem of aggression and violence offers one potentially effective approach to drug abuse and violence prevention. On the basis of an understanding of the etiological factors and developmental mechanisms of drug abuse and violence, we recognized that modifications to the current LST drug abuse prevention model were necessary. These modifications included adding self-management skills for dealing with anger and frustration and including domain-specific material concerning violence-related knowledge and attitudes, norms, and skills for resisting media and peer influences that promote aggression and violence. Beyond the components of a school-based preventive intervention, we suggest that practitioners include a parent intervention that incorporates videotape, written materials, homework assignments, and training workshops. Although not yet subjected to empirical testing with respect to aggression and violence, this combined school and parent approach to drug abuse and violence prevention would appear to offer considerable promise. Future research should be undertaken to test the effect of this prevention approach on aggression and violence, drug use, and risk factors associated with both types of behavior.

REFERENCES

Arkin, R. M., Roemhild, H. J., Johnson, C. A., Luepker, R. V., & Murray, D. M. (1981). The Minnesota smoking prevention program: A seventh grade health curriculum supplement. *Journal of School Health, 51,* 616–661.

Bangert-Drowns, R. L. (1988). The effects of school-based substance abuse education: A meta-analysis. *Journal of Drug Education, 18,* 243–265.

Barnes, G. M., & Welte, J. W. (1986). Adolescent alcohol abuse: Subgroup differences and relationships to other problem behaviors. *Journal of Adolescent Research, 1,* 79–94.

Bell, R. M., Ellickson, P. L., & Harrison, E. R. (1993). Do drug prevention effects persist into high school? *Preventive Medicine, 22,* 463–483.

Bettes, B. A., Dusenbury, L., Kerner, J., James-Ortiz, S., & Botvin, G. J. (1990). Ethnicity and psychosocial factors in alcohol and tobacco use in adolescence. *Child Development, 61,* 557–565.

Botvin, G. J., Baker, F., Dusenbury, L. S., Botvin, E. M., & Diaz, T. (1995). Long-term follow-up results of a randomized drug abuse prevention trial in a White middle-class population. *Journal of the American Medical Association, 273,* 1106–1112.

Botvin, G. J., Batson, H., Witts-Vitale, S., Bess, V., Baker, E., & Dusenbury, L. (1989). A psychosocial approach to smoking prevention for urban Black youth. *Public Health Reports, 104,* 573–582.

Botvin, G. J., & Botvin, E. M. (1992). School-based and community-based prevention approaches. In J. H. Lowinson, P. Ruiz, & R. B. Millman (Eds.), *Substance abuse: A comprehensive textbook* (2nd ed., pp. 910–927). Baltimore: Williams & Wilkins.

Botvin, G. J., & Cardwell, J. (1992). Primary prevention (smoking) of cancer in Black populations (Grant No. N01-CN-6508; Final Report to National Cancer Institute). Ithaca, NY: Cornell University Medical College.

Botvin, G. J., Dusenbury, L., Baker, E., James-Ortiz, S., Botvin, E. M., & Kerner, J. (1992). Smoking prevention among urban minority youth: Assessing effects on outcome and mediating variables. *Health Psychology, 11,* 290–299.

Botvin, G. J., Dusenbury, L., Baker, E., James-Ortiz, S., & Kerner, J. (1989). A skills training approach to smoking prevention among Hispanic youth. *Journal of Behavioral Medicine, 12,* 279–296.

Botvin, G. J., Epstein, J. A., Schinke, S. P., & Diaz, T. (1994). Correlates and predictors of smoking among inner city youth. *Developmental and Behavioral Pediatrics, 15,* 67–73.

Botvin, G. J., Goldberg, C. J., Baker, E., Dusenbury, L., & Botvin, E. M. (1992). Correlates and predictors of smoking among Black adolescents. *Addictive Behaviors, 17,* 97–103.

Botvin, G. J., Schinke, S. P., Epstein, J. A., & Diaz, T. (1994). The effectiveness of culturally-focused and generic skills training approaches to alcohol and drug abuse prevention among minority youth. *Psychology of Addictive Behaviors, 8,* 116–127.

Botvin, G. J., Schinke, S. P., Epstein, J. A., Diaz, T., & Botvin, E. M. (1995). Effectiveness of culturally focused and generic skills training approaches to alcohol and drug abuse prevention among minority adolescents: Two-year follow-up results. *Psychology of Addictive Behaviors, 9,* 183–194.

Botvin, G. J., & Tortu, S. (1988). Peer relationships, social competence, and substance abuse prevention: Implications for the family. *Journal of Chemical Dependency Treatment, 1,* 245–273.

Brook, J. S., Brook, D. W., Gordon, A. S., Whiteman, M., & Cohen, P. (1990). The psychological etiology of adolescent drug use: A family interactional approach. *Genetic, Social and General Monographs, 116,* 111–267.

Bruvold, W. H., & Rundall, T. G. (1988). A meta-analysis and theoretical review of school based tobacco and alcohol intervention programs. *Psychology and Health, 2,* 53–78.

Centers for Disease Control and Prevention (CDC). (1985). Homicides among young black males: United States, 1970–1982. *Mortality and Morbidity Weekly Report, 34,* 629–633.

Coie, J. D., & Koeppl, G. (1990). Adapting intervention to the problems of aggressive and disruptive children. In S. Asher & J. Coie (Eds.), *Peer rejection in childhood* (pp. 309–337). Cambridge, England: Cambridge University Press.

Coie, J. D., Lochman, J. E., Terry, R., & Hyman, C. (1992). Predicting early adolescent disorder from childhood aggression and peer rejection. *Journal of Consulting and Clinical Psychology, 60,* 783–792.

Coie, J. D., Watt, N. F., West, S. G., Hawkins, J. D., Asarnow, J. R., Markman, H. J., Ramey, S. L., Shure, M. B., & Long, B. (1993). A conceptual framework and some directions for a national research program. *American Psychologist, 48,* 1013–1022.

Comstock, G., & Strasburger, V. C. (1990). Deceptive appearances: Television violence and aggressive behavior. *Journal of Adolescent Health Care, 11,* 31–42.

Coombs, R. H., Paulson, M. J., & Richardson, M. A. (1991). Peer vs. parental influence in substance use among Hispanic and Anglo children and adolescents. *Journal of Youth and Adolescence, 20,* 73–88.

Dawkins, R., & Dawkins, M. (1983). Alcohol use and delinquency among Black, White and Hispanic offenders. *Adolescence, 18,* 639–645.

Dembo, R., Blount, W. R., Schmeidler, J., & Burgos, W. (1986). Perceived environmental drug use risk and the correlates of early drug use or nonuse among inner-city youths: The motivated actor. *International Journal of the Addictions, 2,* 977–1000.

Dodge, K. A. (1980). Social cognition and children's aggressive behavior. *Child Development, 51,* 162–170.

Dodge, K. A. (1986). A social information-processing model of social competence in children. In *Minnesota symposium on child psychology* (pp. 77–125). Hillsdale, NJ: Erlbaum.

Dodge, K. A., Price, J., Bachorowski, J., & Newman, M. (1990). Hostile attributional biases in severely aggressive adolescents. *Journal of Abnormal Psychology, 99,* 385–392.

Donovan, J. E., & Jessor, R. (1985). Structure of problem behavior in adolescence and young adulthood. *Journal of Consulting and Clinical Psychology, 56,* 762–765.

Donovan, J. E., Jessor, R., & Costa, F. M. (1988). Syndrome of problem behavior in adolescence: A replication. *Journal of Consulting and Clinical Psychology, 56,* 762–765.

Dusenbury, L., Kerner, J. F., Baker, E., Botvin, G. J., James-Ortiz, S., & Zauber, A. (1992). Predictors of smoking prevalence among New York Latino youth. *American Journal of Public Health, 82,* 55–58.

Ellickson, P. L., Bell, R. M., & McGuigan, K. (1993). Preventing adolescent drug use: Long term results of a junior high program. *American Journal of Public Health, 83,* 856–861.

Elliott, D. S. (1994, February). *Youth violence: An overview.* Paper presented for the Aspen Institute's Children's Policy Forum, Children and Violence Conference, Queenstowne, MD.

Elliott, D. S., Huizinga, D., & Menard, S. (1989). *Multiple problem youth: Delinquency, substance use and mental health problems.* New York: Springer-Verlag.

Epstein, J. A., Botvin, G. J., Diaz, T., & Schinke, S. P. (1994). The role of social factors and individual characteristics in promoting alcohol among inner-city minority youth. *Journal of Studies on Alcohol, 56,* 39–46.

Evans, R. I., Hansen, W. B., & Mittlemark, M. B. (1977). Increasing the validity of self-reports of smoking behavior in children. *Journal of Applied Psychology, 62*, 521–523.

Evans, R. I., Rozelle, R. M., Mittlemark, M. B., Hansen, W. B., Bane, A. L., & Havis, J. (1978). Deterring the onset of smoking in children: Knowledge of immediate physiological effects and coping with peer pressure, media pressure, and parent modeling. *Journal of Applied Social Psychology, 8*, 126–135.

Farrell, A. D., Danish, S. J., & Howard, C. W. (1992). Relationship between drug use and other problem behaviors in urban adolescents. *Journal of Consulting and Clinical Psychology, 60*, 705–712.

Federal Bureau of Investigation. (1992). *Crime in the United States: 1991*. Washington, DC: U.S. Government Printing Office.

Flannery, D. J., Vazsonyi, A. T., Torquati, J., & Fridrich, A. (1994). Ethnic and gender differences in risk for early adolescent substance use. *Journal of Youth and Adolescence, 23*, 195–213.

Flay, B. R., Keopke, D., Thomson, S. J., Santi, S., Best, J. A., & Brown, K. S. (1989). Long-term follow-up of the first Waterloo smoking prevention trial. *American Journal of Public Health, 79*, 1371–1376.

Flynn, B. S., Worden, J. K., Secker-Walker, S., Badger, G. J., Geller, B. M., & Costanza, M. C. (1992). Prevention of cigarette smoking through mass media intervention and school programs. *American Journal of Public Health, 82*, 827–834.

Garrison, C. Z., McKeown, R. E., Valois, R. F., & Vincent., M. L. (1993). Aggression, substance use, and suicidal behaviors in high school students. *American Journal of Public Health, 83*, 179–184.

Hammond, W. R., & Yung, B. R. (1991). Preventing violence in at-risk African-American youth. *Journal of Health Care for the Poor and Underserved, 2*, 359–373.

Hammond, W. R., & Yung, B. R. (1993). Psychology's role in the public health response to assaultive violence among young African-American men. *American Psychologist, 48*, 142–154.

Hansen, W. B. (1992). School based substance prevention: A review of the state-of-the-art in curriculum. *Health Education Research, 7*, 403–430.

Hawkins, J. D., Catalano, R. F., & Miller, J. Y. (1992). Risk and protective factors for alcohol and other drug problems in adolescence and early adulthood: Implications for substance abuse prevention. *Psychological Bulletin, 112*, 64–105.

Hurd, P., Johnson, C. A., Pechacek, T., Bast, C. P., Jacobs, D., & Luepker, R. (1980). Prevention of cigarette smoking in seventh grade students. *Journal of Behavioral Medicine, 3*, 15–28.

Jessor, R., & Jessor, S. L. (1977). *Problem behavior and psychosocial development: A longitudinal study of youth*. San Diego, CA: Academic Press.

Johnston, L. D., O'Malley, P. M., & Bachman, J. G. (1994). *National survey results on drug use from the Monitoring the Future Study, 1975–1993: Volume I. Secondary School Students*. Rockville, MD: U.S. Department of Health and Human Services.

Kandel, D., Simcha-Fagan, R., & Davies, M. (1986). Risk factor for delinquency and illicit drug use from adolescence to young adulthood. *Journal of Drug Issues, 16,* 67–90.

Kann, L., Warren, W., Collins, J. L., Ross, J., Collins, B., & Kolbe, L. J. (1993). Results from the national school-based 1991 Youth Risk Behavior Survey and progress toward achieving related health objectives for the nation. *Public Health Reports, 108,* 47–55.

Kazdin, A. E. (1987). Treatment of antisocial behavior in children: Current status and future directions. *Psychological Bulletin, 102,* 187–203.

Kazdin, A. E. (1993). Adolescent mental health: Prevention and treatment programs. *American Psychologist, 48,* 127–141.

Kingery, P. M., Pruitt, B. E., & Hurley, R. S. (1992). Violence and illegal drug use among adolescents: Evidence from the U.S. national adolescent student health survey. *International Journal of the Addictions, 27,* 1445–1464.

Kumpfer, K. L., & Alvarado, R. (1995). Strengthening families to prevent drug use in multi-ethnic youth. In G. J. Botvin, S. Schinke, & M. A. Orlandi (Eds.), *Drug abuse prevention with multiethnic youth* (pp. 255–294). Newbury Park, CA: Sage.

Lochman, J. E. (1987). Self- and peer perceptions and attributional biases of aggressive and nonaggressive boys in dyadic interactions. *Journal of Consulting and Clinical Psychology, 55,* 404–410.

Lochman, J. E. (1992). Cognitive–behavioral intervention with aggressive boys: Three-year follow-up and preventive effects. *Journal of Consulting and Clinical Psychology, 60,* 426–432.

Lochman, J. E., Coie, J. D., Underwood, M. K., & Terry, R. (1993). Effectiveness of a social relations interventions program for aggressive and nonaggressive, rejected children. *Journal of Consulting and Clinical Psychology, 61,* 1053–1058.

Luepker, R. V., Johnson, C. A., Murray, D. M., & Pechacek, T. F. (1983). Prevention of cigarette smoking: Three year follow-up of educational programs for youth. *Journal of Behavioral Medicine, 6,* 53–61.

MacKinnon, D. P., Johnson, C. A., Pentz, M. A., Dwyer, J. H., Hansen, W. B., Flay, B. R., & Wang, E. Y. I. (1991). Mediating mechanisms in a school-based drug prevention program: First-year effects of the Midwestern Prevention Project. *Health Psychology, 10,* 164–172.

Maddahian, E., Newcomb, M. D., & Bentler, P. M. (1985). Single and multiple patterns of adolescent substance use: Longitudinal comparisons of four ethnic groups. *Journal of Drug Education, 15,* 311–326.

Maddahian, E., Newcomb, M. D., & Bentler, P. M. (1988). Risk factors for substance use: Ethnic differences among adolescents. *Journal of Substance Abuse, 1,* 11–23.

McAlister, A., Perry, C., & Maccoby, N. (1979). Adolescent smoking: Onset and prevention. *Pediatrics, 63,* 650–658.

McAlister, A., Puska, P., Koskela, K., Pallonen, U., & Maccoby, N. (1980). Mass communication and community organization for public health education. *American Psychologist, 35,* 375–379.

McGee, L., & Newcomb, M. D. (1992). General deviance syndrome: Expanded hierarchical evaluations at four ages from early adolescence to adulthood. *Journal of Consulting and Clinical Psychology, 60,* 766–776.

Murray, D. M., Davis-Hearn, M., Goldman, A. I., Pirie, P., & Luepker, R. V. (1988). Four- and five-year follow-up results from four seventh-grade smoking prevention strategies. *Journal of Behavioral Medicine, 11,* 395–405.

National Institute on Drug Abuse. (1991). *National household survey on drug abuse: Population estimates, 1991* (DHHS Pub. No. ADM 92-1887). Rockville, MD: Author.

National Institute on Drug Abuse. (1993). *National household survey on drug abuse: Population estimates, 1993* (DHHS Pub. No. SMA-94-3017). Rockville, MD: Author.

Newcomb, M. D., & Bentler, P. M. (1988). *Consequences of adolescent drug use: Impact on the lives of young adults.* Newbury Park, CA: Sage.

Newcomb, M. D., Maddahian, E., Skager, R., & Bentler, P. M. (1987). Substance abuse and psychosocial risk factors among teenagers: Associations with sex, age, ethnicity, and type of school. *American Journal of Drug and Alcohol Abuse, 13,* 413–433.

New York City Department of Health. (1993). *Injury mortality in New York City.* New York: Author.

Patterson, G. R. (1986). Performance models for antisocial boys. *American Psychologist, 41,* 432–444.

Pentz, M. A., Dwyer, J. H., MacKinnon, D. P., Flay, B. R., Hansen, W. B., Wang, E. Y., & Johnson, C. A. (1989). A multicommunity trial for primary prevention of adolescent drug abuse: Effects on drug prevalence. *Journal of the American Medical Association, 261,* 3259–3266.

Perry, C., Killen, J., Slinkard, L. A., & McAlister, A. L. (1983). Peer teaching and smoking prevention among junior high students. *Adolescence, 9,* 277–281.

Rodriguez, J. (1990). Childhood injuries in the United States. *American Journal of Diseases of Childhood, 144,* 627–646.

Ross, L., Greene, D., & House, P. (1977). The "false consensus effect": An egocentric bias in social perception and attribution processes. *Journal of Experimental Social Psychology, 13,* 279–301.

Snow, D. L., Tebes, J. K., Arthur, M. W., & Tapasak, R. C. (1992). Two-year follow-up of a social–cognitive intervention to prevent substance use. *Journal of Drug Education, 22,* 101–114.

Snyder, J. J., Dishion, T. J., & Patterson, G. R. (1986). Determinants and consequences of association with deviant peers during preadolescence and adolescence. *Journal of Early Adolescence, 6,* 20–43.

Sussman, S., Dent, C. W., Stacy, A. W., & Sun, P. (1993). Project Towards No Tobacco Use: One-year behavior outcomes. *American Journal of Public Health, 83,* 1245–1250.

Tardiff, K., & Gross, E. (1986). Homicide in New York City. *Bulletin of the New York Academy of Medicine, 62,* 413–426.

Telch, M. J., Killen, J. D., McAlister, A. L., Perry, C. L., & Maccoby, N. (1982). Long-term follow-up of a pilot project on smoking prevention with adolescents. *Journal of Behavioral Medicine, 5,* 1–8.

Wallace, J. M., Bachman, J. G., O'Malley, P. M., & Johnston, L. D. (1995). Racial/ethnic differences in adolescent drug use: Exploring possible explanations. In G. J. Botvin, S. Schinke, & M. A. Orlandi (Eds.), *Drug abuse prevention with multiethnic youth* (pp. 59–80). Newbury Park, CA: Sage.

White, H. R., Pandina, R. J., & LaGrange, R. L. (1987). Longitudinal predictors of serious substance abuse and delinquency. *Criminology, 25,* 715–740.

4

Health Promotion in Minority Adolescents: Emphasis on Sexually Transmitted Diseases and the Human Immunodeficiency Virus

James R. Rodrigue, Kenneth P. Tercyak, Jr., and Celia M. Lescano

Nicque, a 15-year-old Hispanic female, saw a physician at the teaching hospital because she had abdominal pain and some cloudy discharge from her vagina. She told the physician that she had experienced these symptoms for a couple of weeks but thought that they would resolve after a few days. The physician questioned her about her sexual history, and she informed the doctor that she had had sex "a few times" in the past, but quickly added that she had been dating the same boy for almost 6 months. Diagnostic testing revealed that Nicque had endocervical gonorrhea, and it was apparent that the condition had gone untreated for some time. Nicque was surprised to learn that she also had pelvic inflammatory disease, which could lead to chronic pelvic pain, infertility, or ectopic pregnancy in the future.

Sexually transmitted diseases (STDs) and the human immunodeficiency virus (HIV) are increasingly more prevalent in adolescents and young adults (Centers for Disease Control and Prevention [CDC], 1995a, 1995b), particularly among minorities (Rosenberg, 1995). Recent studies have indicated that multiple, serial sexual partners characterize the patterns of sexual relationships in adolescents and young adults (Seidman & Rieder, 1994), yet condom use is inconsistent and infrequent (Boyer & Kegeles, 1991). Programs targeting increased awareness of STDs and HIV have generally failed to produce lasting behavioral change because they have failed to account for relevant intrapersonal, situational, and environmental variables (Auerbach, Wypijewska, & Brodie, 1994). Furthermore, few health-promotion programs have specifically tailored their efforts to meet the needs of minority adolescents. In this chapter, we selectively review the nature of adolescent sexual activity and condom use as well as the prevalence of STDs and HIV with specific reference to minority adolescents, providing examples of prevention programs that have been empirically validated with this population.

Adolescent Sexual Behaviors

Onset and Frequency of Sexual Activity

Adolescence is a time of initiation of several risk-taking behaviors. The age of initiation of sexual intercourse varies by gender and ethnicity; however, there is no question that sexual activity among adolescents has increased significantly during the past 2 decades. According to a recent review, approximately 10% of adolescents have had intercourse by the age of 13, nearly 25% of females and 33% of males have engaged in sexual activity by age 15, and up to 75% of females and 86% of males have had intercourse by age 19 (Seidman & Rieder, 1994). Although males are still more likely than females to engage in sexual activity during adolescence, proportional estimates indicate that more females have become sexually active in recent years (Brooks-Gunn & Paikoff, 1993).

Initiation of sexual activity during adolescence also varies by ethnicity. For instance, surveys during the past several years indicate that

69% of Black males, 26% of White females and males, and 24% of Black females have had sexual intercourse at least once before the age of 15 (CDC, 1995b; Sonenstein, Pleck, & Klu, 1989). These percentages rise to 98% (Black males), 76% (White females), 86% (White males), and 83% (Black females) by the age of 19. Estimates of initial sexual intercourse among Hispanic adolescents are similar. However, more recent data have revealed that Black adolescent males are approximately 2 years ahead of White and Hispanic males in the proportion who report having initiated sexual intercourse at a specified age (Sonenstein, Pleck, & Klu, 1991).

Number of sexual partners during adolescence may play an important role in understanding the risk of STDs and HIV transmission. Females 15 to 19 years old who reported having two or more sexual partners increased from 38% in 1971 to 59% in 1988 (Miller, Christopherson, & King, 1993). Moreover, Black adolescent males reported an average of two to three more lifetime sexual partners than White or Hispanic adolescent males (Sonenstein et al., 1991). These figures may reflect the episodic nature of relationships during the teenage years and may be highly correlated with onset of sexual activity at an early age. Adolescents who first had intercourse at age 13 are likely to have more lifetime sexual partners by age 18 in comparison with those whose first sexual encounter was at age 15. Because Black adolescent males are often younger than White or Hispanic adolescent males at time of first intercourse, it is not surprising that their number of lifetime sexual partners at age 19 is higher. It also is noteworthy that the nature of adolescent relationships is generally monogamous and, despite evidence of multiple sexual partners during the teenage years, relationships are characterized by sequential rather than simultaneous sexual partnerships (Zabin & Hayward, 1993). Only 20% of adolescent males, for instance, reported having more than one sexual partner in the same month (Sonenstein et al., 1991).

Current Trends in STDs and HIV Among Minority Adolescents

Incidence estimates of STDs—including chlamydia, gonorrhea, human papillomavirus, genital herpes, hepatitis B, and syphilis—indicate that these diseases are more prevalent than HIV infection (Braverman & Strasburger, 1994). However, STD statistics are a marker for HIV-related high-risk behavior, in that they represent disease transmission from unprotected sexual intercourse. Over 12 million cases of STD are diagnosed each year in the United States, and many of these cases lead to serious medical and psychosocial consequences, including infertility, ectopic pregnancy, and adjustment disorder (Seidman & Rieder, 1994).

The rate of STDs among adolescents in the United States is very high. Specifically, national statistics show that the most common STDs among adolescents are candidiasis (38% of total STDs), chlamydia (37%), gonorrhea (19%), and HIV (4%; Office of Technology Assessment, 1991). Gonorrhea rates, for instance, are highest in the adolescent female age groups of 10–14 and 15–19, with 3,500 diagnosed cases per 100,000 sexually active adolescent females (DiClemente, 1990). Also, syphilis and pelvic inflammatory disease (PID) occur much more frequently in adolescents than in all other age groups. STDs are 2 to 3 times more common in inner-city minority adolescent populations (J. B. Jemmott, Jemmott, & Fong, 1992). Furthermore, it has been estimated that Black adolescents are as much as 15 times more likely than Whites to acquire gonorrhea (DiClemente, 1990) and 5 times more likely to acquire HIV. Black adolescent females are nearly 11 times more likely to have an AIDS diagnosis compared with White adolescent females, and significantly more adolescents with AIDS (53%) are members of ethnic minority groups compared with adult figures (38%; Boyer & Kegeles, 1991; DiClemente, 1993). Death attributable to syphilis and PID also is more likely for Black adolescents (Grimes, 1986).

Condom Use by Adolescents

Sexual activity increases the risk of pregnancy, STDs, and HIV transmission during adolescence. Regular use of condoms can prevent these health problems. However, the CDC (1995a) has reported that in 1991 and 1993 less than 50% of sexually active ethnic and racial minority high school students used condoms at last intercourse. Recent trends indicate an increase in condom use for adolescents of all races from 1991 to 1993: for example, White, non-Hispanic (from 47% to 52%); Black, non-Hispanic (48% to 57%); and Hispanic (38% to 46%). Although these trends are positive, the regular use of condoms continues to be at an unacceptable level in terms of preventing the transmission of STDs and HIV. It also is noteworthy that there is a strong association between age and condom use, with adolescents who are younger at the time of first sexual contact less likely to use any contraceptive than older adolescents (Mosher & McNally, 1991). Furthermore, minority adolescents are generally unaware that spermicides and sponges, particularly those with nonoxynol-9, have been shown to be effective in preventing STD and HIV transmission.

Understanding why adolescents do not regularly use condoms or other contraceptives has been the focus of considerable attention by researchers, clinicians, and health policy analysts in recent years. Consensus has been that the failure of adolescents to regularly use condoms is multicausal in nature. Barriers to condom use include a lack of knowledge about sexual biology and STDs (e.g., "I thought I was too young to get gonorrhea" or "I didn't have sex enough times to get it"), the nature of partner relationships ("I never thought my boyfriend had been with anyone before" or "He said a condom would spoil the mood"), privacy issues ("I was embarrassed to buy them because someone might recognize me" or "What if my parents ever found them?"), procrastination ("I just didn't get around to it"), and practical considerations ("I don't have the money to buy them"; Brooks-Gunn & Furstenberg, 1989).

Communication and interpersonal factors play a central role in condom use. Communicating one's desire to engage in sexual activity safely by using a condom is an important yet infrequent event in the context of sexual intimacy during adolescence. Negotiating condom use with a sexual partner who does not recognize or share the same commitment to sexual responsibility or similar perceptions of risk requires confidence, assertiveness, and effective sexual communication skills. In addition to these skills, adolescents must learn to cope effectively with potential embarrassment, vulnerability of their self-image (perhaps more common for adolescent females) or of the sexual encounter itself (perhaps more common for adolescent males), and possible rejection. Unfortunately, the link between sexual negotiation skills and condom use, although empirically validated among adults (e.g., Catania et al., 1994), has not been studied in adolescents.

STD and HIV Intervention Research

Perhaps nowhere in recent times has the need for HIV intervention been as saliently portrayed as in the film *Kids*, written by Harmony Korine and directed by Larry Clark. The film, which takes place on the streets of New York City, follows a young girl in her desperate and tragic search for the sexual partner she knows infected her with HIV in an effort to notify him of her seropositivity. *Kids* highlights the pressing need for the dissemination of prevention programs out of research labs and into real-world practice. This cinematic glimpse into the lives of inner-city youth reflects a growing population of underserved and highly at-risk children.

STD and HIV prevention programs for minority adolescent youths are as multifaceted as the population to which they pertain. Clinicians and researchers actively involved in this type of endeavor must thoughtfully formulate and ask questions in an effort to systematically address the growing needs for effective programs ultimately aimed at stopping disease transmission. For example, precisely who is being targeted in this intervention may likely dictate the strategy used in the intervention as well as affect the generalizability of its findings. For our purposes, we have quite broadly identified adolescents of minority background to be the population of interest. Yet, within this clinical research area, the descriptor *minority* simultaneously applies to many different subgroups (i.e., racial, ethnic, and sociocultural). These terms are not mutually exclusive of other intrapersonal variables by which members of these groups may be further classified (i.e., by gender, age, and sexual orientation). Because minority status is traditionally defined in relative terms when a smaller population is compared with the majority, so too we attempt to confine our discussion in this relative manner predominantly to ethnocultural issues and, where data are available, to sexual orientation as well.

As mentioned, the issues associated with minority adolescent STD and HIV prevention are multidimensional. In the actual practice of prevention, this often translates into the design and implementation of programs by many different professionals, paraprofessionals, and laypeople. At the individual level, this may include psychologists, physicians, nurses, social and public health workers, counselors, educators, members of the clergy, and even peers. At a broader systematic level, one encounters school districts; juvenile offices of national, state, and local branches of government; and organized parent groups. Exhibit 1 illustrates an intervention model proposed for practicing nurses, yet these guidelines can also be selectively used by other professionals involved in prevention work (L. S. Jemmott, 1993).

Exhibit 1

Individual Intervention Strategies With Minority Youth

Provide correct AIDS knowledge by teaching
- correct and concrete information about AIDS
- specific information about AIDS prevention
- about intravenous drug use
- about the reproductive system

Increase the perception of personal vulnerability to AIDS through
- statistics and prevalence data
- highlighting ramifications of contracting STDs and AIDS

Change negative attitudes regarding condom use by
- assessing attitudes toward condoms
- discussing positive attitudes toward condoms

Increase condom-use behavior and reduce other high-risk sexual behaviors by
- discussing the youth's sexual history
- teaching how condoms can prevent sexual transmission of HIV infection
- teaching how to use condoms properly
- teaching methods of communicating and negotiating condom use with a partner
- scheduling follow-up appointments with youth

From "AIDS Risk Among Black Male Adolescents: Implications for Nursing Interventions," by L. S. Jemmott, 1993, *Journal of Pediatric Health Care, 7*, p. 6. Copyright 1993 by Mosby-Yearbook. Adapted with permission.

Individuals may act alone or as part of a multidisciplinary team. The access to resources and attendant domains of expertise vary widely from provider to provider and prevention site to prevention site. Inner-city school-based programs often call on classroom teachers to educate students about the risks of AIDS. Hospital clinics conducting prevention classes may recruit members of their medical and health staffs, each sharing their own unique perspective on the problem. Alternatively, religiously based youth groups are likely to emphasize self-esteem, moral values, and personal resilience to social pressures through peer leadership and spiritual guidance.

Some public school districts have adopted psychosocially minded and health-related content areas directly into lower and middle school curricula with good success (Weissberg, Caplan, & Harwood, 1991). These programs attempt to synergistically combine the efforts of professionals to permit progress along interdisciplinary lines. A significant portion of this education is related to the prevention of STDs and HIV before these children engage in sexual activity. Recently, popular cultural icons have been tapped to promote HIV prevention. These approaches have typically been used in conjunction with mass media resources to reach a wide audience (Donovan, Jason, Gibbs, & Kroger, 1991). Basketball star Magic Johnson's seropositive status has been publicized in part to send a message to youth of their own particular vulnerability to HIV infection.

In reviewing the current literature on reducing minority adolescents' risk to HIV, we identified several common trends. Generally, the work can be split among those programs targeted at preventing high-risk behaviors before they occur and those that seek to promote the change of risky behaviors already initiated. Developmentally older children are often the focus of the latter strategy. Interventions typically involve revising sexual behaviors (i.e., increasing condom usage) as a primary means to reduce one's risk. Other methods include education, health promotion, early detection, and partner notification (D'Angelo, Brown, English, Hein, & Remafedi, 1994). In one study (Sellers, McGraw, & McKinlay, 1994), investigators examined the actual effect of promoting condom use among Latino youth. Contrary to concerns that the distribution of condoms may promote sexual promiscuity in the sample, the study showed that this fear was unfounded. Additionally, work by J. B. Jemmott, Jemmott, Spears, Hewitt, and Cruz-Collins (1992), in which Black adolescent males were engaged in open discussions of safer sex practices, also drew a similar conclusion.

Asking where interventions can take place is also important. In this respect, practitioners are very fortunate because the possibilities seem as limitless as the number of locations in which one routinely encounters minority youth: in the schools, community centers, and hospital clinics, just to name a few. Yet, one must also keep in mind the locations in which infections may spread. These less well-controlled locales often pose a multitude of programmatic challenges to people involved in conducting prevention work. However, working through these issues has led to new possibilities for increased prevention sites. For instance, Rotheram-Borus, Koopman, Haignere, and Davies (1991) successfully provided runaway youth living in a shelter with group discussions, education, counseling, and training in AIDS issues. Both condom use and safer sex increased as a result of the work, and effects were maintained at 3- and 6-month follow-ups. Work with runaways has also shown the need to target reductions in alcohol and drug use (Koopman, Rosario, & Rotheram-Borus, 1994). More research is needed to further evaluate the long-term efficacy of these prevention efforts, but they represent an innovative approach to addressing the sexual risk taking of adolescents who are otherwise difficult to reach.

Knowledge, Motivation, and Behavioral Skills Acquisition

Accomplishing lasting behavior change is known to be more difficult than simply having an impact on knowledge. For instance, Norris and Ford (1991) described the results of face-to-face interviews conducted with at-risk Black and Hispanic male and female adolescents. Both AIDS and condom knowledge were explored as well as sexual behavior and condom and intravenous needle use. With regard to knowledge, a high percentage of both Black and Hispanic participants were accurate in their knowledge of AIDS transmission by sex or needles and that condoms provide some protection. However, a prominent subset of both ethnicities reported being unaware that nonlatex condoms provided ineffective protection. The researchers analyzed AIDS sexual risk behaviors and found that although many sexually active participants reported using condoms, the majority reported having unprotected vaginal intercourse. Hispanic women were highly represented in this latter sample. Similarly, Rotheram-Borus and Koopman (1991) described sexual risk behavior, AIDS knowledge, and beliefs about AIDS prevention among Black and Hispanic gay and bisexual adolescent males. They described this population as having moderately high AIDS knowledge and positive attitudes toward AIDS prevention. However, despite these two positive indicators, the actual sex practices of these youth placed them at high risk for contracting HIV, thus underscoring the gap between knowledge and behavior in minority adolescents.

Indeed, the knowledge–prevention relationship remains elusive within the behavioral sciences, and several conceptual and methodological limitations of studies have been offered to explain the failure to observe a more consistent link (Fisher & Fisher, 1992). A solid information base about risk factors and disease may affect initial behavior change in some instances, but it is generally insufficient for maintenance of such behavior over extended time periods. As noted by Fisher and Fisher, the maintenance of behavioral change over time requires the dissemination of behaviorally relevant information (e.g., modes of disease transmission) in prevention programs targeting STDs and HIV. Also, particularly relevant to interventions with adolescent minority groups is the need for efforts to identify "group-specific gaps" in knowledge and then focus program activities on enhancing knowledge and awareness in those areas. Such elicitation research might include the use of open-ended questions and focus groups, in which minority adolescents may be more likely to discuss real-life situations, attitudes, and beliefs about sexual behavior and disease transmission, and what they do or do not know about prevention.

Numerous conceptual models have been used in the design and implementation of prevention programs, including the health belief model, theory of reasoned action, protection motivation theory, and theory of planned behavior. These models emphasize the need to consider individuals' attitudes and beliefs toward STD and HIV prevention and to incorporate such constructs into risk-reduction programs. However, despite the relationship between preventive behaviors and such variables as attitudes, perceived vulnerability, perceived costs and benefits of prevention, and the presence or absence of cue stimuli, researchers generally agree that adolescents must be highly motivated to initiate and subsequently maintain STD and HIV prevention behaviors (Fisher & Fisher, 1992). Therefore, intervention programs should include a motivational component to promote greater sexual responsibility by adolescents.

STD and HIV prevention programs, to be effective, must not only fill information gaps and increase motivation to engage in preventive behavior but also provide ample opportunity for the acquisition and practice of behavioral skills. These include sexual communication skills, assertiveness skills, condom use and purchasing skills, and self- and partner-reinforcement skills. Some additional skill building may also be necessary to meet the prevention needs of specific minority groups, specifically in cultures where significant gender–power issues are involved (Mays & Cochran, 1988). However, possessing certain behavioral skills may not lead to behavior change if youth do not believe that they can use them effectively. Therefore, the enhancement of self-efficacy and the opportunity to practice using new behavioral skills are considered essential ingredients in any STD and HIV prevention program.

Effective Interventions With Minority Adolescents: A Few Examples

Most intervention approaches for STD are embedded within interventions developed for HIV prevention. In fact, by preventing HIV transmission, interventions are essentially promoting effective preventive practices for STDs. J. B. Jemmott, Jemmott, and Fong (1992) designed their intervention to reduce the HIV risk of Black adolescent males. Participants were randomly assigned to an AIDS risk-reduction condition or a control, career opportunities condition. In the risk-reduction group, participants received a 5-hr intervention that was designed to increase AIDS and STD knowledge and to decrease attitudes toward risky sexual practices. The intervention used videotapes, games, exercises, and other materials to foster learning and participation. For example, one videotape had a multiethnic cast, and an "AIDS basketball" game was played, in which opposing small groups earned points by correctly answering AIDS-related questions. A condom exercise focused on correct usage, and role-playing was performed to depict problems encountered in implementing safer sex practices. The facilitators for the groups were Black men and women with health-related professional backgrounds. Results indicated that the intervention group had lower intentions of engaging in sexual behaviors related to HIV posttreatment. Less favorable attitudes toward risky sex practices and greater AIDS knowledge were also evidenced. At the 3-month follow-up evaluation, the intervention group reported engaging in less risky sexual behavior than those in the control condition, with fewer intentions to engage in such behavior at all. Interestingly, the effects of male facilitators were initially stronger than those of female facilitators with the group of male adolescents, although this was not so at follow-up. Jemmott et al. stated that their research provides some empirical rationale for matching facilitators and group members by gender.

Schinke, Gordon, and Weston (1990) described a self-instruction program designed to prevent HIV infection among Black and Hispanic adolescents. All participants in this study completed questionnaires about their drug use, sexual activity, HIV-infection knowledge, attitudes, and risks and then received an informational sheet on AIDS and AIDS prevention. Participants were subsequently randomly assigned either to receive a self-instructional guidebook with or without group instruction or to a control group. At outcome measurement 1 month later, participants in both guidebook conditions significantly improved in their retest scores over pretest. This intervention strategy was particularly unique because the guidebook was written in comic book form:

> Written in rap music verse, the guide informed participants about AIDS risks, myths, and prevention strategies. . . . Lyrics were presented by a cartoon character drawn to mirror participants' age and ethnic–racial backgrounds. Throughout the guide, the character described how adolescents can contract AIDS and how they can avoid it through behavior change. (Schinke et al., 1990, p. 433)

Schinke et al.'s study implies that the self-instructional technique can help to reduce Black and Hispanic adolescents' risk behaviors for infection. In addition, the youth involved in the group discussion improved more in their willingness to talk with friends about sexual matters. Other work has also focused on the possibility of using video technology as a means of confidential, home-based intervention (Schinke, Orlandi, Schilling, & Parms, 1992; Winett et al., 1992).

In 1992, L. S. Jemmott and Jemmott described their intervention designed to increase the intention to use condoms among Black female adolescents. The study showed that skill building and self-efficacy combined were successful strategies for procuring the sexual partners of these girls to support condom use as well as for achieving higher levels of both participants' knowledge regarding STDs and AIDS and their intentions to use condoms. Separately, Langer, Zimmerman, Warheit, and Duncan (1993) showed that AIDS-related knowledge, attitudes, beliefs, and behaviors associated with lower risk were more prevalent in self-directed students than more peer-directed students, a finding that further highlights the importance of incorporating individuals' frames of reference into an intervention.

Quirk, Godkin, and Schwenzfeier (1993) described an HIV prevention program that targeted adolescent and young adult minority females at an inner-city family health center. Over 200 adolescents and young adults (including 101 Black and Latino participants) were randomly assigned to receive either provider-delivered HIV counseling or peer-delivered HIV education. The provider-delivered counseling occurred in the context of the office visit, lasted about 10 min, and addressed several issues, including past sexual activity and IV drug use, motivation to change behavior, identifying support services, developing a plan for safer sex, and relapse prevention. Providers received appropriate training before participating in the study. The peer-delivered program included a review of HIV brochures (e.g., risk factors, pathogenesis, and prevention actions) by a trained peer educator. Most interesting about this intervention was the viewing of a 5-min videotape with rap lyrics speaking out against HIV and the actions one can take to prevent its transmission. The video had been written and performed by local adolescents.

The researchers found that, although attitudes and self-reported behavior (i.e., intercourse frequency) did not change, adolescents in both groups reported significant improvements in AIDS facts, how to use a condom effectively, and appropriate preventive behaviors that were maintained at the 1-month follow-up. Moreover, the provider-delivered program was slightly more effective than the peer-delivered intervention in improving knowledge. Despite the lack of behavioral change, this study provides an innovative effort to train health care providers to deliver low-cost, pragmatic prevention programs to minority adolescents who are at high risk for STDs and HIV infection. Training that involves provisions for basic counseling techniques, role-playing exercises, and opportunities to discuss cultural issues indigenous to the local population may prove beneficial to health care providers in their struggle to reduce high-risk sexual activity among adolescents.

Exhibit 2 highlights Winett and Anderson's (1994) guidelines for disease prevention interventions designed for use with adolescents. These guidelines emphasize the need for a culturally sensitive approach to intervention, particularly in working with minority youth. In addition, Boyer and Kegeles (1991) recommended six programmatic strategies that each program should follow to effectively enhance AIDS risk reduction among adolescents:

1. Focus on the most recent medical information available, including cause, transmission, and prevention as well as dispelling myths about HIV and AIDS.
2. Present information within the context of comprehensive health education (i.e., sexuality, sexual intercourse, pregnancy, and STDs).
3. Use many communication strategies (i.e., peer discussions, role-playing, theater, videos, and music).
4. Pay attention to cultural values, religious beliefs, and social customs as well as to language and communication styles of participants.

Exhibit 2

Guidelines for Disease-Prevention Interventions With Youth

- Effective programs are culturally sensitive and developmentally appropriate.
- Brief, singular programs do not promote long-term behavior changes, whereas longer, more comprehensive, and multilevel programs do.
- Programs emphasizing only information and knowledge do not yield behavior changes.
- Generic skills training (i.e., problem solving) does not necessarily reduce specific risk behaviors. Specific training for specific problems should be combined with generic skills training.
- Effective programs appear to be multiyear efforts and may need to include 40 to 50 hr of skills training.
- Ecological interventions should be included where possible, involving both teachers and parents.
- Competency-based interventions must be carefully implemented to maintain their integrity. This means including well-trained staff, organizational resources and support, and ongoing monitoring of the program.

From "HIV Prevention in Youth: A Framework for Research and Action," by R. A. Winett and E. S. Anderson. In T. H. Ollendick and R. J. Prinz (Eds.), *Advances in Clinical Child Psychology, Volume 16* (p. 11), 1994, New York: Plenum. Copyright 1994 by Plenum. Adapted with permission.

---

5. Engage in an ongoing evaluation process of the effectiveness of the program's strategies in light of achieving set goals (i.e., formally assess the program's impact on participants' lives).
6. Obtain the cooperation and financial support of public organizations as well as assemble knowledgeable teams of educators and researchers.

Guidelines to Successful Interventions

Interventions with minority youth often take place over a period of time; they cannot be accomplished successfully in one session. Well-designed programs are meant to be both informative and educational and to promote skill building and mastery of the STD and HIV prevention behaviors themselves. Various programs have accomplished this in multimodal formats and through the use of written materials, videotapes, role-plays, games, exercises, and facilitated group discussions. The actors in videos, or those characters otherwise portrayed, are often depicted in ways that emulate the appearance, mannerisms, and behaviors of the targeted population. With minority adolescents, this has involved multiethnic casting and the incorporation of lesbian, gay, and bisexual sexual orientations and plot lines as well as the settings in which the behaviors are likely to occur.

Demonstrations and discussions are often an important component to interventions: Both seek to grab the attention of the participants to facilitate their learning. For example, high school and college AIDS educators not only teach the proper act of putting on a condom by demonstrating, but amusingly do so on such phallic objects as bananas or baseball bats, or even on more lifelike anatomical models. Educators may also emphasize the eroticism of condom usage by suggesting that it be incorporated into foreplay and that condoms generally enable a man to maintain an erection for a longer period of time (J. B. Jemmott, Jemmott, Spears, et al., 1992). Preventionists are also aware that too much fear induced by STDs and HIV awareness and risk statistics can make audience members defensive and, therefore, unlikely to benefit from the program in the intended manner (Richard, van der Pligt, & de Vries, 1995).

Beyond the components described above, what factors further increase the likelihood of sexual behavior change among minority adolescents? This has not been an easy question to answer, and the different factors assessed within various studies have often not been consistent. As mentioned previously, increased knowledge does not always lead to behavior change, although it may lead to increased intentions to use condoms or decreased intentions to engage in risky behavior (J. B. Jemmott, Jemmott, & Fong, 1992; Rotheram-Borus & Koopman, 1991). DiClemente (1993) pointed to the need to increase adolescents' social competence, including communication, negotiation, assertiveness, and refusal skills. Furthermore, increasing self-efficacy and outcome expectancies regarding condom use may assist in increasing intentions to use condoms (J. B. Jemmott, Jemmott, Spears, et al., 1992; L. S. Jemmott & Jemmott, 1992).

Conclusion

With some exceptions, adolescents form sexual partnerships and do not regularly use condoms. Consequently, STDs are more common in adolescents than in adults and, extrapolating backward from HIV infection rates among young adults, one can assume that a significant proportion of adolescents are infected with the AIDS virus. Minority adolescents are especially at risk considering that they engage in sexual activity at an early age and tend to have more partners during their teenage years.

In addition to the decisions to engage in sexual activity, developmental research has shown that adolescents commonly deny or underestimate their personal susceptibility to STDs or HIV infection and may experience guilt over planning sexual intercourse. These developmental issues and attitudinal barriers, which may be reinforced within certain cultural groups, highlight the need for prevention programs that are more personal and targeted to specific minority groups. Unfortunately, few programs designed to promote sexual responsibility and prevent STD and HIV transmission have targeted interventions to meet the needs of minority adolescents.

We have briefly highlighted the sexual behaviors of minority adolescents and the associated health consequences (i.e., STDs and HIV). Furthermore, we have reviewed guidelines that are considered essential for effective interventions with adolescents, including establishing a culturally sensitive knowledge base, increasing motivation to engage in prevention behaviors, and the acquisition and implementation of effective behavioral skills. Clearly, additional programmatic research is needed to empirically examine the ecological validity of STD and HIV prevention programs in ethnically diverse groups of adolescents.

REFERENCES

Auerbach, J. D., Wypijewska, C., & Brodie, H. K. H. (Eds.). (1994). *AIDS and behavior: An integrated approach*. Washington, DC: National Academy Press.

Boyer, C. B., & Kegeles, S. M. (1991). AIDS risk and prevention among adolescents. *Social Science and Medicine, 33*, 11–23.

Braverman, P. K., & Strasburger, V. C. (1994). Sexually transmitted diseases. *Clinical Pediatrics, 33*, 26–37.

Brooks-Gunn, J., & Furstenberg, J. J., Jr. (1989). Adolescent sexual behavior. *American Psychologist, 44*, 249–257.

Brooks-Gunn, J., & Paikoff, R. L. (1993). "Sex is a gamble, kissing is a game": Adolescent sexuality and health promotion. In S. G. Millstein, A. C. Peterson, & E. O. Nightingale (Eds.), *Promoting the health of adolescents: New directions for the twenty-first century* (pp. 180–208). New York: Oxford University Press.

Catania, J. A., Coates, T. J., Golden, E., Dolcini, M. M., Peterson, J., Kegeles, S., Siegel, D., & Fullilove, M. T. (1994). Correlates of condom use among Black, Hispanic, and White heterosexuals in San Francisco: The AMEN longitudinal survey. *AIDS Education and Prevention, 6,* 12–26.

Centers for Disease Control and Prevention. (1995a). Trends in sexual risk behavior among high school students—United States, 1990, 1991, and 1993. *Morbidity and Mortality Weekly Report, 44,* 124–125.

Centers for Disease Control and Prevention. (1995b). U.S. HIV and AIDS cases reported through June 1995. *HIV/AIDS Surveillance Report, 7,* 1–34.

D'Angelo, L. J., Brown, R., English, A., Hein, K., & Remafedi, G. (1994). HIV infection and AIDs in adolescents: A position paper of the Society for Adolescent Medicine. *Journal of Adolescent Health, 15,* 427–434.

DiClemente, R. J. (1990). The emergence of adolescents as a risk group for human immunodeficiency virus infection. *Journal of Adolescent Research, 5,* 7–17.

DiClemente, R. J. (1993). Confronting the challenge of AIDS among adolescents: Directions for future research. *Journal of Adolescent Research, 8,* 156–166.

Donovan, R. J., Jason, J., Gibbs, D. A., & Kroger, F. (1991). Paid advertising for AIDS prevention: Would the ends justify the means? *Public Health Reports, 106,* 645–651.

Fisher, J. D., & Fisher, W. A. (1992). Changing AIDS-risk behavior. *Psychological Bulletin, 111,* 455–474.

Grimes, D. A. (1986). Deaths due to sexually transmitted diseases. *Journal of the American Medical Association, 255,* 1727–1729.

Jemmott, J. B., III, Jemmott, L. S., & Fong, G. T. (1992). Reductions in HIV risk-associated sexual behaviors among Black male adolescents: Effects of an AIDS prevention intervention. *American Journal of Public Health, 82,* 372–377.

Jemmott, J. B., III, Jemmott, L. S., Spears, H., Hewitt, N., & Cruz-Collins, M. (1992). Self-efficacy, hedonistic expectancies, and condom-use intentions among inner-city Black adolescent women: A social cognitive approach to AIDS risk behavior. *Journal of Adolescent Health, 13,* 512–519.

Jemmott, L. S. (1993). AIDS risk among Black male adolescents: Implications for nursing interventions. *Journal of Pediatric Health Care, 7,* 3–11.

Jemmott, L. S., & Jemmott, J. B., III. (1992). Increasing condom-use intentions among sexually active Black adolescent women. *Nursing Research, 41,* 273–279.

Koopman, C., Rosario, M., & Rotheram-Borus, M. J. (1994). Alcohol and drug use and sexual behaviors placing runaways at risk for HIV infection. *Addictive Behaviors, 19,* 95–103.

Langer, L. M., Zimmerman, R. S., Warheit, G. J., & Duncan, R. C. (1993). Decision-making orientation and AIDS-related knowledge, attitudes, and behaviors of Hispanic, African-American, and White adolescents. *Health Psychology, 12,* 227–234.

Mays, V. M., & Cochran, S. D. (1988). Issues in the perception of AIDS risk and risk reduction activities by Black and Hispanic/Latina women. *American Psychologist, 43,* 949–957.

Miller, B. C., Christopherson, C. R., & King, P. K. (1993). Sexual behavior in adolescence. In T. P. Gullotta, G. R. Adams, & R. Montemayor (Eds.), *Adolescent sexuality* (pp. 57–76). Newbury Park, CA: Sage.

Mosher, W. D., & McNally, J. W. (1991). Contraceptive use at first premarital intercourse: United States, 1965–1988. *Family Planning Perspectives, 23,* 108–116.

Norris, A. E., & Ford, K. (1991). AIDS risk behaviors of minority youth living in Detroit. *American Journal of Preventive Medicine, 7,* 416–421.

Office of Technology Assessment. (1991). *Adolescent Health, Vol. 1: Summary and policy options.* Washington, DC: U.S. Government Printing Office.

Quirk, M. E., Godkin, M. A., & Schwenzfeier, E. (1993). Evaluation of two AIDS prevention interventions for inner-city adolescent and young adult women. *American Journal of Preventive Medicine, 9,* 21–26.

Richard, R., van der Pligt, J., & de Vries, N. (1995). Anticipated affective reactions and prevention of AIDS. *British Journal of Social Psychology, 34,* 9–21.

Rosenberg, P. S. (1995). Scope of the AIDS epidemic in the United States. *Science, 270,* 1372–1375.

Rotheram-Borus, M. J., & Koopman, C. (1991). Sexual risk behavior, AIDS knowledge, and beliefs about AIDS among predominantly minority gay and bisexual male adolescents. *AIDS Education and Prevention, 3,* 305–312.

Rotheram-Borus, M. J., Koopman, C., Haignere, C., & Davies, M. (1991). Reducing HIV sexual risk behaviors among runaway adolescents. *Journal of the American Medical Association, 266,* 1237–1241.

Schinke, S. P., Gordon, A. N., & Weston, R. E. (1990). Self-instruction to prevent HIV infection among African-American and Hispanic-American adolescents. *Journal of Consulting and Clinical Psychology, 58,* 432–436.

Schinke, S. P., Orlandi, M. A., Schilling, R. F., & Parms, C. (1992). Feasibility of interactive videodisc technology to teach minority youth about preventing HIV infection. *Public Health Reports, 107,* 323–330.

Seidman, S. N., & Rieder, R. O. (1994). A review of sexual behavior in the United States. *American Journal of Psychiatry, 151,* 330–341.

Sellers, D. E., McGraw, S. A., & McKinlay, J. B. (1994). Does the promotion and distribution of condoms increase teen sexual activity? Evidence from an HIV prevention program for Latino youth. *American Journal of Public Health, 84,* 1952–1959.

Sonenstein, F. L., Pleck, J. H., & Klu, L. C. (1989). Sexual activity, condom use and AIDS awareness among adolescent males. *Family Planning Perspectives, 21,* 152–158.

Sonenstein, F. L., Pleck, J. H., & Klu, L. C. (1991). Levels of sexual activity among adolescent males in the United States. *Family Planning Perspectives, 23*, 162–167.

Weissberg, R. P., Caplan, M., & Harwood, R. L. (1991). Promoting competent young people in competence-enhancing environments: A systems-based perspective on primary prevention. *Journal of Consulting and Clinical Psychology, 59*, 830–841.

Winett, R. A., & Anderson, E. S. (1994). HIV prevention in youth: A framework for research and action. In T. H. Ollendick & R. J. Prinz (Eds.), *Advances in clinical child psychology, volume 16* (pp. 1–43). New York: Plenum.

Winett, R. A., Anderson, E. S., Moore, J. F., Sikkema, K. J., Hook, R. J., Webster, D. A., Taylor, C. D., Dalton, J. E., Ollendick, T. H., & Eisler, R. M. (1992). Family/media approach to HIV prevention with a home-based, parent-teen video program. *Health Psychology, 11*, 203–206.

Zabin, L. S., & Hayward, S. C. (1993). *Adolescent sexual behavior and childbearing*. Newbury Park, CA: Sage.

Chapter 5

Increasing Physical Activity Levels Among Youth: A Public Health Challenge

Wendell C. Taylor, Bettina M. Beech,
and Sharon S. Cummings

Researchers have documented that physical activity in youth can have physical and psychological effects. Both Baranowski et al. (1992) and Sallis (1994) have presented reviews investigating physical activity among youth and its favorable influence on aerobic fitness, blood lipids, blood pressure, body composition, glucose, insulin, skeletal health, and injuries, as well as on psychological variables. In spite of such well-documented benefits, however, evidence shows that during adolescence, the amount of time an individual spends in physical activity often decreases with age (Rowland, 1990). This decline raises an important challenge for those who work with adolescents: to en-

We gratefully acknowledge the assistance of Ms. Betty Goodrum in typing the manuscript and in reviewing it for APA style requirements.

courage physically inactive children to become active and encourage active children to remain active as they become adults.

In response to this challenge, the objectives of determinants and intervention research have been to identify both facilitators and barriers to physical activity and then develop and implement effective programs to increase activity. In this chapter, we focus on physical activity levels, determinants of activity levels, and potential interventions with youth. Our primary focus is on individuals from 10 to 19 years of age. We devote one part of the chapter to the role of health care professionals in promoting physical activity among youth. Throughout, we identify the knowledge and information available that specifically pertains to ethnic minority youth.

Levels of Physical Activity Among Youth

The distinctions among *physical activity, exercise,* and *physical fitness* are important because studies in each of these areas focus on different concepts. In their 1985 study, Caspersen, Powell, and Christenson defined *physical activity* as bodily movement produced by skeletal muscles that results in energy expenditure above the resting level. According to these researchers, *exercise* is a subset of physical activity associated with higher levels of intensity and exertion; that is, exercise is planned, structured, and repetitive bodily movement to improve or maintain physical fitness. Alternatively, *physical fitness* is a set of attributes that a person has that influences his or her ability to perform physical activity. Such attributes or fitness components include agility, balance, body composition, cardiorespiratory endurance, flexibility, muscular endurance, muscular strength, and anaerobic power (Baranowski et al., 1992). Individually and combined, these three major components enhance or impede one's capacity to perform activities, to exercise, to participate in sports, or to accomplish occupational tasks. Overall then, physical activity is movement, exercise is a specific type of activity, and fitness is the ability to perform activity.

Physical activity includes recreational and leisure-time interests as well as sport involvement. The high end of the physical activity spectrum is vigorous activity, such as running. The low end of the activity spectrum is inactivity or sedentary behaviors, such as television viewing. In addition, physical activity can vary in frequency, intensity, duration, and type. Approaches to measuring physical activity include self-reports (e.g., frequency questionnaires and diaries) and objective assessments (e.g., motion sensors, heart rate monitors, and observation). In population-based studies, objective assessments are typically not financially practical or easy to administer. Recent reviews (Baranowski et al., 1992; Pate, Long, & Heath, 1994; Sallis & McKenzie, 1991) of physical activity levels among youth have included studies using both self-report and objective methods of assessing activity.

Several consistent findings have been reported from reviews of studies assessing the physical activity behavior of youth. For example, Rowland (1990) reported a 50% decline in physical activity for youth between the ages of 6 and 16 years. In addition, Sallis (1993) noted that boys are about 15% to 25% more active than girls. During the school-age years, activity levels decline at a rate of approximately 2.7% per year in boys and 7.4% per year in girls (Sallis, 1993).

The majority of physical activity by youth occurs outside of school (Pate et al., 1994). Most adolescents spend more than 3 hours per week in leisure-time activities outside of school (Pate et al., 1994). The top five activities for boys are bicycling, basketball, football, baseball or softball, and swimming, whereas for girls, the top five are swimming, bicycling, dancing, rollerskating, and walking (Pate et al., 1994). In school, activity during physical education class is frequently limited. During physical education classes, elementary school students spend less than 10% of class time and middle school students spend less than 17% of class time in moderate-to-vigorous physical activity (Simons-Morton, Taylor, Snider, & Huang, 1993; Simons-Morton, Taylor, Snider, Huang, & Fulton, 1994).

National medical and professional organizations have issued recommendations, opinion statements, objectives, and guidelines for youth physical activity (Sallis & Patrick, 1994). For example, two of the objectives that arose out of Healthy People 2000 (Department of Health and Human Services, 1990) were to increase to at least 30% the proportion of people who engage regularly, preferably daily, in light-to-moderate physical activity for at least 30 min and to increase to at least 75% the proportion of children and adolescents aged 6–17 years of age who engage in vigorous physical activity 3 or more days per week (for 20 min or more per session). Additional recommendations from the American Academy of Family Physicians, the American Academy of Pediatrics, the American College of Sports Medicine, and the American Medical Association have addressed physical activity counseling for youth as well as physical activity guidelines for this age group (U.S. Public Health Service, 1994). However, because many of the existing guidelines for physical activity by youth were based on studies of adult behavior, the International Consensus Conference on Physical Activity Guidelines for Adolescents was convened in June 1994 in San Diego, California, to review the literature on health effects of youth physical activity and to develop physical activity guidelines specifically for adolescents (Sallis, 1994). Thirty-four experts from scientific, medical, and governmental organizations were invited to participate in the conference. Two guidelines arose from the conference:

1. All adolescents should be physically active daily, or nearly every day, as part of play, games, sports, work, transportation, recreation, physical education, or planned exercise, in the context of family, school, and community activities.
2. Adolescents should engage in three or more sessions per week of activities that last 20 minutes or more at a time and that require moderate to vigorous levels of exertion. (Sallis, 1994, pp. 307–308)

Using the two guidelines developed specifically for adolescents and comparing estimates from a comprehensive review of adolescent activity patterns, Pate et al. (1994) determined that most of these youth are meeting the standard for the first guideline (80%) and a much smaller percentage (50%) are meeting the standard for the second guideline. Other researchers have shown that: (a) age and physical activity are inversely related during adolescence (Rowland, 1990; Sallis, 1993); (b) boys are more active than girls, and the discrepancy increases with age (Sallis, 1993); (c) a sizable percentage of adolescents are not meeting either of the recommended guidelines; and (d) many adolescents report little or no participation in physical activity (Pate et al., 1994). Given the consequences that may result if today's youth grow from adolescence into adulthood with low levels of physical activity, it is clear that improving the physical activity levels of young people represents an important public health challenge.

Activity Among Ethnic Minority Youth

Several studies have investigated ethnic differences in youth activity levels, and their findings have been mixed. In a large sample of ninth-grade boys and girls, African Americans reported watching more television and being more physically active than other ethnic groups (i.e., Asians, Pacific Islanders, Latinos or Hispanics, and Whites; Robinson & Killen, 1995). In another study of ninth- and eleventh-grade students, Zakarian, Hovell, Hofstetter, Sallis, and Keating (1994) noted that, when levels of vigorous exercise are compared, minority adolescents may not differ greatly from White adolescents. Studies such as these show no consistent pattern in youth activity according to ethnic group.

Alternatively, another group of studies have reported that ethnic minorities, particularly African American girls, are less physically active than their White counterparts. In studying African American girls from fifth through twelfth grades, Wolf et al. (1993) reported that almost 50% of the girls viewed 5 or more hours of television per day, in comparison with more than 25% of the Asian American girls and approximately 20% of the White and Hispanic girls. Additionally, in a national survey of American high school students, Heath, Pratt, Warren, and Kann (1994) reported that African American students were significantly less likely (28.8%) to be vigorously active than were either White (39.3%) or Hispanic students (34.5%). In the same study, African American female students were shown to be the least active of all subgroups (with 38.0% classified as sedentary). Heath et al. concluded that the low levels of physical activity found in women and African Americans are evident by the ninth grade. Other studies (e.g., Ainsworth, Berry, Schnyder, & Vickers, 1992; Ford & Goode, 1994) have also indicated that African American female college students are less physically active than their African American male peers.

Overall, if one takes into account all of these studies, it becomes apparent that a consistent and clear pattern of youth physical activity levels and ethnic differences has not been firmly established. The discrepant findings may be related to the types of questions posed, the intensity of activity, regional differences, types of activities, economic factors, activity preferences, or age differences. Ethnic differences and activity levels may be related, and their link remains an interesting hypothesis. Furthermore, activity preferences can vary across age, gender, and ethnic groups (Gottlieb & Chen, 1985). More research is needed to explore these issues.

Determinants of Physical Activity Among Youth

Determinants are factors and variables positively or negatively associated with physical activity. Because the data are primarily correlational, *determinant*, as we use the word in this chapter, does not imply a cause-and-effect relationship. The value of determinants research is that results can be used to guide the design of interventions to promote physical activity.

Determinants of youth physical activity are different from those for adult activity. Age, maturity, and control of the environment are characteristics that distinguish youth from adult activity. In youth, age (i.e., childhood or early, middle, or late adolescence) in combination with maturation and developmental levels can influence capability, opportunity, and interest in types of activity. Moreover, in many circumstances, young people may not have independent control of their environments. Parents, relatives, teachers, coaches, and other adults can exert the dominant influence on a young person's environment and opportunities. Youth is a unique time period, and a better understanding of activity determinants for this age group can help develop effective interventions to promote and sustain activity from childhood to adulthood.

The literature on determinants of youth physical activity comprises less than 100 studies. These studies have used a variety of theoretical approaches, including the expectancy-value model (Dempsey, Kimiecik, & Horn, 1993), personal investment theory (Tappe, Duda, & Menges-Ehrnwald, 1990), problem behavior theory (Donovan, Jessor, & Costa, 1991), protection–motivation theory (Fruin, Pratt, & Owen, 1991), the theory of motivation and emotion (Duncan, 1993), the theory of reasoned action (Theodorakis, Doganis, Bagiatis, & Gouthas, 1991), and social–cognitive theory (Stucky-Ropp & DiLorenzo, 1993). The different approaches reflect the diversity of influence by individual characteristics, social factors, and the physical environment on the targeted population. The extent to which particular variables or theories may have greater relevance for adolescent minority populations than other variables or theories has not been sufficiently investigated.

Overall, a broad range of variables has been studied, and comparative theoretical studies have been limited.

Review of the Literature

This part of the chapter updates two previous reviews (Sallis et al., 1992; Taylor, Baranowski, & Sallis, 1994) on determinants of physical activity among young people. Twenty-one additional studies from 1990 to 1994, not included in the two earlier reviews, are referenced here (e.g., Aaron et al., 1993; Armstrong & McManus, 1994; Biddle & Armstrong, 1992; Dempsey et al., 1993; Donovan et al., 1991; Douthitt, 1994; Duncan, 1993; Eck, Klesges, Hanson, & Slawson, 1992; Faucette et al., 1995; Felton & Parsons, 1994; Fruin et al., 1991; McMurray et al., 1993; Nader et al., 1995; Robinson et al., 1993; Sallis et al., 1993; Stucky-Ropp & DiLorenzo, 1993; Tappe et al., 1990; Terre, Ghiselli, Taloney, & DeSouza, 1992; Theodorakis et al., 1991; Wolf et al., 1993; Zakarian et al., 1994). We included only studies with some measure of physical activity as the dependent variable. For example, studies that investigated attitudes toward physical activity and did not relate the attitudes to some actual measure of physical activity were not reviewed.

The determinants of physical activity patterns in youth are many and diverse. We identified six domains that reflect this diversity: demographic and biological; psychological, cognitive, and emotional; behavioral attributes and skills; social and cultural; physical environment; and characteristics of physical activity.

Enjoyment (Biddle & Armstrong, 1992; Duncan, 1993; Stucky-Ropp & DiLorenzo, 1993) and physical competence (Dempsey et al., 1993; Tappe et al., 1990) are two determinants in the youth activity literature that have received strong and consistent support. Enjoyment can be thought of, simply as fun or, conceptually, as seeking the balance between challenge and skill (Petlichkoff, 1992). To motivate youth participation in physical activity one must create environments, situations, and conditions that provide enjoyable experiences. The enjoyment may emanate from the social context (e.g., being with others), from involvement in a particular activity (e.g., tennis), or from expressing oneself physically (e.g., through dance). From another perspective, competence, ability, and skills in physical activity have been tied to activity participation among youth. Learning to improve and becoming more competent in an activity (e.g., swimming, tennis, or basketball) may lead to mastery experiences, feelings of success and competence, intrinsic motivation, and consistent participation in such activity. Thus, an environment that permits and encourages skill-building and mastery experiences may promote activity participation by youth.

Activity Among Ethnic Minority Youth

Several studies that we describe below have investigated cultural and ethnic differences and determinants of physical activity among youth. One study (Greendorfer & Ewing, 1981) reported that the location of facilities (e.g., parks and schools), opportunities to participate in games or sports, and stronger values about sports (e.g., importance to the child or the child's father that he or she be good in sports) had more influence on African American children than on White children, whose sports involvement was influenced more by teachers and fathers. One national survey (Wilson Sporting Goods Company, 1988) revealed that African American and White girls were equally as likely to be involved in sports and that their reasons for participating in and quitting sports were the same. The ethnic differences in this survey stemmed from the fact that African American girls participated more often through their schools than did White girls (65% vs. 50%), and White girls participated more often through private organizations (21% vs. 7%). African American girls were more likely than their White counterparts to feel that "boys make fun of girls who play sports" (25% vs. 1%) and more often had parents who felt that sports participation was more important for boys than for girls (30% vs. 11%). Both of these studies reported differences between African American and White youths and their determinants of activity.

In recent studies, Nader et al. (1995) and Sallis et al. (1993) compared activity levels of Mexican American and White children. In children ages 4 to 7 years, Mexican American children had more indoor and outdoor play rules from parents, made fewer requests for activity, and received fewer activity prompts from parents than did White children. Among 4 year olds, Mexican American children were less active than White children at home and during recess. Moreover, as reported elsewhere (McKenzie, Sallis, Nader, Broyles, & Nelson, 1992), Mexican American children spent more time in the presence of adults and had access to fewer toys for activity at home and during recess than did White children. Such differences can influence later activity patterns.

Zakarian et al. (1994) examined factors related to vigorous exercise among low socioeconomic status ninth- and eleventh-grade adolescents, predominantly minorities (e.g., Asian Americans, African Americans, and Mexican Americans). In their sample, self-efficacy, support of friends, perceived benefits of exercise, perceived barriers to exercise, and body image were significantly related to vigorous exercise outside of school. Ethnic differences were not a focus of the study, and no such differences were reported.

Overall, ethnic differences related to determinants of youth activity have been reported in the literature. However, the findings have not shown a clear and consistent pattern related to ethnic and cultural influences. More research is needed to identify cultural factors and to determine cultural influences independent of socioeconomic status, environmental conditions, and school setting. Our perspective is that other relevant determinants of activity may diminish the influence of ethnic and cultural differences. Another perspective (e.g., Melnyk & Weinstein, 1994) is that an increasing awareness is needed of the role that cultural diversity plays in people's attitudes and behaviors toward health. For example, as Melnyk and Weinstein suggested, instead of poor motivation, perhaps lack of access to exercise facilities, preference for social versus individual exercise regimens, and culturally based attitudes toward exercise are reasons for low levels of physical activity among African American women. In fact, good compliance has been demonstrated with exercise components in a weight control program designed primarily for African American women. In addition, children of various ethnic backgrounds may be socialized into sports differently. Boys with above-average athletic skills from different racial and ethnic backgrounds may be socialized into sports through different forms of encouragement, particularly from the family (Oliver, 1980). Some families may stress athletic competition as a viable channel to upward mobility, whereas other families may stress sports as an opportunity to develop as an individual and believe that seeking a professional career in sports is a "treadmill to nowhere." Another potential factor influencing physical activity may be safety in the neighborhood or at the playground, park, school, or community center. We recommend that researchers undertake systematic and well-designed studies to identify these unique cultural influences on physical activity among youth.

Interventions for Increasing Physical Activity Among Youth

Regular physical activity can improve adolescents' health (Sallis, 1994). Interventions, guided by determinants research, can provide opportunities for youth to become more active. To date, interventions for increasing youth physical activity have involved either single-factor (i.e., physical activity only) or multiple-risk-factor reduction programs (i.e., promoting activity, smoking cessation, and good nutrition). Settings for these interventions have included schools, homes (family), communities, and health care facilities. For an overview and critique of physical activity interventions with youth, refer to the 1992 review by Sallis et al. The purpose of the next part of this chapter is to describe interventions designed specifically for ethnic minority youth.

Increasing Activity Among Ethnic Minority Youth

From 1983 to 1995, at least five prominent interventions aimed at increasing physical activity in ethnic minority youth were developed, implemented, and evaluated. One prominent intervention, the Know Your Body (KYB) program (Bush et al., 1989), was started in 1983 in nine Washington, DC, public elementary schools. The participants were African American students in fourth through sixth grades, and researchers reported both a physical activity component and a fitness assessment.

The KYB program is classroom based and teacher delivered; its three primary intervention components are improving nutrition, increasing physical activity, and preventing cigarette smoking. The KYB curriculum is guided by social learning theory; behavior changes in students were expected as a result of values clarification, goal setting, modeling, rehearsal, feedback of screening results, and reinforcement. The physical activity component promoted the adoption of a regular program of endurance activity to supplement skills and strength activities. The students received an annual personalized health screening and completed surveys to measure knowledge, behavior, attitudes, and psychosocial factors (Bush et al., 1989). The postexercise pulse recovery rate (fitness index) was used to measure changes in physical activity.

In the 4-year Washington, DC, study (Bush et al., 1989), three schools were each randomly selected from three socioeconomic levels (low, middle, or high) and assigned to a treatment condition ($n = 9$) or control condition ($n = 9$). A 5-year evaluation (including an evaluation 1 year after the intervention) indicated that the intervention group was significantly more fit than the control group at Year 3 ($p <$ .01). No significant differences in fitness were reported for Years 2, 4, and 5 (Bush et al., 1989).

In the late 1980s and early 1990s, researchers reported on three additional interventions intended to increase the physical activity levels among ethnic minority youth. Nader et al. (1989) investigated the effectiveness of a family-based intervention to reduce the risk of cardiovascular disease in 206 healthy Mexican American and White families. Each family had a fifth- or sixth-grade child and low-to-middle income. Families were randomly assigned to a year-long educational intervention to improve their eating habits and increase regular physical activity; each was measured at a 24-month follow-up. The intervention used social learning theory strategies to promote such behavior as self-monitoring, goal setting, behavioral rehearsal, modeling, and self-regulation skills. Intervention families received 3 months of intensive weekly interventions, followed by 9 months of monthly or bimonthly maintenance sessions. Intra- and interfamilial interactions and support were encouraged; learning activities were experiential or through games and discussion. Nader et al. assessed physical activity by 7-day recall and measured fitness with a cycle ergometer test. Results showed that Whites and Mexican Americans in the experimental groups gained significantly more knowledge of the skills required to change activity habits than did those in the control groups. In reported physical activity and tested fitness, there were no differences between the groups. Nader et al. attributed the minimal effect of the physical activity intervention to unrealistic goals (e.g., instead of advocating aerobic exercise, walking would have been more appropriate), insufficient intervention, and the difficulty of changing people's activity patterns.

Baranowski et al. (1990) designed and implemented a center-based program to promote activity among healthy African American families with children in the sixth through seventh grades. Ninety-four families were randomly assigned to either an experimental or a control group. In the experimental group, families participated in one education session and two fitness sessions per week for 14 weeks. Educational sessions included individual counseling, small group education, and aerobic activity. Free transportation and babysitting were provided, as well as reminders to promote attendance. Following the 14th week of the program, the researchers conducted a postprogram assessment. They assessed activity using a 7-day recall and a "frequency of aerobic activity" form. They assessed cardiovascular fitness with bicycle submaximal stress tests. Additionally, pulse and blood pressure were taken as cardiovascular measures. In children, activity increased in the control group and decreased in the experimental group. Among children in the experimental group who attended more than half of the fitness sessions, the frequency of postprogram aerobic activity was highest. No significant differences were detected among cardiovascular fitness indicators. Baranowski et al. concluded that low participation rates ($M = 28\%$) were the primary reason for lack of consistent program effects. Participants cited conflicts with work and school schedules (for adults and children, respectively) as their main reasons for low attendance. The authors concluded that, given the barriers to participation in center-based activities, emphasizing activities that families can participate in without a center (e.g., walking or bicycling) may be a more effective intervention strategy.

In a third study, Johnson et al. (1991) designed an intervention program for 19 fourth and fifth graders and their families (predominately African American). The children had elevated risk factors (blood pressure and ponderosity). The program included eight 90-min sessions (of presentations, activities, and group aerobic exercise) and three nutrition, exercise, and smoking counseling sessions over 12 weeks. Children's physical activity levels were evaluated on the basis of a 1-mile run–walk performance. All children significantly improved their run times, showing an average decrease of 1.5 min (14.9 vs. 13.4 min; $p < .01$). Johnson et al. concluded that, as a result of their program, families demonstrated positive changes in eating habits, physical activity, and cardiovascular health knowledge.

More recently, Ewart, Loftus, and Hagberg (1995) evaluated the efficacy of school-based aerobic exercise program for lowering blood pressure in a high-risk urban sample of ninth-grade African American girls. Girls in the intervention group received a one-semester aerobics class of fitness instruction and training designed to be enjoyable and engaging for high-risk girls. Eighteen 50-min class periods involved lecture and discussion, and 60 class periods were spent performing aerobic exercise. Girls assigned randomly to the control group received the standard physical education curriculum. After completing the aerobics class, 81% of the girls expressed a desire to participate in a supervised exercise maintenance program for at least one additional semester. Ewart et al. concluded that the participants generally enjoyed aerobic exercise and most expressed a desire to continue exercising regularly.

In addition to these five studies, two other intervention studies are noteworthy. Flores (1995) reported on a small-scale controlled trial called Dance for Health, which tested an aerobic program designed for African American and Hispanic adolescents to improve aerobic capacity, maintain or decrease weight, and improve attitudes toward physical activity and physical fitness. This 12-week school-based intervention was combined with a culturally sensitive health curriculum for 110 boys and girls aged 10 to 13 years. Girls in the Dance for Health program significantly decreased their body mass index and resting heart rates compared with girls in the usual physical activity program. There were no significant differences between the intervention and control groups for boys. Another intervention, the Child and Adolescent Trial for Cardiovascular Health (CATCH; Luepker et al., 1995) was a large-scale controlled field trial that evaluated a 3-year school and home program for the primary prevention of cardiovascular disease in an ethnically diverse sample of third to fifth graders (13% African American, 69% White, 14% Hispanic, and 4% other). CATCH was implemented in four sites comprising 56 intervention and 40 control elementary schools. After 3 years of the program, intervention school students reported significantly more daily vigorous activity than did control school students. Furthermore, during physical education classes, the intensity of activity increased significantly in intervention schools compared with control schools.

Behavioral research on physical activity among youth is in an early stage of development. Consistently effective methods of increasing physical activity in healthy youth are not yet available (see Sallis et al., 1992). Not surprisingly, the literature on promoting physical activity among ethnic minority and underserved youth is not extensive or well developed. The available literature does indicate more success in promoting physical activity in high-risk ethnic minority youth (e.g., those with high blood pressure) than among otherwise healthy ethnic minority youth (Johnson et al., 1991; Nader et al., 1989). In addition, studies with smaller samples and more intensive interventions have reported greater success in improving the physical activity levels of ethnic minority youth (Flores, 1995; Luepker et al., 1995). School-based interventions have also been more effective than interventions in other settings. More research is needed to determine optimal strategies of involving ethnic minority families in health behavior change programs. Interventions to improve muscular strength and flexibility merit further study, as do those promoting aerobic exercise.

Given the paucity of data and mixed findings in existing studies, we recommend that more research be undertaken to establish effective, optimal, and culturally appropriate interventions for ethnic minority youth. In designing an effective program encouraging physical activity among these populations, one should carefully investigate such issues as safety in neighborhoods, activity preferences, peer norms, family values and expectations, and physical status (e.g., weight, fitness levels, and chronic conditions). Overall, the limited success of physical activity interventions with ethnic minority youth further supports the difficulty and complexity of altering physical activity patterns irrespective of age, gender, and ethnic background.

Health Care Professionals and Physical Activity in Youth

One of the recommendations from the American Medical Association's (1994) Guidelines for Adolescent Preventive Health Services is that all adolescents should annually receive health guidance about the benefits of exercise and should be encouraged to engage in safe exercise on a regular basis. Also, one of the objectives from Healthy People 2000 was to increase to at least 50% the proportion of primary care providers who routinely assess and counsel their patients regarding the frequency, duration, type, and intensity of their physical activity practices.

Physical activity counseling with children has been recommended by many medical and sports organizations, including the American Academy of Family Physicians, the American Academy of Pediatrics, the American College of Sports Medicine, and the American Medical Association (U.S. Public Health Service, 1994). Accordingly, several approaches have been published to guide health care professionals in promoting activity among youth. DuRant and Hergenroeder (1994) presented principles to promote changes in health behavior (specifically, physical activity in youth) that were based on social–cognitive theory. They recommended the GAPS model (gather information, assess further, problem identification, and self-efficacy and solving barriers) as a method to implement these principles in a health care setting. Rowland (1990) described clinical approaches to the sedentary child, including the diagnosis of exercise deficiency, a sample activity questionnaire, early exercise interventions, motivational factors, and exercise recommendations. He concluded with a section titled "Physicians Can Do More." Another strategy, named *PACE* (Physician Based Assessment and Counseling for Exercise; Pender, Sallis, Long, & Calfas, 1994) offers an approach to physical activity counseling that is innovative, theoretically based, and empirically tested. This approach is structured and easy to adopt by health care professionals. PACE was created for adults, so age-appropriate strategies still need to be developed for its use with young people. The majority of the population has some contact with a physician during the year. Potentially, the advice given by a health care professional, given his or her credibility as an information source, may have high relevance for youth in spite of the low frequency of well visits by youth.

Health Care Professionals and Activity in Ethnic Minority Youth

The potential influence of health care providers among minority youth is substantial. Unfortunately, this potential is not being fulfilled. In a national survey of pediatricians' practices and attitudes, Nader, Taras, Sallis, and Patterson (1987) categorized the ethnic composition of the practices into two groups: those where African Americans numbered fewer than 25% of patients or those where African American patients were equal to or greater than 25% of patients in practice. Differences emerged between these two practices. For example, pediatricians with many African American patients were less likely to routinely recommend dietary sodium or fat reduction in 6- to 12-year-old children, believed it was less important to discuss exercise with adolescents, and more often felt ineffective in promoting exercise as a lifestyle change with their patients compared with pediatricians who had fewer African American patients (Nader et al., 1987). Increasing the number of health care professionals who confidently and effectively address and encourage physical activity among minority youths may bring about lifestyle changes that decrease the prevalence in such conditions as obesity, hypertension, and diabetes.

White (1993) has suggested clinical strategies for promoting exercise among ethnic minority patients. One strategy is to draw on resources and program initiatives targeted to the special needs of patients' communities. Organizations such as the National Coalition of Hispanic Health and Human Services Organizations, American Indian Health Care Association, Asian American Health Forum, National Black Women's Health Project, and the Office of Minority Health Resource Center can provide materials, resources, and publications, as well as assist health care professionals in becoming familiar with the customs and values of a particular culture. Furthermore, White recommended that health care professionals examine the preconceptions, assumptions, and cultural biases that they bring to their sessions. As an example, because of individual biases and assumptions, the psychologist and patient may not share the same concept of what exercise involves. Similarly, not all cultures share the same concept of competitive play and sport. The professional needs to explore the patients' attitudes about exercise and physical activity and get his or her own cultural perspective.

Understanding the costs of exercise and recognizing differences in cross-cultural interactions requires sensitivity on the part of the practitioner (White, 1993). Careful attention should always be paid to these variables during interventions. Difficulties in cross-cultural interactions can lead to misunderstandings and, thus, ineffective patient care. Alternatively, when cultural values are incorporated into service delivery, greater compliance can be expected (White, 1993).

Building on strength and creating community are important approaches for promoting activity in ethnic minority communities (White, 1993). For example, in some communities, the family plays a central role in the culture (e.g., Hispanic community values), and so getting the whole family involved in an activity program is important. Various types of aerobics use traditional Native American music, jazz, and other music strongly reflecting cultural influences. In creating community, the National Black Women's Health Project's Walking for

Wellness program illustrates the benefits in the African American community by promoting activity within a relevant, cultural framework. The program revolves around peer support groups. Among many African American women, weight control programs that include close interaction with a group leader will tend to be more effective than programs emphasizing an individualistic approach and a learning orientation (White, 1993). Working within a community can therefore offer an effective approach.

In summary, a health care professional can be immensely more effective in promoting physical activity among ethnic minority youth by being culturally aware and sensitive to the needs of the patient. This awareness and sensitivity means taking the time to learn about and work with a culture's potentially different communication style and health care beliefs while keeping in mind the commonalities and basics of activity promotion (White, 1993).

Conclusion and Recommendations

Physical activity is a health-enhancing behavior. Increasing the physical activity levels of individuals at a young age requires creative efforts, and reaching more diverse populations of youth is a public health challenge. In this chapter, we have presented research on the levels and determinants of physical activity, as well as on potential interventions with ethnic minority youth. Communities, educators, individuals, families, and health care professionals have unique opportunities to promote physical activity in ethnic minority youth. Professionals can seize these opportunities with knowledge, training, skillful counseling, and cultural sensitivity and awareness to help achieve the objective of transforming inactive youths to active youth and active youth to active adults. Even modestly effective health care professional counseling could have a substantial public health impact (Pate et al., 1995). Therefore, commitment and ongoing collaboration are needed among behavioral scientists, health care professionals, and all those concerned with youth. Working together, these individuals can effectively confront the public health challenge of developing and implementing effective programs to promote physical activity for minority youth.

REFERENCES

Aaron, D. J., Kriska, A. M., Dearwater, S. R., Anderson, R. L., Olsen, T. L., Cauley, J. A., & Laporte, R. E. (1993). The epidemiology of leisure physical activity in an adolescent population. *Medicine and Science in Sports and Exercise, 25,* 847–853.

Ainsworth, B. E., Berry, C. B., Schnyder, V. N., & Vickers, S. R. (1992). Leisure-time physical activity and aerobic fitness in African-American young adults. *Journal of Adolescent Health, 13,* 606–611.

American Medical Association. (1994). *AMA guidelines for adolescent preventive health services (GAPS): Recommendations and rationale.* Baltimore: Williams & Wilkins.

Armstrong, N., & McManus, A. (1994). Children's fitness and physical activity: A challenge for physical education. *The British Journal of Physical Education, 25,* 20–26.

Baranowski, T., Bouchard, C., Bar-Or, O., Bricker, T., Heath, G., Kimm, S. Y., Malina, R., Obarzanek, F., Pate, R., Strong, W. B., Truman, B., & Washington, R. (1992). Assessment, prevalence, and cardiovascular benefits of physical activity and fitness in youth. *Medicine and Science in Sports and Exercise, 24*(Suppl.), S237–S247.

Baranowski, T., Simons-Morton, B., Hooks, P., Henske, J., Tiernan, K., Dunn, J. K., Burkhalter, H., Harper, J., & Palmer, J. (1990). A center-based program for exercise change among Black-American families. *Health Education Quarterly, 17,* 179–196.

Biddle, S., & Armstrong, N. (1992). Children's physical activity: An exploratory study of psychological correlates. *Social Science and Medicine, 34,* 325–331.

Bush, P. J., Zuckerman, A. E., Taggart, V. S., Theiss, P. K., Peleg, E. O., & Smith, S. A. (1989). Cardiovascular risk factor prevention in Black school children: The "Know Your Body" evaluation project. *Health Education Quarterly, 16,* 215–227.

Caspersen, C. J., Powell, K. E., & Christenson, G. M. (1985). Physical activity, exercise, and physical fitness: Definitions and distinctions for health-related research. *Public Health Reports, 100,* 126–131.

Dempsey, J. M., Kimiecik, J. C., & Horn, T. S. (1993). Parental influence on children's moderate-to-vigorous physical activity participation: An expectancy-value approach. *Pediatric Exercise Science 5,* 151–167.

Department of Health and Human Services. (1990). *Healthy People 2000: National health promotion and disease prevention objectives* (DHHS Publication No. [PHS] 91-50212). Washington, DC: U.S. Government Printing Office.

Donovan, J. E., Jessor, R., & Costa, F. M. (1991). Adolescent health behavior and conventionality–unconventionality: An extension of problem-behavior theory. *Health Psychology, 10,* 52–61.

Douthitt, V. L. (1994). Psychological determinants of adolescent exercise adherence. *Adolescence, 29,* 711–722.

Duncan, S. C. (1993). The role of cognitive appraisal and friendship provisions in adolescents' affect and motivation toward activity in physical education. *Research Quarterly for Exercise and Sport, 64,* 314–323.

DuRant, R. H., & Hergenroeder, A. C. (1994). Promotion of primary activity among adolescents by primary care providers. *Pediatric Exercise Science, 6,* 448–463.

Eck, L. H., Klesges, R. C., Hanson, C. L., & Slawson, D. (1992). Children at familial risk for obesity: An examination of dietary intake, physical activity and weight status. *International Journal of Obesity, 16,* 71–78.

Ewart, C. K., Loftus, K. S., & Hagberg, J. M. (1995). School-based exercise to lower blood pressure in high-risk African-American girls: Project design and baseline findings. *Journal of Health Education, 26*(Suppl. 2), S99–S105.

Faucette, N., Sallis, J. F., McKenzie, T., Alcaraz, J., Kolody, B., & Nugent, P. (1995). Comparison of fourth grade students' out-of-school physical activity levels and choices by gender: Project SPARK. *Journal of Health Education, 26*(Suppl. 2), S82–S90.

Felton, G. M., & Parsons, M. A. (1994). Factors influencing physical activity in average-weight and overweight young women. *Journal of Community Health Nursing, 11,* 109–119.

Flores, R. (1995). Dance for health: Improving fitness in African American and Hispanic adolescents. *Public Health Reports, 110,* 189–193.

Ford, D. S., & Goode, C. R. (1994). African American college students' health behaviors and perceptions of related health issues. *Journal of American College Health, 42*(5), 206–210.

Fruin, D. J., Pratt, C., & Owen, N. (1991). Protection motivation theory and adolescents' perceptions of exercise. *Journal of Applied Social Psychology, 22,* 55–69.

Gottlieb, N. H., & Chen, M. S. (1985). Sociocultural correlates of childhood sporting activities: Their implications for heart health. *Social Science in Medicine, 21,* 533–539.

Greendorfer, S. L., & Ewing, M. E. (1981). Race and gender differences in children's socialization into sport. *Research Quarterly for Exercise and Sport, 52,* 301–310.

Heath, G. W., Pratt, M., Warren, C. W., & Kann, L. (1994). Physical activity patterns in American high school students. *Archives of Pediatrics and Adolescent Medicine, 148,* 1131–1136.

Johnson, C. C., Nicklas, T. A., Arbeit, M. L., Harsha, D. W., Mott, D. S., Hunter, S. M., Wattigney, W., & Berenson, G. S. (1991). Cardiovascular intervention for high-risk families: The Head Smart Program. *Southern Medical Journal, 84,* 1305–1312.

Luepker, R. V., Perry, C. L., McKinlay, S. M., Nader, P. R., Parcel, G. S., Stone, E. J., Webber, L. S., Elder, J. P., Feldman, H. A., Johnson, C. C., Kelder, S. H., & Wu, M., for the CATCH Collaborative Group. (1995). *Outcomes of a field trial to improve children's dietary patterns and physical activity: The Child and Adolescent Trial for Cardiovascular Health (CATCH).* Manuscript submitted for publication.

McKenzie, T. L., Sallis, J. F., Nader, P. R., Broyles, S. L., & Nelson, J. A. (1992). Anglo- and Mexican-American preschoolers at home and at recess: Activity patterns and environmental influences. *Journal of Developmental and Behavioral Pediatrics, 13,* 173–180.

McMurray, R. G., Bradley, C. B., Harrell, J. S., Bernthal, P. R., Frauman, A. C., & Bangdiwala, S. I. (1993). Parental influences on childhood fitness and activity patterns. *Research Quarterly for Exercise and Sport, 64,* 249–255.

Melnyk, M. G., & Weinstein, E. (1994). Preventing obesity in Black women by targeting adolescents: A literature review. *Journal of the American Dietetic Association, 94,* 536–540.

Nader, P. R., Sallis, J. F., Broyles, S. L., McKenzie, T. L., Berry, C. C., David, T. B., Zive, M. M., Elder, J. P., & Frank-Spohrer, G. C. (1995). Ethnic and gender trends for cardiovascular risk behaviors in Anglo- and Mexican-American children, ages four–seven. *Journal of Health Education, 26,* S27–S35.

Nader, P. R., Sallis, J. F., Patterson, T. L., Aabramson, I. S., Rupp, J. W., Senn, K. L., Atkins, C. J., Roppe, B. E., Morris, J. A., Wallace, J. P., & Vega, W. A. (1989). A family approach to cardiovascular risk reduction: Results from the San Diego Family Health Project. *Health Education Quarterly, 16,* 229–244.

Nader, P. R., Taras, H. L., Sallis, J. F., & Patterson, T. L. (1987). Adult heart disease prevention in childhood: A national survey of pediatricians' practices and attitudes. *Pediatrics, 79,* 843–850.

Oliver, M. L. (1980). Race, class and the family's orientation to mobility through sport. *Sociological Symposium, 30,* 62–86.

Pate, R. R., Long, B. J., & Heath, G. (1994). Descriptive epidemiology of physical activity in adolescents. *Pediatric Exercise Science, 6,* 434–447.

Pate, R. R., Pratt, M., Blair, S. N., Haskell, W. L., Macera, C. A., Bouchard, C., Buchner, D., Ettinger, W., Heath, G. W., King, A. C., Kriska, A., Leon, A. S., Marcus, B. H., Morris, J., Paffenbarger, R. S., Patrick, K., Pollock, M. L., Rippe, J. M., Sallis, J., & Wilmore, J. H. (1995). Physical activity and public health. A recommendation from the Centers for Disease Control and Prevention and the American College of Sports Medicine. *Journal of the American Medical Association, 273,* 402–407.

Pender, N. J., Sallis, J. F., Long, B. J., & Calfas, K. J. (1994). Health-care provider counseling to promote physical activity. In R. K. Dishman (Ed.), *Advances in exercise adherence* (pp. 213–235). Champaign, IL: Human Kinetics.

Petlichkoff, L. M. (1992). Youth sport participation and withdrawal: Is it simply a matter of fun? *Pediatric Exercise Science, 4,* 105–110.

Robinson, T. N., Hammer, L. D., Killen, J. D., Kraemer, H. C., Wilson, D. M., Hayward, C., & Taylor, C. B. (1993). Does television viewing increase obesity and reduce physical activity? Cross-sectional and longitudinal analyses among adolescent girls. *Pediatrics, 91,* 273–280.

Robinson, T. N., & Killen, J. D. (1995). Ethnic and gender differences in the relationships between television viewing and obesity, physical activity, and dietary fat intake. *Journal of Health Education, 26*(Suppl. 2), S91–S98.

Rowland, T. W. (1990). *Exercise and children's health*. Champaign, IL: Human Kinetics.

Sallis, J. F. (1993). Epidemiology of physical activity and fitness in children and adolescents. *Critical Reviews in Food Science and Nutrition, 33*(4–5), 403–408.

Sallis, J. F. (Ed.). (1994). Physical activity guidelines for adolescents [Special issue]. *Pediatric Exercise Science, 6*(4).

Sallis, J. F., & McKenzie, T. L. (1991). Physical education's role in public health. *Research Quarterly for Exercise and Sport, 62*, 124–137.

Sallis, J. F., Nader, P. R., Broyles, S. L., Berry, C. C., Elder, J. P., McKenzie, T. L., & Nelson, J. A. (1993). Correlates of physical activity at home in Mexican-American and Anglo-American preschool children. *Health Psychology, 12*, 390–398.

Sallis, J. F., & Patrick, K. (1994). Physical activity guidelines for adolescents: Consensus statement. *Pediatric Exercise Science, 6*, 302–314.

Sallis, J. F., Simons-Morton, B. G., Stone, E. J., Corbin, C. B., Epstein, L. H., Faucetts, N., Iannotti, R. J., Killen, J. D., Klesges, R. C., Petray, C. K., Rowland, T. W., & Taylor, W. C. (1992). Determinants of physical activity and interventions in youth. *Medicine and Science in Sports and Exercise, 24*(Suppl.), S248–S257.

Simons-Morton, B. G., Taylor, W. C., Snider, S. A., & Huang, I. W. (1993). The physical activity of fifth-grade students during physical education classes. *American Journal of Public Health, 83*, 262–264.

Simons-Morton, B. G., Taylor, W. C., Snider, S. A., Huang, I. W., & Fulton, J. E. (1994). Observed levels of elementary and middle school children's physical activity during physical education classes. *Preventive Medicine, 23*, 437–441.

Stucky-Ropp, R. C., & DiLorenzo, T. M. (1993). Determinants of exercise in children. *Preventive Medicine, 22*, 880–889.

Tappe, M. K., Duda, J. L., & Menges-Ehrnwald, P. (1990). Personal investment predictors of adolescent motivational orientation toward exercise. *Canadian Journal of Sport Sciences, 15*, 185–192.

Taylor, W. C., Baranowski, T., & Sallis, J. F. (1994). Family determinants of childhood physical activity: A social–cognitive model. In R. K. Dishman (Ed.), *Advances in exercise adherence* (pp. 319–342). Champaign, IL: Human Kinetics.

Terre, L., Ghiselli, W., Taloney, L., & DeSouza, E. (1992). Demographics, affect, and adolescents' health behaviors. *Adolescence, 27*(105), 12–24.

Theodorakis, Y., Doganis, G., Bagiatis, K., & Gouthas, M. (1991). Preliminary study of the ability of the reasoned action model in predicting exercise behavior of young children. *Perceptual and Motor Skills, 72*, 51–58.

U.S. Public Health Service. (1994). Physical activity in children. *American Family Physician, 50*, 1285–1288.

White, J. (1993). Minority patients: Clinical strategies to promote exercise. *Physician and Sports Medicine, 21*(5), 136–144.

Wilson Sporting Goods Company. (1988). *The Wilson report: Moms, dads, daughters, and sports*. River Grove, IL: Author.

Wolf, A. M., Gortmaker, S. L., Cheung, L., Gray, H. M., Herzog, D. B., & Colditz, G. A. (1993). Activity, inactivity, and obesity: Racial, ethnic, and age differences among schoolgirls. *American Journal of Public Health, 83,* 1625–1627.

Zakarian, J. M., Hovell, M. F., Hofstetter, C. R., Sallis, J. F., & Keating, K. J. (1994). Correlates of vigorous exercise in a predominantly low SES and minority high school population. *Preventive Medicine, 23,* 314–321.

Chapter 6

The Role of Diet in Minority Adolescent Health Promotion

Dawn K. Wilson, Susan C. Nicholson, and Jenelle S. Krishnamoorthy

The promotion of healthy dietary habits is especially important for minority adolescents, who are at increased risk for developing cardiovascular diseases, obesity, diabetes mellitus, and cancer in early adulthood (Garb & Stunkard, 1975; Harris, Hadden, Knowler, & Bennett, 1987; Stern, Pugh, Gaskill, & Hazuda, 1982; Stone, Baranowski, Sallis, & Cutler, 1995; U.S. Department of Health and Human Services [U.S. DHHS], 1986). Intake of specific nutrients such as dietary fat, cholesterol, and sodium have been linked to major risk factors of elevated blood cholesterol, obesity, and high blood pressure, among others (American Heart Association, 1988). These risk factors have been

The project reported in this chapter was supported by a National Institutes of Health FIRST Award Grant HL-46736 to Dawn K. Wilson.

detected among children (Newman, Freedman, & Berenson, 1986) and have been shown to track from childhood into the adult years (Nicklas, Webber, Johnson, Srinivasan, & Berenson, 1995). Previous research has indicated that dietary modification can reduce the risk and incidence of chronic illness in adolescent populations (Gliksman, Lazarus, & Wilson, 1993). Promoting a healthy diet among adolescents can help to normalize body weight (Epstein, 1986) and may reduce their risk of chronic illness. Preliminary research has begun to address these issues in minority adolescent populations, yet much more research is needed. In this chapter, we review ethnic differences in dietary intake among minority adolescents and highlight research that has been successful in promoting healthy eating habits among this population. The studies we review were selected to illustrate the significance of environmental influences (i.e., family, school, community, and media), individual influences (i.e., self-efficacy and locus of control), and genetic influences (i.e., family history and gender) on the development of dietary interventions for specific adolescent minority populations.

The Year 2000 health objectives outlined by the U.S. Public Health Service (U.S. DHHS, 1991) advocate specific dietary recommendations for adolescents. They recommend that adolescents limit their intake of dietary fat to 30% and of saturated fat to 10% of their total calories. The guidelines also suggest that adolescents eat at least five vegetables and fruits, six or more servings of grains, and three servings of calcium enriched foods per day. Adolescents should reduce their sodium intake by eliminating the use of table salt, preparing foods without salt, and purchasing more low sodium foods. Specifically, the Year 2000 health objectives propose that these recommendations be met by requiring more informative nutritional labeling of foods; by increasing the availability of reduced-fat foods; by encouraging restaurants to offer low-fat, low-calorie foods; and by modifying school lunch and breakfast programs. These guidelines are particularly relevant for minority adolescents, who are at increased risk for developing chronic illness in early adulthood.

Ethnic Differences in Dietary Intake

Research on dietary intake across ethnic groups has been limited; however, some evidence has suggested that there are ethnic differences in nutrient intake. African Americans, Mexican Americans,

Siouan Indians, and Asian Americans have been the primary focuses of these studies. Overall, adolescents of all ethnicities appear to be eating more fat and sodium and fewer vegetables, fruits, and whole grains than the recommended daily guidelines reviewed above (Simons-Morton, Baranowski, Parcel, O'Hara, & Matteson, 1990; Subar et al., 1992). A number of studies have indicated that sodium intake is especially high among African American adolescents. For example, Frank et al. (1992) found that African American adolescents ate significantly more lunch meat and pork and significantly fewer vegetables than did White peers. Frank, Zive, Nelson, Broyles, and Nader (1991) also reported that Mexican American children (preschoolers) consumed significantly more high-fat foods, such as whole milk, refried beans, lard, and eggs, than did White children. These patterns of consumption were similar among Mexican American parents, suggesting that eating habits established in young children may continue through adolescence and into adulthood. Although studies including Siouan Indians have not examined differences in nutrient intake compared with other ethnic groups, Harland, Smith, Ellis, O'Brien, and Morris (1992) did find Sioux diets to be characterized by high levels of carbohydrates and sodium intake, especially among males. Dietary research among Asian Americans has not specifically compared their intake to other ethnic groups. One study (Kirby, Baranowski, Reynolds, Taylor, & Binkley, 1995) that included Asian American children (ages 9–11 years) with children of other ethnic minority groups found that lower income families ate very few fresh fruits and vegetables and more fast foods than did higher income families. Such studies have highlighted some of the important nutritional distinctions across ethnic groups; however, further research is needed to better illuminate these differences from a cultural perspective.

Conceptual Framework of Dietary Behavior in Minority Adolescents

In this chapter, we propose a conceptual framework for specifically understanding dietary behaviors among minority adolescent populations (see Figure 1). We begin by highlighting aspects of the environmental, individual, and genetic factors that are particularly relevant to promoting healthy diets among minority adolescents. Environmen-

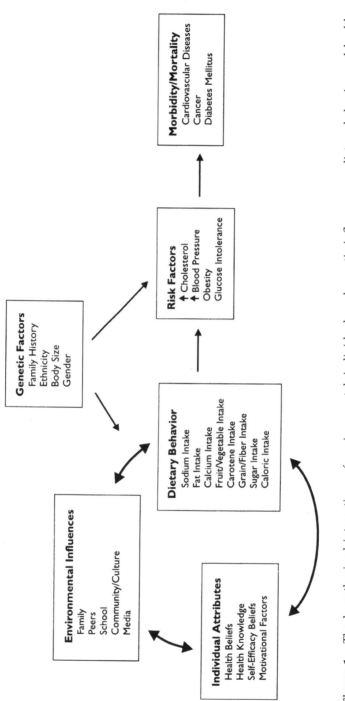

Figure 1. The hypothesized interactions of environmental, individual, and genetic influences on dietary behavior and health risk factors.

tal influences, individual attributes, and dietary behavior are proposed to reciprocally interact in the development of health risk factors that ultimately lead to increased morbidity and mortality. In addition, genetic factors such as family history may indirectly influence this reciprocal relationship while directly influencing the development of risk factors. With the clinician in mind, we expand on each of these factors from an intervention perspective in the discussion that follows. Environmental influences include the role of family, peers, school, community, culture, and the media. Individual attributes include health beliefs, self-efficacy beliefs, health knowledge, and motivational factors. Although these individual attributes have not been examined much among minority adolescents, we argue that specific individual factors may be important for future research in certain minority populations. Genetic factors include family history of dietary-related risk factors, gender, ethnicity, and body size. Because minority adolescents are at increased risk for developing chronic illness, knowledge of genetic risk may be used as a motivational cue for encouraging adolescents at risk to engage in healthy dietary habits.

Dietary health behaviors are culturally influenced, in that food choices, methods of cooking, and traditions all reflect cultural values. Thus, it is important to have knowledge of and respect for the target community's culture and language when developing dietary interventions. The specific content of a dietary intervention may vary across ethnic groups. For example, within the Mexican American community, an intervention might target reducing the use of lard in food preparation, whereas, within the African American community the target of an intervention might be lowering sodium consumption. The specific components of interventions—the use of community leaders and liaisons as staff, the inclusion of culturally meaningful activities, and the integration of the culture's language—will vary across ethnic groups. In contrast, the conceptual framework shown in Figure 1 and the overall structure of the dietary program are applicable across all groups. For example, the influences of the environment may be particularly relevant to minority groups because of the emphasis in their cultures on family and community or the collective, as opposed to in White culture, where the emphasis is on the individual.

Environmental Influences

Family-based approaches. Several lines of evidence suggest that targeting families, especially among minority adolescent populations, may be important for promoting healthy dietary habits. First, research has demonstrated a moderate aggregation of dietary variables among younger minority adolescents and their parents (Patterson, Rupp, Sallis, Atkins, & Nader, 1988), suggesting that parents may influence their children's eating habits. Furthermore, because minority families share a genetic predisposition to health risk factors, family involvement may be especially important in motivating adolescents to alter their long-term eating habits. Finally, parents and peers may serve as role models for adolescents by consuming foods that are healthy and by reinforcing dietary knowledge and behaviors learned in schools (Perry et al., 1988).

Parental involvement in dietary programs has been shown to be a critical aspect of promoting healthy dietary habits in minority adolescents. Nader et al. (1989) randomly assigned Mexican American and White families with adolescent children either to a 1-year educational intervention designed to decrease sodium and fat intake or to a no-treatment control group. The participants included younger adolescents who were recruited from schools that were matched according to social economic status. Treatment families of both ethnicities gained significantly more knowledge of the skills required to change their dietary habits, improved their diets, and had lower blood pressures than those in the control group. Wadden et al. (1990) examined the effects of a 16-week weight-loss program for African American adolescent females who received differing levels of parent participation. Forty-seven adolescent females were randomly assigned to participate alone, participate with their mothers in the same session, or participate with their mothers in concurrent sessions. Results showed that the greater the number of sessions attended by mothers, the greater the weight loss of the adolescents. Baranowski et al. (1990) examined the effects of a cardiovascular disease prevention program on lowering sodium and fat intake in African American families. Ninety-six families with adolescent children were randomly assigned to either a 14-week intervention or a control group. Intervention participants reported lower sodium intake, especially among boys. All of these studies suggest that parental involvement may substantially enhance the outcomes of minority adolescent dietary programs.

Social support from family members may be one way in which parental involvement influences adolescents' compliance with dietary interventions. Parents may encourage adolescents to adopt healthy dietary behaviors, which may in turn decrease their health risks. Preliminary research by our group has demonstrated that such social support may facilitate dietary compliance among African American adolescents. For example, we (Wilson, Moody, Harshfield, & Alpert, 1991) studied the relationship between dietary social support from parents and reductions in sodium intake in African American adolescents. We assigned healthy adolescents and their parents to either a 6-week low-sodium diet group or a standard-diet control group. Participants who complied with the dietary program showed a significant increase in dietary social support from family members and a decrease in systolic blood pressure from pre- to posttreatment. In another study (Wilson et al., 1996), African American adolescents and their parents were randomly assigned to either a high-potassium diet group or a usual diet control group. Adolescents in the high-potassium group demonstrated a greater increase in potassium excretion and dietary social support than did adolescents in the control group. In a study by Nader et al. (1983), White, African American, and Mexican American families were randomly assigned to a 3-month low-sodium, low-fat diet program, or a no-treatment control group. The treatment group showed a greater increase in social support specific to diet than the no-treatment control group. Each of the studies reviewed above provides evidence that familial support may be especially important for increasing minority adolescents' compliance with dietary programs.

Another way that parents and peers may influence adolescents' eating behaviors is through role-modeling. Sallis and Nader (1988) found that, among Mexican American families, parent–child fat and calorie intakes were highly correlated. This suggests that children may at an early age learn from their parents about the social cues, expectations, and consequences of eating habits. Oei and Baldwin (1992) have proposed that, for younger adolescents, peer education that uses role models may also be an important influence in dietary intervention programs. In addition, they suggest that as adolescents become older, hero figures may affect their attitudes and health behaviors. In another study, Cohen, Felix, and Brownell (1989) randomly assigned adolescents to either peer-led or teacher-led groups promoting a low-sodium, low-fat dietary intervention. At posttreatment, both groups were shown to be equally effective for changing nutritional habits, however, the peer-led group was more effective in reducing blood pressure. Although Cohen et al. did not specifically indicate whether they included minority adolescents, their data provides preliminary evidence for the importance of peer role-modeling.

School-based approaches. School-based programs are another type of approach for promoting healthy dietary habits among minority adolescents. The school setting can be a particularly strong resource for minority adolescents, who may have a limited home environment (i.e., limited access to parks and playgrounds). School-based dietary programs that have been successful with minority adolescent populations have usually included several key components: (a) incorporating directly observable behavioral objectives, (b) obtaining support from school staff and cafeteria workers, and (c) incorporating culturally relevant information into the intervention.

School-based programs that have incorporated behavioral objectives that are directly observable have been effective in promoting and maintaining healthy dietary change. Coates et al. (1985) examined the effectiveness of a 4-week school-based intervention for decreasing consumption of salty snack foods and increasing consumption of "heart-healthy" snacks among African American adolescents. One hundred fifty-four students from one high school received the treatment program, whereas 130 students from another high school served as the no-treatment control group. The program incorporated parental involvement, a schoolwide media program, and a classroom instruction program. The classroom instruction program included setting written goals for substituting heart-healthy snacks for salty snacks. The treatment program was effective in producing reductions in salty snack foods, however, long-term changes were only significant for students who participated in the classroom instruction program that incorporated written objectives. Relatedly, Bush et al. (1989) examined the effects of a 4-year program for reducing coronary heart disease risk factors among 1,041 African American adolescents. Participants were randomly assigned to either a treatment program or a control program (no treatment). The treatment program involved goal setting, modeling, rehearsal, feedback of screening results, and reinforcement of healthful eating behaviors. Treatment participants showed significant decreases in cholesterol and blood pressure, which were maintained over a 2-year follow-up. Finally, in Perry et al.'s (1989) study, younger children (ages 8–9 years) participated in either a treatment or control school-based program designed to increase healthy eating habits. The intervention program included modeling through stories and role-playing, self-monitoring of behaviors, behavioral contracting, and material rewards. Treatment participants showed significant reductions in the use of salt (it was not stated whether minorities were included). Together, these studies reviewed above provide evidence that incorporating directly observable behavioral objectives—such as setting written goals, modeling behaviors, and providing feedback—can successfully result in long-term dietary change.

Another important aspect of school-based interventions has been obtaining support from school staff (e.g., teachers) and school cafeteria providers. Bush et al. (1989) reported that young African American adolescents who were part of a coronary heart disease prevention program and were judged to have the best teachers showed significant decreases in total serum cholesterol at a 2-year follow-up. Resnicow, Cross, and Wynder (1991) also examined the effects of a comprehensive school health education program designed to decrease total cholesterol in young adolescents. They conducted three studies with a combined sample of Whites, African Americans, and Hispanics. The program incorporated a teacher component, a health-screening component, and extracurricular activities. The teacher component advocated decision making, goal setting, and communication skills. The extracurricular activities included modifying the school cafeteria, developing recipe books, and holding heart-healthy bake sales. The intervention schools reported significantly less consumption of high-fat foods in comparison with no-treatment schools. The intervention participants also showed 4%–7% decreases in total cholesterol level across all ethnic groups. Although Bush et al. and Resnicow et al. did not specifically determine which components of their programs were most effective in creating dietary change, their findings do provide evidence for the importance of obtaining support from school staff and cafeteria providers when designing dietary interventions for adolescents.

Other investigators have more specifically modified school cafeteria programs to provide healthier food options. Parcel, Simons-Morton, O'Hara, Baranowski, and Wilson (1989) worked with the food service personnel to institute specific goals for dietary change in several school cafeterias in Houston, Texas. Their study sample was 62% White, 21% Mexican, 15% African American, and 2% Asian American and Native American. Participants ranged in age from 5 to 10 years.

School lunches were modified to decrease the sodium content to less than 600 mg per average school lunch and to decrease the total fat to 30% and saturated fat to 10% or less of the total calories per day. New recipes were tested for taste, texture, appearance, and appeal. The results demonstrated significant decreases in the use of salt. Similarly, in a recent review by Stevens and Davis (1988) it was found that effective dietary programs modified the offerings of school cafeterias to include salad bars, fresh fruit, and whole grain breads. Continued research is needed to better understand how programs such as these might affect specific adolescent minority groups.

More recently, investigators have integrated culturally relevant information into their school-based dietary interventions. For example, Schinke, Moncher, and Singer (1994) developed a cancer risk-reduction program that included a nutrition focus on reducing fat intake and increasing such nutrients as fiber and carotene. The study included 368 Native American adolescents whose schools participated in either an intervention or a control program. The intervention involved using an interactive computer program to present information in the context of a Native American story. The story emphasized the culturally relevant traditional advantages of sound nutrition (e.g., natural and whole foods). A second aspect of the computer program focused on problem solving and helping adolescents to offset negative pressures within the context of the story. The students received positive feedback on what they had learned through a computerized posttest. Students in the intervention program showed a greater increase in knowledge regarding positive dietary changes than students from schools who did not receive the intervention. This study did not include behavioral measures to determine if this acquired knowledge would generalize to adolescents' behavior. Nevertheless, this type of program may be especially effective with minority adolescents because it is culturally and developmentally appropriate and has a game-like quality.

Community and cultural influences. Community-based dietary interventions may be particularly effective in addressing the specific cultural perspectives of different minority groups (see chap. 12 in this volume for a comprehensive review). Preliminary evidence suggests that dietary programs that integrate ethnic cultural values and traditions may be the most effective in promoting healthy eating habits (Kumanyika & Bonner, 1985). In addition, studies that have incorporated community leaders and resources (i.e., churches, grocery stores, and restaurants) have also been successful in shaping minority adolescents' dietary habits (Nader et al., 1989). Finally, researchers have demonstrated that media, especially television, may influence minority adolescent food choices (Dietz & Gortmaker, 1985).

Kumanyika and Bonner (1985) proposed that culture is particularly important as an influence of dietary behavior. Cultural traditions and values have been shown to affect an individual's food selections, preparation styles, and eating patterns. For example, certain tastes or food themes are associated with specific feelings and meanings within a culture (e.g., *soul food* may denote fried and barbecued meats within the African American community; Kumanyika & Bonner, 1985). This phenomenon is further exemplified by Schinke et al.'s (1994) program, already described above, which encouraged culturally based, natural, whole foods such as fruits, vegetables, and grains in a Native American adolescent population. Cultural values may also influence the approach an investigator uses in trying to alter eating behaviors. For example, Foreyt, Ramirez, and Cousins (1991) incorporated an approach that highlighted the importance of losing weight for the entire family into their program targeted at Mexican American women, because women of this culture are often uncomfortable with focusing on themselves as individuals. Davis, Gomez, Lambert, and Skipper (1993) also found that Navajo and Pueblo Indian families who had limited access to fresh produce, fish, poultry, and low-calorie foods benefited from a community-based approach. Families were linked with members of the community who helped them gain better access to foods and showed them how to adapt their current food preparation techniques into a more heart-healthy diet.

Investigators have also incorporated cultural values within the context of their programs by including community leaders, such as consultants, liaisons, and staff members. For example, Nader et al. (1989) hired bilingual Spanish-speaking community members as part of their family-based dietary intervention. In this study, families were also encouraged to prepare heart-healthy snacks that were consistent with their cultural food preferences as part of the weekly dietary intervention. Before initiating their dietary program, Baranowski et al. (1990) met with the community advisory council to discuss its development and implementation for African American families. The authors also hired African American community members to serve as educators and incorporated pictures and articles from African American magazines as part of their intervention. Such culturally sensitive approaches to community-based dietary programs may be especially crucial for minority populations (Kumanyika & Bonner, 1985).

Researchers have demonstrated that community resources such as churches, supermarkets, and restaurants can also be effective in influencing minority adolescents' eating behaviors. Church-based dietary interventions may be particularly helpful among minority populations because of the central role of the church in providing communication and support networks (Hatch & Lovelace, 1980). Kumanyika and Charleston (1992) implemented a weight-loss program for African American families that included older adolescents as part of a church-based program. Their program incorporated nutritional education, behavioral counseling, social support networks, adherence monitoring, fees, and incentives. The results demonstrated an average weight loss of 6 lb posttreatment for each participant who completed the program.

Supermarkets may be another important community resource for changing adolescents' eating behaviors. Mayer, Dubbert, and Elder (1989) reported that supermarkets use specific point-of-choice strategies to influence children's and adolescents' food preferences. Many of these strategies have targeted foods with low nutritional value (e.g., such as candy in the checkout aisles), so Mayer et al. recommended that supermarkets implement specific nutritional targets to promote more nutritionally sound food choices among children and adolescents. In another study, Winett et al. (1991) tried to directly influence shoppers by placing a kiosk with an interactive computer program (Nutrition for a Lifetime System) in a supermarket to promote healthy food selections. The program incorporated nutritional information, food preparation suggestions, goal setting, and motivational information. Shoppers were given feedback about their food choices and positive praise for making healthy selections. Results indicated that shoppers that used the interactive computer program increased their purchase of low-fat and high-fiber foods. Similarly, Colby, Elder, Peterson, Knisley, and Carleton (1987) examined the influence of three different messages on selection of menu items in a family-style restaurant. Customers were more likely to choose healthy entrees when they were described as both healthy and delicious as opposed to being described only as healthy or when no description was given. These studies provide good examples of incorporating innovative approaches for improving diet within the context of commercially based community settings.

The media, especially television, is another source of influence on adolescent dietary behavior. Television advertisements that promote fast foods high in fat, cholesterol, sodium, and sugar often specifically target adolescents. In a study by Dietz and Gortmaker (1985), children's television viewing was positively correlated with snacking behavior and attempts to influence parents' shopping selections. Bowen, Tomoyasu, and Cauce (1991) also found that television viewing was highly correlated with obesity in children. Furthermore, African American children have reported watching significantly more television than have other ethnic subgroups of children (Hispanics, Asians, Whites, and Native Americans), according to Robinson and Killen (1995). These authors also found dietary fat intake to be significantly related to weekly hours of television watching among Asian Pacific Islander boys and African American girls. Together, results of these studies suggest that the media may negatively affect minority adolescents' dietary behaviors.

Individual Attributes

There are a number of individual factors that may be important to consider in developing dietary health-promotion programs targeted at minority adolescents. These variables include health beliefs, self-efficacy beliefs (confidence that one can perform a targeted dietary behavior), health knowledge, and motivational factors. We review each of these variables in turn below.

Health beliefs. Investigators have examined health beliefs among minority populations with regard to diet and health-risk factors. Kumanyika et al. (1989) interviewed African American and Hispanic adults about their awareness of specific dietary prevention strategies, which included lowering sodium intake and lowering ideal weight. Less than half of the respondents to their survey thought that decreasing sodium intake would prevent high blood pressure. An even smaller number of respondents believed that maintaining ideal body weight would prevent high blood pressure.

Some evidence suggests that health beliefs such as locus of control may also be related to dietary adherence. The locus of control construct is based on Rotter's (1966) social learning theory, which states that the occurrence of a specific behavior in a given situation is a function of both outcome expectancy and reinforcement value. Houts and Warland (1989) examined the relationship between locus of control and reinforcement values as a predictor of nutritious food behavior. The authors hypothesized that individuals with an internal locus of control would report more nutritious food behavior than those who had an external locus of control, and their results confirmed this hypothesis. Other investigators have also suggested that the greater incidence of obesity among individuals of low socioeconomic status, such as minorities, may be due to their beliefs in an external locus of control (Bowen et al., 1991). Native American adolescents (Tyler & Holsinger, 1975) and African American adolescents (Wilson, Williams, Arheart, Bryant, & Alpert, 1994) have also been shown to have greater beliefs in external locus of control in comparison with White adolescents, suggesting that minority adolescents may feel they have less control over their health outcomes than their white counterparts.

Dietary self-efficacy. Several studies have provided evidence that dietary self-efficacy beliefs can affect an individual's compliance with various dietary interventions (see chap. 9, by Resnicow et al., in this volume). Wilson et al. (1996) examined changes in dietary self-efficacy as part of a 4-week dietary program. Forty-three African American adolescents and their parents were randomly assigned to either a high-potassium-diet group or a usual diet control group. The intervention was also designed to increase self-efficacy by having the children practice dietary behavioral techniques. Adolescents in the high-potassium group demonstrated a greater increase in potassium excretion and dietary potassium intake than did those in the control group. Adolescents in the treatment (vs. control) group also showed greater increases in dietary self-efficacy, specifically with regard to behavioral skills. In a subsequent study, Wilson and Bayer (1995) examined changes in dietary self-efficacy during a low-sodium diet intervention. Dietary self-efficacy increased in children who complied with the sodium protocol from pre- to posttreatment. Parcel et al. (1989) also examined the effects of a school-based dietary intervention on changing early adolescents' dietary self-efficacy beliefs. The participants included Whites (62.3%), Mexicans (20.9%), African Americans (14.8%), and Asian Americans or Native Americans (2%). When the student was the unit of analysis, an increase in dietary self-efficacy was evident in response to the intervention. In contrast to the abovementioned studies, Baranowski et al. (1990) found that a general measure of self-efficacy was not related to behavioral change in a sample of African American families that included adolescent children. In general, the studies we have described provide preliminary evidence suggesting that dietary self-efficacy may be an important psychosocial variable for practitioners to consider when designing dietary interventions.

Health knowledge. Although some studies have shown that health knowledge is unrelated to dietary change, others have suggested that enhancing health education may be important, especially among low-income minority populations. Specifically, some data suggest that health knowledge is related to dietary choices among minority adolescents. Burdine, Chen, Gottlieb, Peterson, and Vacalis (1984) examined the relationship of ethnicity, sex, and fathers' occupation on heart-health knowledge and nutritional behavior in 2,695 seventh- and eighth-grade students. The sample was 62% White, 13% African American, 21.6% Mexican American, and 3.3% "other." A regression analysis demonstrated that knowledge about heart health was one of the strongest predictors for children who made healthier food choices. Other investigators have also reported that, compared with the general population, minority populations tend to be less well educated (U.S. DHHS, 1986), suggesting that increasing health knowledge in these groups could increase motivation for eating healthy foods. However, in general, studies have shown that increasing dietary health knowledge is unrelated to changing dietary habits in adolescents (Perry et al., 1987). Further research is needed that specifically examines this relationship in low-income minority populations and focuses on adolescents.

Motivational factors. Factors such as concern about physical appearance and taste preferences may be strong motivational forces for shaping eating behaviors among adolescents. Research has demonstrated that certain minority groups have an ideal body image that may weaken their motivation to comply with healthy dietary regimens. For example, Cohn et al. (1987) found that the ideal body images of Asian American adolescents were heavier than their actual body weights. Furthermore, adolescent females have been shown to be more concerned about being thin than adolescent males (Cohn et al., 1987). However, Huenemann, Shapiro, Hampton, and Mitchell (1966) found that African American adolescents in particular were less likely to think of themselves as overweight and needing to diet compared with White adolescents. Similar findings were also demonstrated for overweight African American female adolescents (Desmond, Price, Hallinan, & Smith, 1989). Thus, African American adolescents in general may not feel they need to lose weight or to change their dietary habits because of having different cultural standards than White adolescents.

Some evidence has also recently indicated that food choices among adolescents may be strongly influenced by taste. In a study of 355 adolescents, Contento, Michela, and Goldberg (1988) examined the relationship between food choices and food attributes. Their study sample was 47% White, 21% African American, 20% Hispanic, and 12% Asian or Native American. The study identified a group of adolescents whose food choices were motivated by taste preference. Other adolescents' food choices were motivated by environmental factors, such as social support provided by peers or family members. The various ethnic groups were evenly distributed among the groups identified by motivational factors. Other investigators have also found that African American, Hispanic, and Asian American adolescents may be motivated by their taste preferences to choose less healthy foods (Michela & Contento, 1986). For example, African Americans (vs. Whites) have been shown to generally enjoy foods that are higher in sugar and caloric content (Bowen et al., 1991; Huenemann et al., 1966). These studies suggest that taste preferences may inhibit minority adolescents from eating healthy foods.

Genetic Factors

Preliminary evidence has suggested that family history of dietary risk factors is important for understanding adolescent food preferences. Other genetic or biological influences may be accounted for by ethnicity, body size, and gender. Although the evidence we present next suggests a genetic role for understanding eating behaviors among adolescents, environmental and individual differences are also important and may interact with genetic influences in complex ways.

Family genetics and history of dietary risk factors. Several studies have provided evidence that family history of dietary risk factors may be related to adolescents' food preferences. Fischer and Dyer (1981) reported that family history of obesity was related to increased intake of sweets, dairy products, and fatty foods in a sample of 116 high school girls. Their results also indicated that having a family history of heart problems was related to decreased consumption of milk, eggs, and salty foods. Levine, Lewy, and New (1976) found a family history of hypertension to be associated with a greater prevalence of obesity among African American adolescents. Some investigators have also analyzed dietary intake among twin populations as evidence of a genetic variance for nutrient intake. In one of these studies, De Castro (1993) found significant heritabilities for identical and fraternal twins with regard to the amount of food energy and macronutrients eaten daily. In contrast, Fabsitz, Garrison, Feinleib, and Hjortland (1978) demonstrated that, in addition to a genetic variance, environmental effects (e.g., how frequently twins saw each other) were important in accounting for similarities in twins' nutrient intakes. These results suggest that there may be an interaction between genetic and environmental factors that influences eating behaviors among adolescents.

Ethnicity and body size. Ethnicity and body size may also be associated with adolescents' eating preferences. From a cultural perspective, African Americans have been shown to view individuals with larger body sizes more favorably than do Whites (Kumanyika, 1993). Research has demonstrated that about 50% of African American women are obese (Wadden et al., 1990). Although obesity is equally prevalent among White and African American females during childhood, by adolescence the rate of obesity increases considerably for African American females (Wadden et al., 1990). According to the National Heart, Lung, and Blood Institute's [NHLBI's] Growth and Health Study (NHLBI Growth and Health Study Research Group, 1992) African American girls (ages 9–10 years) were significantly taller, heavier, and had greater central body skinfold measures than did White girls. Such differences in body size have been linked to earlier physical maturation in African American girls (NHLBI Growth and Health Study Research Group, 1992). For Mexican Americans, the prevalence of obesity is greater than in the general population and approximately 4 to 6 times higher than in Whites (Stern et al., 1982). Garb and Stunkard (1975) have also reported the prevalence of obesity to be very high among Navajo children. These data suggest that certain ethnic groups may be at greater risk for obesity; however, the specific influences of genetic and environmental factors are not yet known.

Gender. The majority of the dietary intervention studies reviewed in this chapter did not examine gender differences in eating behaviors. Robinson and Killen (1995) found that adolescent boys of all ethnic groups (Hispanics, Asian Americans, African Americans, and Whites) ate significantly more high-fat foods than did adolescent girls. A number of environmental factors may differentially influence male and female eating behaviors, such as gender role stereotypes and their relationship to dietary behaviors. For example, Perry et al. (1987) found that a program design that emphasized weight and physical appearance as secondary benefits of healthy eating was more relevant for adolescent girls (compared with boys). They suggested that involvement of boys may be enhanced by incorporating male sports role models and increasing emphasis on improved strength, endurance, and performance as a result of healthy eating habits. Similarly, Kumanyika and Charleston (1992) found that females were much more likely to volunteer for their church-based weight-loss program than males. These studies suggest that additional research is needed to better understand how genetic and environmental factors may differentially affect male versus female adolescent eating behaviors.

Summary and Recommendations

In this chapter we have highlighted principles of dietary intervention strategies that may be particularly helpful for reaching minority adolescents. The most effective interventions across ethnic groups incorporated a similar overall structure that included directly observable dietary behaviors; involved parents, school, and community members; and integrated culturally relevant information. In contrast, the specific content and components of successful interventions were individually designed for each targeted ethnic community. Many of the studies included African Americans and Hispanic populations, whereas few of the studies focused on Pacific Islander, Asian American, or Native American populations. Community resources such as churches, grocery stores, and media sources (e.g., television) have also played a role in shaping minority adolescent dietary behaviors. Although such resources may have traditionally advocated foods with low nutritional value, they could be encouraged to modify messages to promote more healthy eating behaviors among minority adolescents. Many of the interventions reviewed in this chapter targeted decreasing sodium, fat, and caloric intake in African American and Hispanic adolescent populations. Further research is needed to better understand the benefits of advocating other nutritional interventions, such as increasing potassium and calcium consumption. Individual attributes such as dietary self-efficacy and motivational factors also seem to be important for understanding minority adolescent food choices, and so additional research is needed in this area as well. Finally, genetic risk factors, such as family history of illness, are potentially strong motivational factors for encouraging increased healthy food consumption among minority adolescents, although only limited studies with respect to these factors exist within the context of dietary health-promotion programs. In summary, the integration of environmental, individual, and genetic influences of dietary behavior is a comprehensive framework that can assist practitioners in their efforts to improve the diets of minority adolescents.

REFERENCES

American Heart Association. (1988). Dietary guidelines for healthy American adults. *Circulation, 77*, 721A–724A.

Baranowski, T., Henske, J., Simons-Morton, B., Palmer, J., Tiernan, K., Hooks, A. C., & Dunn, J. K. (1990). Dietary change for cardiovascular disease prevention among Black American families. *Health Education Research, 5*, 433–443.

Bowen, D. J., Tomoyasu, N., & Cauce, A. M. (1991). The triple threat: A discussion of gender, class, and race differences in weight. *Women and Health, 17*, 123–143.

Burdine, J. N., Chen, M. S., Gottlieb, N. H., Peterson, F. L., & Vacalis, T. D., (1984). The effects of ethnicity, sex and father's occupation on heart health knowledge and nutrition behavior of school children: The Texas Youth Health Awareness Survey. *Journal of School Health, 54*, 87–90.

Bush, P. J., Zuckerman, A. E., Taggart, V. S., Theiss, P. K., Peleg, E. O., & Smith, S. A. (1989). Cardiovascular risk factor prevention in Black school children: The "Know Your Body" evaluation project. *Health Education Quarterly, 16*, 215–227.

Coates, T. J., Barofsky, I., Saylor, K. E., Simons-Morton, B., Huster, W., Sereghy, E., Straugh, S., Jacobs, H., & Kidd, L. (1985). Modifying the snack food consumption patterns of inner-city high school students: The Great Sensations Study. *Preventive Medicine, 14*, 234–247.

Cohen, R. Y., Felix, M. R. J., & Brownell, K. D. (1989). The role of parents and older peers in school-based cardiovascular prevention programs: Implications for program development. *Health Education Quarterly, 16*, 245–253.

Cohn, L. D., Adler, N. E., Irwin, C. E., Millstein, S. G., Kegeles, S. M., & Stone, G. (1987). Body-figure preferences in male and female adolescents. *Journal of Abnormal Psychology, 96*, 276–279.

Colby, J. J., Elder, J. P., Peterson, G., Knisley, P. M., & Carleton, R. A. (1987). Promoting the selection of healthy food through menu item description in a family-style restaurant. *American Journal of Preventive Medicine, 3,* 171–177.

Contento, I. R., Michela, J. L., & Goldberg, C. J. (1988). Food choice among adolescents: Population segmentation by motivations. *Journal of Nutrition Education, 20,* 289–298.

Davis, S., Gomez, Y., Lambert, L., & Skipper, B. (1993). Primary prevention of obesity in American Indian children. *Annals of the New York Academy of Sciences, 699,* 167–180.

De Castro, J. M. (1993). Genetic influences on daily intake and meal patterns of humans. *Physiology and Behavior, 53,* 777–782.

Desmond, S. M., Price, J. H., Hallinan, C., & Smith, D. (1989). Black and White adolescents' perceptions of their weight. *Journal of School Health, 59,* 353–358.

Dietz, W. H., Jr., & Gortmaker, S. L. (1985). Do we fatten our children at the television set? Obesity and television viewing in children and adolescents. *Pediatrics, 75,* 807–812.

Epstein, L. H. (1986). Treatment of childhood obesity. In K. D. Brownell & J. P. Foreyt (Eds.), *Handbook of eating disorders* (pp. 159–179). New York: Basic Books.

Fabsitz, R. R., Garrison, R. J., Feinleib, M., & Hjortland, M. (1978). A twin analysis of dietary intake: Evidence for a need to control for possible environmental differences in MZ and DZ twins. *Behavior Genetics, 8,* 15–25.

Fischer, C. A., & Dyer, E. D. (1981). Blood-pressure correlates of adolescent girls. *Psychological Reports, 49,* 683–693.

Foreyt, J. P., Ramirez, A. G., & Cousins, J. H. (1991). Cuidando El Corazon—A weight reduction intervention for Mexican-Americans. *American Journal of Clinical Nutrition, 53*(Suppl. 6), 1639S–1641S.

Frank, G. C., Nicklas, T. A., Webber, L. S., Major, C., Miller, J. F., & Berenson, G. S. (1992). A food frequency questionnaire for adolescents: Defining eating patterns. *Journal of the American Dietetic Association, 92,* 313–318.

Frank, G. C., Zive, M., Nelson, J., Broyles, S. L., & Nader, P. R. (1991). Fat and cholesterol avoidance among Mexican-American and Anglo preschool children and parents. *Journal of the American Dietetic Association, 91,* 954–961.

Garb, J. L., & Stunkard, A. J. (1975). Social factors and obesity in Navaho Indian children. In A. Howard (Ed.), *Recent advances in obesity research* (pp. 37–39). London: Newman.

Gliksman, M. D., Lazarus, R., & Wilson, A. (1993). Differences in serum lipids in Australian children: Is diet responsible? *International Journal of Epidemiology, 22,* 247–254.

Harland, B. F., Smith, S. A., Ellis, R., O'Brien, R., & Morris, E. R. (1992). Comparison of the nutrient intakes of Blacks, Siouan Indians, and Whites in Columbus County, North Carolina. *Journal of the American Dietetic Association, 92,* 348–351.

Harris, M. I., Hadden, W. C., Knowler, W. C., & Bennett, P. H. (1987). Prevalence of diabetes and impaired glucose tolerance and plasma glucose levels in U.S. population aged 20–74 years. *Diabetes, 36*, 523–534.

Hatch, J. W., & Lovelace, K. A. (1980). Involving the southern rural church and students of the health professions in health education. *Public Health Reports, 95*, 23–25.

Houts, S. S., & Warland, R. H. (1989). Rotter's social learning theory of personality and dietary behavior. *Journal of Nutrition Education, 21*, 172–179.

Huenemann, R. L., Shapiro, L. R., Hampton, M. C., & Mitchell, B. W. (1966). A longitudinal study of gross body composition and body conformations and their association with food and activity in a teenage population: View of teenage subjects on body conformation, food, and activity. *American Journal of Clinical Nutrition, 18*, 325–338.

Kirby, S. D., Baranowski, T., Reynolds, K. D., Taylor, G., & Binkley, D. (1995). Children's fruit and vegetable intake: Regional, adult–child, socioeconomic, and urban–rural influences. *Journal of Nutrition Education, 27*, 1–11.

Kumanyika, S. K. (1993). Ethnicity and obesity development in children. *Annals of the New York Academy of Sciences, 699*, 81–92.

Kumanyika, S. K., & Bonner, M. (1985). Toward a lower-sodium lifestyle in Black communities. *Journal of the National Medical Association, 77*, 969–975.

Kumanyika, S. K., & Charleston, J. B. (1992). Lose weight and win: A church-based weight loss program for blood pressure control among Black women. *Patient Education and Counseling, 19*, 19–32.

Kumanyika, S. K., Savage, D. D., Ramirez, A. G., Hutchinson, J., Trevino, F. M., Adams-Campbell, L. L., & Watkins, L. O. (1989). Beliefs about high blood pressure prevention in a survey of Blacks and Hispanics. *American Journal of Preventive Medicine, 5*, 21–26.

Levine, L. S., Lewy, J. E., & New, M. I. (1976). Hypertension in high school students. *New York State Journal of Medicine, 76*, 40–44.

Mayer, J. A., Dubbert, P. M., & Elder, J. P. (1989). Promoting nutrition at the point of choice: A review. *Health Education Quarterly, 16*, 31–43.

Michela, J. L., & Contento, I. R. (1986). Cognitive, motivational, social, and environmental influences on children's food choices. *Health Psychology, 5*, 209–230.

Nader, P. R., Baranowski, T., Vanderpool, N. A., Dunn, K., Dworkin, R., & Ray, L. (1983). The Family Healthy Project: Cardiovascular risk reduction education for children and parents. *Developmental and Behavioral Pediatrics, 4*, 3–10.

Nader, P. R., Sallis, J. F., Patterson, T. L., Abramson, I. S., Rupp, J. W., Senn, K. L., Atkins, C. J., Roppe, B. E., Morris, J. A., Wallace, J. P., & Vega, W. A. (1989). A family approach to cardiovascular risk reduction: Results from the San Diego Family Health Project. *Health Education Quarterly, 16*, 229–244.

National Heart, Lung, and Blood Institute Growth and Health Study Research Group. (1992). Obesity and cardiovascular disease risk factors in Black and White girls: The NHLBI Growth and Health Study. *American Journal of Public Health, 82*, 1613–1620.

Newman, W. P., Freedman, D. S., & Berenson, G. (1986). Relation of serum lipoprotein levels and systolic blood pressure to early atherosclerosis: The Bogalusa Heart Study. *New England Journal of Medicine, 314,* 138–144.

Nicklas, T. A., Webber, L. S., Johnson, C. C., Srinivasan, S. R., & Berenson, G. S. (1995). Foundations for health promotion with youth: A review of observations from the Bogalusa Heart Study. *Journal of Health Education, 26*(Suppl. 2), 18–26.

Oei, T. P., & Baldwin, A. R. (1992). Smoking education and prevention: A developmental model. *Journal of Drug Education, 22,* 155–181.

Parcel, G. S., Simons-Morton, B., O'Hara, N. M., Baranowski, T., & Wilson, B. (1989). School promotion of healthful diet and physical activity: Impact on learning outcomes and self-reported behavior. *Health Education Quarterly, 16,* 181–199.

Patterson, T. L., Rupp, J. W., Sallis, J. F., Atkins, C. J., & Nader, P. R. (1988). Aggregation of dietary calories, fats, and sodium in Mexican-American and Anglo families. *American Journal of Preventive Medicine, 14,* 75–82.

Perry, C. L., Klepp, K. I., Halper, A., Dudovitz, B., Golden, D., Griffin, G., & Smyth, M. (1987). Promoting healthy eating and physical activity patterns among adolescents: A pilot study of "Slice of Life." *Health Education Research, 2,* 93–103.

Perry, C. L., Luepker, R. V., Murray, D. M., Hearn, M. D., Halper, A., Dudvitz, B., Maile, M. C., & Smyth, M. (1989). Parent involvement with children's health promotion: A one-year follow-up of the Minnesota Home Team. *Health Education Quarterly, 16,* 171–180.

Perry, C. L., Luepker, R. V., Murray, D. M., Kurth, C., Mullis, R., Crockett, S., & Jacobs, D. R. (1988). Parent involvement with children's health promotion: The Minnesota Home Team. *American Journal of Public Health, 78,* 1156–1160.

Resnicow, K., Cross, D., & Wynder, E. (1991). The role of comprehensive school-based interventions. *Annals of the New York Academy of Sciences, 623,* 285–298.

Robinson, T. N., & Killen, J. D. (1995). Ethnic and gender differences in the relationship between television viewing and obesity, physical activity, and dietary fat intake. *Journal of Health Education, 26*(Suppl. 2), S91–S98.

Rotter, J. B. (1966). Generalized expectancies for internal versus external control of reinforcement. *Psychological Monographs, 80* (Whole No. 609).

Sallis, J. F., & Nader, P. R. (1988). Family determinants of health behaviors. In D. S. Gochman (Ed.), *Health behavior* (pp. 107–124). New York: Plenum Press.

Schinke, S. P., Moncher, M. S., & Singer, B. R. (1994). Native American youths and cancer risk reduction. *Journal of Adolescent Health, 15,* 105–110.

Simons-Morton, B. G., Baranowski, T., Parcel, G. S., O'Hara, N. M., & Matteson, R. C. (1990). Children's frequency of consumption of foods high in fat and sodium. *American Journal of Preventive Medicine, 6,* 218–227.

Stern, M. P., Pugh, J. A., Gaskill, S. P., & Hazuda, H. P. (1982). Knowledge, attitudes, and behavior related to obesity and dieting in Mexican Americans and Anglos: The San Antonio Heart Study. *American Journal of Epidemiology, 115,* 917–927.

Stevens, N. H., & Davis, L. G. (1988). Exemplary school health education: A new charge from HOT districts. *Health Education Quarterly, 15,* 63–70.

Stone, E. J., Baranowski, T., Sallis, J. F., & Cutler, J. A. (1995). Review of behavioral research for cardiopulmonary health: Emphasis on youth, gender, and ethnicity. *Journal of Health Education, 26*(Suppl.), 9–17.

Subar, A. F., Heimendinger, J., Krebs-Smith, S. M., Patterson, B. H., Kessler, R., & Pivonka, E. (1992). *Five a day for better health: A baseline study of American's fruit and vegetable consumption.* Rockville, MD: National Cancer Institute.

Tyler, J. D., & Holsinger, D. N. (1975). Locus of control differences between rural American Indian and White children. *Journal of Social Psychology, 95,* 149–155.

U.S. Department of Health and Human Services. (1986). *Report of the secretary's task force on Black and minority health.* Washington, DC: U.S. Government Printing Office.

U.S. Department of Health and Human Services. (1991). *Healthy people 2000.* Washington, DC: U.S. Government Printing Office.

Wadden, T. A., Stunkard, A. J., Rich, L., Rubin, C. J., Sweidel, G., & McKinney, S. (1990). Obesity in Black adolescent girls: A controlled clinical trial of treatment by diet, behavior modification, and parental support. *Pediatrics, 85,* 345–352.

Wilson, D. K., & Bayer, L. A. (1995, August). *Compliance to a low sodium diet in African-American adolescents.* Paper presented at the 103rd Annual Convention of the American Psychological Association, New York.

Wilson, D. K., Krishnamoorthy, J. S., Williams, Z. L., Holmes, S. D., Eck, L. H., & Alpert, B. S. (1996). Gender differences in cardiovascular reactivity following a high potassium diet in Black adolescents. Manuscript submitted for publication.

Wilson, D. K., Moody, K., Harshfield, G., & Alpert, B. S. (1991, August). *Dietary social support augments sodium reduction in Black children.* Paper presented at the 99th Annual Convention of the American Psychological Association, San Francisco, CA.

Wilson, D. K., Williams, Z. L., Arheart, K., Bryant, E. S., & Alpert, B. S. (1994). Race and sex differences in health locus of control beliefs and cardiovascular reactivity. *Journal of Pediatric Psychology, 19,* 769–778.

Winett, R. A., Moore, J. F., Wagner, J. L., Hite, L. A., Leahy, M., Neubauer, T. E., Walberg, J. L., Walker, W. B., Lombard, D., Geller, E. S., & Mundy, L. L. (1991). Altering shoppers' supermarket purchases to fit nutritional guidelines: An interactive information system. *Journal of Applied Behavior Analysis, 24,* 95–105.

Minority Adolescent Female Health: Strategies for the Next Millennium

Barbara J. Guthrie, Cleopatra Howard Caldwell, and Andrea G. Hunter

According to the Healthy People 2000 mid-decade review (U.S. Department of Health and Human Services [U.S. DHHS], 1995), there still remains a significant challenge regarding the health of minority groups. Specifically, this population continues to experience disproportionately worse health outcomes than other Americans. To actualize the vision of healthy people in healthy communities, researchers must begin to develop unique strategies that have the potential to close these disproportionate health gaps. To this end, in this chapter we provide an approach for promoting health with minority adolescent females.

Our purpose in writing this chapter was to examine the antecedents and correlates of several health problems currently affecting minority adolescent females. Our approach to considering the health status and health behaviors of this population incorporates a perspective that highlights how gender, race, social class, and environment interact to influence health outcomes. To be effective, health-promotion interventions that target minority adolescent females must be sensitive to these integral relationships as well as to the values, beliefs, resources, and developmental status of these females (Millstein, Irwin, & Brindis, 1991). This perspective has the potential to guide the development of viable health interventions that are gender-specific and culturally responsive to minority adolescent females needs.

In this chapter, we first give an overview of minority adolescent females' health status and some of the associated factors. We then provide a framework for understanding the interplay between situations in which girls are vulnerable (i.e., unsupervised parties at which alcohol and other drugs are available) and the likelihood of adolescent females engaging in health-compromising behaviors (i.e., early initiation of sexual activity). We identify social, cultural, and psychological contextual factors and their relationship to minority adolescent female health. We conclude by offering strategies to operationalize the components of our framework for future health-promotion research and intervention projects.

Uncritical characterization of minority adolescent females as "at risk" or "at higher risk" assumes uniformity in the distribution of risky behaviors across cohorts and contexts (regions, class, and residences). Furthermore, risk status associated with such population characteristics as age, gender, and race is static in nature. Instead of focusing on risk status, in the framework we propose we focus on health-compromising behaviors. *Health-compromising behavior* refers to actions that increase vulnerability to negative health outcomes. For two reasons, it is important to distinguish between risk status and health-compromising behaviors, particularly when one is focusing on minority adolescents. First, the labeling of minority adolescents as at risk because of racial or ethnic group membership wrongly assumes homogeneity in behavior and experience. Second, adolescents are likely to experiment with a range of health-compromising behaviors, some of which are more likely to lead to negative health outcomes than others. As others have noted (e.g., Millstein, Petersen, & Nightingale, 1993), engaging in a health-compromising behavior does not always lead directly to a negative health outcome. Therefore, the development of effective health-promotion interventions must address the different levels and patterns of health-compromising behaviors as well as the course, persistence, and context in which these types of behaviors occur.

To fully understand the health status of adolescents in general, and minority adolescent females in particular, researchers must consider the developmental issues associated with adolescence. A key developmental factor during this time is the need for emancipation or independence from families. This need often leads adolescents to test and stretch the boundaries imposed by adults. For adolescent females, however, this task is further complicated by the paradoxical experience of simultaneously striving for independence and connectedness (Llewellyn & Osborne, 1990). Another developmental factor is cognition, which plays a role in young adolescent females' inability to project themselves into the future. Thus, their health-related decisions are often made without any consideration for accountability, responsibility, or future consequences (Howard, 1993). For minority adolescents, Fullilove (1991) has argued, personal invulnerability is accompanied by a loss of hope for the future. Therefore, minority adolescent females who engage in health compromising behaviors are likely to need interventions that focus on reframing hopelessness and despair while highlighting alternative opportunities related to facilitating a healthy maturational process.

Health Status Among Minority Adolescent Females

In this part of the chapter, we provide a brief overview of selected health statistics for African American, Hispanic or Latina, Asian American, and Pacific Islander adolescent females that have been reported in national, regional, or local databases or studies. The specific health statistics we present focus on data that have been closely aligned with adolescent females' health status. These include eating disorders, sexual activity, pregnancy, sexually transmitted diseases (STDs), HIV and AIDS, and substance abuse. Before we present these health statistics, it is important to note some of the limitations of these data.

Currently, information on U.S. adolescent females in general, and minority adolescent females in particular, has been unavailable or inadequate. The most significant problem with available data sources is that they rarely consider adolescents as a distinct group (Millstein et al., 1991). In addition, when ethnic groups are included, they often comprise a small portion of the sample, which makes it impossible to estimate prevalence by gender in any ethnic group with reasonable confidence. Furthermore, African Americans, Hispanics or Latinas, Asian Americans, and Pacific Islanders have been considered as homogeneous groups. This is untrue and is especially inappropriate for Hispanics or Latinas, Asian Americans, and Pacific Islanders (Aoki, Ngin, Mo, & Ja, 1989; Brindis, 1992).

Eating Disorders

In 1993, Abrams, Allen, and Gray reported the prevalence of eating disorders in the United States to be 3.26 in 100,000, among European American adolescent females but only 0.42 in 100,000 among minority adolescent females. The reason for the low prevalence rate among minority adolescent females has been attributed to lack of acculturation or assimilation of mainstream values by minority adolescents as well as to underreporting. Minority adolescent females are exposed to two standards of beauty: one dictated by their own culture and the other based on European American standards. Many chose not to assimilate European American standards of beauty. This lack of assimilation appears to provide a protective factor against the internalization of the importance of thinness (Abrams et al., 1993; Osvold & Sodowsky, 1993). Ultimately, African American adolescent females, followed by Hispanics or Latinas, tend to be more comfortable and satisfied with their bodies than are their White counterparts.

Another plausible explanation for the low prevalence of eating disorders among minority adolescent females compared with Whites is underreporting due to unequal access to health care (Dolan, 1991). The fact that 45% of African American adolescent females were referred for treatment from the emergency room whereas only 4% of White adolescent females were referred from the same setting suggests that minority adolescent females were more likely than other adolescent females to receive treatment for eating disorders at a more advanced stage in an emergency setting. Thus, for minorities, it is likely that only the extreme cases are reported. This may help to explain the reported low prevalence rate of eating disorders among minority adolescent females (Dolan, 1991).

Sexual Activity, Pregnancy, HIV and AIDS, and Other STDs

Over the past several decades, adolescents in general and African American and Hispanic or Latina adolescent females in particular have begun to engage in sexual activity at an earlier age (National Center for Health Statistics [NCHS], 1993; Vega & Amaro, 1994). The median age for the first sexual experience for females declined from age 19 in 1971, to about age 16½ in 1988, and to 15½ in 1990 (U.S. DHHS, 1994b). Data from several national studies have indicated that African American females between the ages of 15 and 19 years are 2 times more likely to be sexually active than European American females of the same age range (Murry, 1992). The Hispanic or Latina female cohort's sexual experience falls between that of European and African American females (Forrest & Singh, 1990). However, a study that focused specifically on adolescent females of Mexican descent found lower rates of early sexual intercourse than among White Americans, although girls of Mexican descent had the highest rate of early births compared with their European American peers (Aneshensel, Becerra, & Fielder, 1990). Although researchers have disagreed over the significance of socioeconomic status as a predictor of sexual behavior among minority adolescent females, a relationship between poverty and sexual behavior has been shown (Murry, 1991).

Most available health data on Asian American and Pacific Islander adolescent females can be found in the area of sexuality and sexual behaviors. Studies (e.g., Erickson & Moore, 1986; Yap, 1986) have reported that Asian American and Pacific Islander females are more sexually conservative, especially in the area of initiation of sexual activity, than adolescent females of other minority groups. However, once sexually active, their sexual behaviors appear to be similar to those of African American and Hispanic or Latina adolescent females (Cochran, Mays, & Leung, 1991). In one of the few studies that disaggregated two Asian American subpopulations (Chinese Americans and Filipino Americans), Horan and DiClemente (1993) found that Chinese American high school students had a lower incidence of sexual activity compared with Filipino American students. However, these authors did not report any gender differences. In another study, Chan (1993) found that Cambodian adolescent females were more likely to report being sexually active in the past year than their Chinese, Vietnamese, or South Asian counterparts. Without disaggregated data, studies cannot generate accurate rates of sexual activity along with the consequences of early initiation of sexual activity among an ethnic group either generally or specifically to adolescent females.

Synonymous with early sexual activity is the issue of consensual or nonconsensual intercourse. Early sexual activity is sometimes a by-product of sexual abuse or forced sex precipitated by a date, stranger, parent, or other relative (McKnight, Nagy, Nagy, & Adcock, 1994). Estimates of survivors of childhood sexual abuse in the United States vary, and even these are likely to be low as a result of underreporting. According to Finkelhor, Hotaling, Lewis, and Smith (1990), almost twice as many women as men have been sexually abused by age 18. Ethnic differences for childhood sexual abuse are not well understood because most studies use aggregate data. Therefore, further study of nonconsensual first intercourse that focuses specifically on young and older minority adolescent females is needed. Regardless of whether a first sexual experience was consensual or nonconsensual, data have shown that the experience, in and of itself, increases the likelihood of females becoming pregnant and acquiring STDs (U.S. DHHS, 1994b).

Concurrent with the increase in adolescent sexual activity is the rate of adolescent pregnancy. In 1974, there were 101 pregnancies per 1,000 adolescent females ages 15–19 years; the number of pregnancies rose to 110, 111, and 116 per 1,000 in 1980, 1988, and 1989, respectively (NCHS, 1993). Regardless of adolescent fertility trends, there has been a consistent 2-to-1 ratio of African American to European American births among adolescent females (Alan Guttmacher Institute, 1994). It should be noted that Hispanic and Latina females fall between their European and African American counterparts. Hispanic and Latina adolescent females, however, are the least likely to effectively use contraceptives compared with their European American female peers (Newacheck, 1989). The fact that African American and Hispanic and Latina adolescent females are least likely to use contraceptives (i.e., condoms), may account for the increasing prevalence of STDs in this population.

The Centers for Disease Control and Prevention (CDC, 1992) reported that there were 4,072 primary and secondary cases of syphilis among 10- to 19-year-olds in 1991. Fifty-five percent of those infected were females. In the same age group, there were 147,471 cases of gonorrhea, and 56% infected were female. African American adolescent females represented a disproportionate number of both syphilis and gonorrhea cases reported (CDC, 1992). The incidence of HIV among adolescents (from 13 to 19 years) had risen from 1% in 1991 to 3% as of June 1994 (CDC, 1994). In conjunction with the growing incidence of HIV is the incidence of AIDS among young and older adolescents. By the end of 1993, the CDC reported 1,628 cases of AIDS among U.S. adolescents aged 12 to 19 years, 13,552 cases among young adults aged 20 to 24 years, and 54,075 cases among adults aged 25 to 29 years. Three quarters of women with AIDS are women of color; 53% are African American and 21% are Hispanic (CDC, 1994). Given the protracted incubation period of HIV and AIDS, it is likely that most of these women acquired the virus during adolescence (CDC, 1994).

Substance Use

Research findings have suggested that premature sexual activity is not an isolated behavior, in that most health-compromising behaviors may co-occur (Fortenberry, 1995). One such co-occurring behavior is substance use. Most research has found that African American adolescent females are less likely to initiate early use of alcohol and cigarette smoking than their Hispanic or Latina and Asian American counterparts (CDC, 1993; Kim, Coletti, Williams, & Hepler, 1995). Guthrie (1990), however, found that context was a key reason for alcohol use among African American adolescent females. In fact, African American females were more likely to drink in situations such as teen parties and while going steady with older boys. Although African American females initiate drinking at an older age than European American females, the consequences of heavy drinking and drinking-related problems (e.g., unprotected sex, truancy, and use of illicit drugs) are disproportionately higher for these females (Castro, Maddahian, Newcomb, & Bentler, 1987; Welte & Barnes, 1987).

Smoking rates have remained steady for all adolescent females over the past decade (Johnston, Bachman, & O'Malley, 1994, 1995). Similar to the pattern of alcohol use, the age of smoking initiation generally is older for minority adolescent females than for European American adolescent females. However, lower income minority adolescent females have experienced increased heavy cigarette usage (U.S. DHHS, 1994a). Finally, African American females are less likely than their European American counterparts to use smoking to control weight (Camp, Klesges, & Relyea, 1993).

Hispanic or Latina adolescent females' rates of any illicit drug use (marijuana, cocaine or crack, and inhalants) over a 1-month period were higher than African American or European American adolescents (Canino, 1994; U.S. DHHS, 1994a). Among African American adolescent females, the use of marijuana has remained steady over the past decade (Botvin, Schinke, & Orlandi, 1995; U.S. DHHS, 1994a). In some urban areas, however, there has been an increase in use of marijuana among eighth-grade minority adolescent females (U.S. DHHS, 1994a; NIDA, 1990).

Racial differences in the correlates and consequences of both marijuana and cocaine or crack use have been reported in several studies. The initiation of drug use by a boyfriend, participation in unsafe sex (Lowry, Holtzman, Truman, & Kann, 1994), and rates of cocaine-related emergency room admissions have been higher for African American and Hispanic or Latina adolescent females than for their White counterparts (National Institute on Drug Abuse, 1994). Furthermore, drug-using African American and Hispanic or Latina females' friends are more likely to be from the same neighborhood (Krohn & Thornberry, 1993) and their use of marijuana is more likely to proceed from marijuana use to cocaine or crack and heroin use, which is often accompanied by heavy alcohol use (Austin & Gilbert, 1989). Amaro, Whitaker, Coffman, and Heeren (1990) also found a positive relationship between acculturation and substance abuse among Hispanic and Latina females. For example, her data revealed that the Hispanic and Latina adolescent females who spoke more fluent English were more likely to use alcohol and tobacco than their counterparts who were not as fluent in English.

Depression and Adolescent Health Problems

Although the causal direction of the relationship between depression, alcohol, tobacco, and other drugs is unclear, researchers (e.g., Chiles, Miller, & Cox, 1980; Puig-Antich, 1982; Rohde, Lewinsohn, & Seeley, 1991) have posited that depression does play a primary etiological role in the development of one or more of these health-compromising behaviors. Studies have found that depression emerges by the age of 14 to 15 years (Petersen, Kennedy, & Sullivan, 1991). With regard to minority adolescents, however, several studies (e.g., Cockerman, 1990) have suggested that race is not associated with depression when combined with socioeconomic status. These studies underscore the fact that minority adolescent females' health problems may co-occur. What remains unclear are the intraethnic differences and the prevalence rates of co-occurring health-compromising behaviors among minority adolescent females. Until more comparative research in the area of intraethnic differences is done, this question will remain unanswered, and the health of minority adolescent females will continue to be compromised. Next, we present a framework for understanding the health needs and behaviors of minority adolescent females.

Gender-Specific Health-Promotion Framework

Health-promotion interventions in the next millennium must consider how gender socialization mediates the interaction of social class, ethnicity, and environment with self-efficacy, which in turn influences behavioral outcomes related to physical and mental health. Gender socialization is the process by which children learn how to think and act as boys or girls in a variety of situations. This process may be facilitated by environmental factors that provide reinforcement of specific gendered behavior (Lips, 1995). Robinson and Ward (1991) postulated that gender socialization has an undeniable influence on the meaning of health as well as on the appropriation of health-related behaviors. Linking gender socialization to health status represents a unique approach to understanding and promoting minority adolescent females' health. Therefore, in the remainder of this part, we focus on issues of gender socialization and self-efficacy as they relate to minority adolescent females' health.

Gender, Sense of Self, and Health Problems

Generally, it is assumed that adolescent females and males proceed through similar stages of development and that autonomy could be understood by using the same model of psychosocial development for both. Current theoretical perspectives on gender and personality argue that adolescent development differs for adolescent females in that females seek to establish their self-identity by balancing their needs for autonomy and attachment (Jordan, 1991; Stern, 1990). Jordan has termed this *self-in-relation*, which connotes a growth through and toward relationships. The struggle inherent in balancing autonomy and attachment may lead to the presence or absence of "voice" in adolescent females. *Voice* refers to an assertion of self and is related to one's visibility and power in social relationships. The presence of an adolescent female's voice is an indicator of adolescent self that is part of creating, maintaining, and re-creating her true self in the social hierarchy (Jack, 1991). The ability to express one's needs, feelings, and experiences is reflective of one's voice being present (Gilligan, 1989; Gilligan, Lyons, & Hanmer, 1990; Hancock, 1989). Conversely, an absence of voice is manifested in the reluctance to speak about one's thoughts and feelings within the context of relationships (Dorney, 1995). According to Gilligan et al. (1990), it is at puberty that females may begin to experience difficulty expressing their unique voices in the face of cultural expectations.

For minority adolescent females, ethnic identity also is a critical component of self-identity. Ethnic identity is formed within the context of family and community and is often affected by negative societal influences such as racism, sexism, and classism. For example, during adolescence, African American adolescent females' thoughts and feelings about how to be female may be in direct conflict with or violate their ethnic convictions (Tolman, 1994; Ward, 1990). This may lead to a lowered self-efficacy, which in turn increases the likelihood of minority adolescent females becoming more vulnerable to dangerous opportunities (e.g., early sexual experiences or use of alcohol and other drugs). Thus, when evaluating the health status of minority adolescent females, it is important to consider how the paradox of autonomy and attachment, coupled with the struggle for an integrated self- and ethnic identity, can manifest itself in health-compromising behaviors. Health-promotion interventions must encourage minority adolescent females to rethink and redefine the quality of their relationships and cultural connectedness in terms of its potential protective influences on their health.

Self-Efficacy

Perceived self-efficacy is concerned with the belief that one can exert control over one's motivation (Bandura, 1992). It is the belief that one has the ability to perform a specific behavior in the context of a social situation and also has appropriate social support for that behavior (Ajzen & Madden, 1986; Bandura, 1994). People who have lower self-efficacy are less able to manage health situations effectively, even when they know what to do and possess the requisite skills. This may lead to discrepancies between knowledge and behavior. Several researchers have found that adolescent females with higher self-efficacy were more able to assert themselves in situations involving sexual negotiation, use of condoms, and refusal of alcohol (Gasch, Fillilove, & Fullilove, 1990; Guthrie, Loveland-Cherry, Frey, & Dielman, 1992; Plight & Richard, 1994). What these findings suggest is that minority adolescent females with higher self-efficacy are more likely to engage in health-enhancing behaviors because they are better able to verbalize needs and values related to their own health. In this sense, self-efficacy creates an essential bridge between a female adolescent's knowing and doing, especially as such actions relate to her health. It follows that any health-promotion intervention should include experiential activities of self-efficacy related to interpersonal attachments and formation of attachments that facilitate enhancement of personal self-efficacy.

In summary, our proposed gender-specific health-promotion framework for minority adolescents considers how gender socialization is influenced by the interaction of social class, ethnicity, and environment. Gender socialization affects self-efficacy. Self-efficacy, in turn, influences outcomes related to health and mental health. The last part of the chapter further delineates this process.

Implications for Future Research and Interventions

Minority adolescent females often experience health problems precipitated by health-compromising behaviors. Consequently, there is a critical need for further study and carefully planned interventions to address these concerns. These efforts must, however, demonstrate an understanding of the multiple contexts within which health-compromising behaviors occur. Effective health services research and interventions targeting minority adolescent populations must be gender-specific and ethnically sensitive and consider the interactive relationships among gender, ethnicity, social class, environment, and health. Our gender-specific health-promotion framework for minority adolescent females, shown in Figure 1, provides a conceptual basis for viewing the nature of these relationships. Next, we provide examples of how we operationalized the components of this framework.

To begin with, health services researchers and providers must speak to minority adolescent females about their health and changing bodies in ways that are cognitively appropriate. Specifically, they must not treat adolescent females as downward extensions of adult women with similar needs and experiences, because this approach fails to rec-

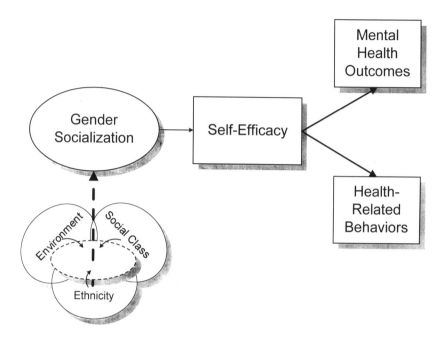

Figure 1. A gender-specific health-promotion framework.

ognize the unique developmental tasks that adolescent females must negotiate. During adolescence, girls may have difficulty coming to terms with the paradox of needing autonomy and needing attachment. This in turn may make them more vulnerable to either excessive relational or self-definitional health problems, such as eating disorders, depression, early sexual activity, pregnancy, and addictive behaviors.

Some level of experimentation with health-compromising behaviors is a normal part of adolescent development; however, more theory-based research and interventions, incorporating the significance of developmental transitions as well as the role of gender and ethnicity within specific contexts, are necessary to precisely identify the factors that facilitate positive change (DiClemente & Peterson, 1994). This approach to adolescent female health promotion is appropriate for two reasons. First, the rapid changes in physiological, social, and emotional development associated with adolescence may exacerbate any potential health problem and impinge on the effectiveness of research or interventions targeting them. Second, prevalence of health problems will vary depending on gender, ethnicity, social class, and environmental contexts. As a result, health-promotion interventions should focus on the integration of relational and self-definitional concerns of minority adolescents. Finally, to fully understand identity formation in minority adolescents, researchers must explore the concept of ethnic identity. As Spencer, Cole, DuPree, and Glymph (1993) suggested, a stable concept of self—both as an individual and as an ethnic group member—is essential to the healthy growth and development of minority adolescent females.

The effectiveness of research or health-promotion strategies will depend on the fit between the intervention and the systems of meaning for the targeted population. For example, in providing for the health needs of a particular Hispanic adolescent female, one must understand her need to fit within a broader peer group as well as her need to remain part of her family. If her family goal is for nonacculturation and her peer-group goal is for assimilation, then the nature of services provided must assist her in understanding this dilemma before effective services can be provided. Critical questions must be addressed: Should communication between the adolescent and providers be in English or Spanish? Because of the importance of interconnectedness within Hispanic family systems, should individual- or family-centered services be the focus of the intervention? What role should peer advisors play in providing services to an adolescent female who may appreciate the affiliative nature of this approach?

Another important component of our framework is the idea that gender socialization influences self-efficacy and self-efficacy affects health and mental outcomes. Because people with lower self-efficacy are less able to manage their health situations effectively, efforts to increase levels of efficacy among minority adolescent females are important for influencing the translation of health-related knowledge into health-enhancing behaviors. Such efforts use experiential activities designed to reach adolescents on their own terms. They might include using small-group discussions, experiential teaching, role-playing, or videotapes to communicate accurate information about health-compromising behaviors while providing empowering experiences based on real-life situations.

The adolescent female who is connected with a larger ethnic community draws on her traditional knowledge and practices. This relationship leads to a reciprocal accountability between the adolescent and the larger ethnic community. Such connectedness continually reinforces the "you can," "we have," or "we will" messages of the ethnic community. These messages help the adolescent female transcend any negative stereotypes communicated by the dominant White culture. Thus, any health-promotion intervention with minority adolescent females must also incorporate the broader context of their community. Special consideration should be given to the role of older women and elders, who may be mirror images of the minority adolescent female. The inclusion of the broader ethnic community in health-promotion activities increases the probability of sustaining the effects of self-efficacy on health for minority adolescent females.

The gendered socialization experiences of adolescent females often include stereotyped attitudes and values (i.e., females are more passive than males) that may have a negative impact on their health (e.g., unprotected sex or male persuasion toward drug use). However, gender socialization plays an important role in mediating the influences of environment, socioeconomic status, and ethnicity on self-efficacy. For example, minority adolescent females who come from a poor school environment and who have been socialized to believe that females will not achieve as much as males will experience lower levels of efficacy than those from the same environment who are taught that females can achieve as much or more than males (Nettles & Pleck, 1993). Thus, one cannot fully understand the influences of gender socialization without examining the interplay between environment, social class, and ethnicity.

To ignore any component of the framework we have proposed will result in less comprehensive and effective services being provided to minority adolescent females. We are currently conducting two empirical projects that incorporate components of this framework. The first study examines the role of gender socialization and self-efficacy in the use and misuse of drugs among pregnant and nonpregnant adolescents (Guthrie, 1995). The second study explores the effects of gender socialization and self-efficacy on mental health outcomes among adolescent mothers in a multigenerational family context (Caldwell, Antonucci, Jackson, Wolford, & Osofsky, 1995). Both of these studies focus on minority adolescent females within specific contexts. Their results will have significant implications for the development of gendered and ethnically relevant health-promotion interventions that incorporate the role of social class and environmental context as important components for positively influencing minority adolescent females' health. We encourage other researchers to empirically test our proposed framework with minority adolescent females.

REFERENCES

Abrams, K., Allen, L., & Gray, J. (1993). Disordered eating attitudes and behaviors, psychological adjustment, and ethnic identity: A comparison of Black and White female college students. *International Journal of Eating Disorders, 14*, 49–57.

Ajzen, I., & Madden, T. J. (1986). Prediction of goal-directed behavior: Attitudes, intentions, and perceived behavioral control. *Journal of Experimental Social Psychology, 22*, 453–474.

Alan Guttmacher Institute. (1994). *Sex and America's teenagers.* New York: Author.

Amaro, H., Whitaker, R., Coffman, M. S., & Heeren, T. (1990). Acculturation and marijuana and cocaine use: Findings from NHANES 1982–1984. *American Journal of Public Health, 80*, 54.

Aneshensel, C. S., Becerra, R. M., & Fielder, E. P. (1990). Onset of fertility-related events during adolescence: A prospective comparison of Mexican American and non-Hispanic White females. *American Journal of Public Health, 80*, 959–963.

Aoki, B., Ngin, C. P. N., Mo, B., & Ja, D. Y. (1989). AIDS prevention models in the Asian American communities. In V. M. Mays, G. W. Albee, & S. F. Schneider (Eds.), *Primary prevention of AIDS: Psychological approaches* (pp. 290–308). Newbury Park, CA: Sage.

Austin, G., & Gilbert, M. (1989). Substance abuse among Latino youth. *Prevention Research Update, 3*(1), 1–26.

Bandura, A. (1992). Self-efficacy mechanism in psychobiologic functioning. In R. Schwarzer (Ed.), *Self-efficacy: Thought control of action* (pp. 355–394). Washington, DC: Hemisphere.

Bandura, A. (1994). Social cognitive theory and exercise of control over HIV infection. In R. J. DiClemente & J. L. Peterson (Eds.), *Preventing AIDS: Theories and methods of behavioral interventions* (pp. 25–59). New York: Plenum Press.

Botvin, G. J., Schinke, S., & Orlandi, M. A. (Eds.). (1995). *Drug abuse prevention with multiethnic youth.* Newbury Park, CA: Sage.

Brindis, C. (1992). Adolescent pregnancy prevention for Hispanic youth: The role of schools, families and communities. *Journal of School Health, 62*, 345–351.

Caldwell, C. H., Antonucci, T. C., Jackson, J. S., Wolford, M. L., & Osofsky, J. D. (1995). *Perceptions of parental support and depressive symptomatology among African American and White adolescent mothers.* Manuscript submitted for publication.

Camp, D. E., Klesges, R. C., & Relyea, G. (1993). The relationship between body weight concerns and adolescent smoking. *Health Psychology, 12,* 24–32.

Canino, G. (1994). Alcohol use and misuse among Hispanic women: Selected factors, processes, and studies. *International Journal of the Addictions, 29,* 1083–1100.

Castro, F. G., Maddahian, E., Newcomb, M. D., & Bentler, P. M. (1987). A multivariate model of the determinants of cigarette smoking among adolescents. *Journal of Health and Social Behavior, 28,* 273–289.

Centers for Disease Control and Prevention. (1992, April). *HIV/AIDS surveillance report.* Atlanta, GA: U.S. Department of Health and Human Services.

Centers for Disease Control and Prevention. (1993). *HIV/AIDS surveillance report.* Atlanta, GA: U.S. Department of Health and Human Services.

Centers for Disease Control and Prevention. (1994). *HIV/AIDS surveillance report.* Atlanta, GA: U.S. Department of Health and Human Services.

Chan, C. S. (1993). Cultural issues in the development of sexuality and sexual expression among Asian American adolescents. In J. Irvine (Ed.), *Sexual cultures: Adolescence, community, and the construction of adolescent identity* (pp. 88–99). Philadelphia: Temple University Press.

Chiles, J. A., Miller, M. L., & Cox, G. B. (1980). Depression in an adolescent delinquent population. *Archives of General Psychiatry, 38,* 15–22.

Cochran, S. D., Mays, V. M., & Leung, L. (1991). Sexual practices of heterosexual Asian-American young adults: Implications for risk of HIV infection. *Archives of Sexual Behavior, 20,* 381–391.

Cockerman, W. (1990). A test of the relationship between race, socioeconomic status, and psychologic distress. *Social Science and Medicine, 31,* 1321–1326.

DiClemente, R., & Peterson, J. (1994). Changing HIV/AIDS risk behaviors: The role of behavioral interventions. In R. J. DiClemente & J. L. Peterson (Eds.), *Preventing AIDS: Theories and methods of behavioral interventions* (pp. 1–4). New York: Plenum Press.

Dolan, B. (1991). Cross-cultural aspects of anorexia nervosa and bulimia: A review. *International Journal of Eating Disorders, 10,* 67–78.

Dorney, J. (1995). Educating toward resistance: A task for women teaching girls. *Youth and Society, 27,* 55–72.

Erickson, P. I., & Moore, D. S. (1986, November). *Sexual activity, birth control use, and attitudes among high school students from three minority groups.* Paper presented at the meetings of the American Public Health Association, Las Vegas, NV.

Finkelhor, D., Hotaling, G., Lewis, I. A., & Smith, C. (1990). Sexual abuse in a national survey of adult men and women: Prevalence, characteristics, and risk factors. *Child Abuse and Neglect, 14,* 19–28.

Forrest, J. D., & Singh, S. (1990). The sexual and reproductive behavior of American women. *Family Planning Perspective, 22,* 206–214.

Fortenberry, J. D. (1995). Adolescent substance use and sexually transmitted diseases at risk: A review. *Journal of Adolescent Health, 16,* 304–308.

Fullilove, M. (1991, March 13). *Testimony before the National Commission on AIDS: Adolescents and HIV disease* (pp. 18–20). Austin, TX: National Commission on AIDS.

Gasch, H., Fullilove, M. T., & Fillilove, R. E. (1990). "Can do" thinking may enable safer sex. *Multicultural Inquiry Research on AIDS Quarterly Newsletter, 4*, 5–6.

Gilligan, C. (1989). Joining the resistance: Psychology, politics, girls and women. *Michigan Quarterly Review, 29*, 501–536.

Gilligan C., Lyons, N., & Hanmer, T. (1990). *Making connections: The rational worlds of adolescent girls at Emma Willard School.* Cambridge, MA: Harvard University Press.

Guthrie, B. (1990). *Race and gender differences in information regarding the meaning attached to adolescent's use and misuse of alcohol.* Ann Arbor: University of Michigan, School of Nursing.

Guthrie, B. (1995). *A model to predict substance abuse among pregnant adolescents.* (Research project funded by the National Institute for Drug Abuse, Grant 1K20-DA00233-01-A). Washington, DC: National Institute for Drug Abuse.

Guthrie, B., Loveland-Cherry, C., Frey, M., & Dielman, T. (1992). [Antecedents to alcohol use and misuse and health outcomes in adolescents]. Unpublished raw data.

Hancock, E. (1989). *The girl within: A groundbreaking new approach to female identity.* New York: Fawcett.

Horan, P. F., & DiClemente, R. J. (1993). HIV knowledge, communication, and risk behaviors among White, Chinese-, and Filipino-American adolescents in a high-prevalence AIDS epicenter: A comparative analysis. *Ethnicity and Diseases, 3*, 97–105.

Howard, M. (1993, March 11). *Testimony before the National Commission on AIDS: Prevention strategies in the workplace and schools: Current challenges.* Austin, TX: National Commission on AIDS.

Jack, D. C. (1991). *Silencing the self: Women and depression.* Cambridge, MA: Harvard University Press.

Johnston, L. D, Bachman, J. G., & O'Malley, P. M. (1994, January 27). *Monitoring the future study* [News release]. Ann Arbor: University of Michigan News and Information Services.

Johnston, L. D., Bachman, J. G., & O'Malley, P. M. (1995, July 17). *Monitoring the future study* [news release]. Ann Arbor: University of Michigan News and Information Services.

Jordan, J. V. (1991). The meaning of mutuality. In J. V. Jordan, A. G. Kaplan, J. B. Miller, I. P Stiver, & J. L. Surrey (Eds.), *Women's growth in connection* (pp. 81–96). New York: Guilford Press.

Kim, S., Coletti, S. D., Williams, C., & Hepler, N. A. (1995). Substance abuse prevention involving Pacific Islander American communities. In G. J. Botvin, S. Schinke, & M. A. Orlandi (Eds.), *Drug abuse prevention with multiethnic youth* (pp. 81–104). Newbury Park, CA: Sage.

Krohn, M., & Thornberry, T. (1993). Network theory: A model for understanding drug abuse among African-American and Hispanic youth. In M. R.

De LaRosa & J. L. Adrodos (Eds.), *Drug abuse among minority youth: Advances in research and methodology* (NIH Pub. No. 93-3479; pp. 102–128). Rockville, MD: National Institutes of Health.

Lips, H. M. (1995). Gender-role socialization: Lessons in femininity. In J. Freeman (Ed.), *Women: A feminist perspective* (pp. 128–148). Mountain View, CA: Mayfield Publishing.

Llewellyn, S., & Osborne, K. (1990). *Women's lives*. London: Routledge.

Lowry, R., Holtzman, D., Truman, B. I., & Kann, L. (1994). Substance use and HIV-related sexual behaviors among U.S. high school students: Are they related? *American Journal of Public Health, 84*, 1116–1120.

McKnight, J. T., Nagy, S., Nagy, M. C., & Adcock, A. (1994). Adolescent sexual activity in Alabama. *Family Practice Research Journal, 14*, 59–65.

Millstein, S. G., Irwin, C. E., & Brindis, C. D. (1991). Sociodemographic trends and projections in the adolescent population. In W. R. Hendee (Ed.), *The health of adolescents* (pp. 1–15). San Francisco: Jossey-Bass.

Millstein, S. G., Petersen, A. C., & Nightingale, E. O. (1993). *Promoting the health of adolescents: New directions for the twenty-first century*. New York: Oxford University Press.

Murry, V. M. (1991). Socio-historical study of Black female sexuality: Transition to first coitus. In R. Staples (Ed.), *The Black family: Essays and studies* (4th ed., pp. 72–87). Belmont, CA: Wadsworth.

Murry, V. M. (1992). Incidence of first pregnancy among Black female adolescents over three decades. *Youth and Society, 23*, 478–506.

National Center for Health Statistics. (1993). Advance report of final natality statistics, 1991. *Monthly Vital Statistics Report, 42*, 3.

National Institute on Drug Abuse. (1990). *National household survey on drug abuse: Main findings, 1988* (DHHS Pub. No. ADM90-1692). Washington, DC: U.S. Government Printing Office.

National Institute on Drug Abuse. (1994). *National household survey on drug abuse: Population estimates, 1993* (DHHS Pub. No. SMA 94–3017). Washington, DC: U.S. Government Printing Office.

Nettles, S. M., & Pleck, J. H. (1993). Risk, resilience, and development: The multiple ecologies of Black adolescents. *Johns Hopkins University, Center for Research on Effective Schooling for Disadvantaged Students, 44*, 28.

Newacheck, P. W. (1989). Adolescents with special health needs: Prevalence, severity, and access to health services. *Pediatrics, 84*, 872–881.

Osvold, L., & Sodowsky, G. (1993). Eating disorders of White American, racial and ethnic minority Americans, and international women. *Journal of Multicultural Counseling and Development, 21*, 143–154.

Petersen, A. C., Kennedy, R. E., & Sullivan, P. (1991). Coping with adolescence. In M. E. Colten & S. Gore (Eds.), *Adolescent stress: Causes and consequences* (pp. 93–110). Chicago: Aldine.

Plight, J., & Richard, R. (1994). Changing adolescents' sexual behaviour: Perceived risk, self-efficacy and anticipated regret. *Patient Education and Counseling, 23*, 187–196.

Puig-Antich, J. (1982). Major depression and conduct disorder in prepuberty. *Journal of the American Academy of Child Psychiatry, 21*, 118–128.

Robinson, T., & Ward, J. V. (1991). A belief in self far greater than anyone's disbelief: Cultivating resistance among African American female adolescents. In C. Gilligan, A. G. Rogers, & D. L. Tolman (Eds.), *Women, girls and psychotherapy* (pp. 87–103). New York: Harrington Park Press.

Rohde, P., Lewinsohn, P. M., & Seeley, J. R. (1991). Comorbidity of unipolar depression, II: Comorbidity with other mental disorders in adolescents and adults. *Journal of Abnormal Psychology, 100,* 214–222.

Spencer, M. B., Cole, S. P., Dupree, D., & Glymph, A. (1993). Self-efficacy among urban African American early adolescents: Exploring issues of risk, vulnerability, and resilience. *Development & Psychopathology, 5,* 719–739.

Stern, L. (1990). Conceptions of separation and connection in female adolescents. In C. Gilligan, N. Lyons, & T. Hanmer (Eds.), *Making connections: The relational worlds of adolescent girls at Emma Willard School* (pp. 73–87). Cambridge, MA: Harvard University Press.

Tolman, D. L. (1994). Listening for cries of connection: Some implications of research with adolescent girls for feminist psychotherapy. *Women and Therapy, 15,* 85–100.

U.S. Department of Health and Human Services. (1994a). *National household survey on drug abuse: Population estimates, 1993* (NIH Pub. No. SMA 94-3017). Rockville, MD: Substance Abuse and Mental Health Sciences Agency, Office of Applied Studies.

U.S. Department of Health and Human Services. (1994b, April/May). *Reducing teenage pregnancy increases life options for youth U.S. Public Health Service Prevention Report,* April/May, pp. 1–4.

U.S. Department of Health and Human Services. (1995). *Healthy People 2000: Midcourse review* (DHHS Pub. No. 91-50212). Washington, DC: Superintendent of Documents, U.S. Government Printing Office.

Vega, W. A., & Amaro, H. (1994). Latino outlook: Good health, uncertain prognosis. *Annual Review in Public Health, 15,* 39–67.

Ward, J. V. (1990). Racial identity formation and transformation. In C. Gilligan, N. Lyons, & T. Hanmer (Eds.), *Making connections: The relational worlds of adolescent girls at Emma Willard School* (pp. 215–232). Cambridge, MA: Harvard University Press.

Welte, J. W., & Barnes, G. M. (1987). Alcohol use among adolescent minority groups. *Journal of Studies on Alcohol, 48,* 329–336.

Yap, J. G. (1986). Philippine ethnoculture and human sexuality. *Journal of Social Work and Human Sexuality, 4,* 121–134.

8

Health Behaviors in the Development of Adult Cardiovascular Disease and Diabetes Among Minorities

Helen P. Hazuda and Ana Monterrosa

A small proportion of adolescents experience chronic conditions that persist into adulthood (e.g., asthma, epilepsy, and insulin-dependent diabetes mellitus). These conditions pose special challenges for affected individuals during both stages of life. The focus of this chapter, however, is chronic diseases that rarely occur among adolescents (i.e., non-insulin dependent diabetes mellitus [NIDDM] and cardiovascular disease [CVD]) but that account for a substantial proportion of premature death and disability among adults, especially among ethnic minorities. Lifestyle plays a major role in the development of these diseases. It is important to realize that although the

This work was supported in part by the Mexican American Medical Treatment Effectiveness Research Center, funded by Grant 1UO1HSO7397 from the Agency for Health Care Policy and Research.

diseases themselves are not usually clinically significant until adult-hood, the lifestyle behaviors that promote their development often begin much earlier, during the critical stage of adolescence. Because adolescents as well as their parents, teachers, and health care provid-ers may feel that these "adult" diseases are of no immediate concern, insufficient attention may be given during adolescence to promoting positive health habits that might reduce risk of these diseases in later life.

We have several objectives in this chapter. First, we establish the relative importance of CVD and NIDDM as causes of death and mor-bidity in the four major minority groups recognized by federal re-porting standards (i.e., African Americans, Hispanics, Native Ameri-cans and Alaska Natives, and Asians and Pacific Islanders). Second, we identify lifestyle factors (i.e., modifiable health behaviors) associ-ated with increased risk of CVD and NIDDM and document their association in the major minority populations. Next, we examine the prevalence of these high-risk health behaviors among minority adults and adolescents, noting the association between adolescent and adult health behavior. We then compare the pattern of risky health behav-iors across minority groups and discuss possible reasons for the sim-ilarities and differences observed. Finally, we make recommendations for designing health promotion interventions to prevent CVD and NIDDM in various minority populations.

CVD and NIDDM as Causes of Mortality in Minorities

Table 1 shows the 1990 rank order for CVD and NIDDM of age-specific crude mortality rates per 100,000 persons among men and women aged 45–64 years old and 65+ years old in the four major ethnic minority groups and among Whites. Data for the table were compiled from death certificates by the National Vital Statistics System (Centers for Disease Control and Prevention [CDC], 1994). A compar-ison of mortality rates for ischemic heart disease, stroke, and NIDDM across ethnic groups (Whites and the four minority groups) results in several generalizations. First, on the basis of rank among causes of death and of absolute mortality rates, CVD and NIDDM constitute substantial public health problems in all four ethnic minorities. Sec-

Table 1

Rank Order of Age-Specific Crude Mortality Rates for Cardiovascular Diseases and Diabetes as Underlying Cause of Death for White and Minority Populations: United States, 1990.

Cause of death	White[a] Men	White[a] Women	African American Men	African American Women	Hispanic[b] Men	Hispanic[b] Women	American Indian & Alaska Native Men	American Indian & Alaska Native Women	Asian & Pacific Islander Men	Asian & Pacific Islander Women
People aged 45–64 years										
Cardiovascular diseases										
Ischemic heart disease	1 (237.1)	1 (75.1)	1 (278.7)	1 (142.0)	1 (180.8)	1 (67.3)	1 (177.3)	1 (69.1)	1 (81.1)	3 (27.9)
Stroke	6 (29.2)	5 (24.0)	3 (99.8)	4 (67.6)	4 (38.1)	3 (29.7)	5 (24.0)	6 (25.4)	3 (29.2)	2 (29.2)
Diabetes	7 (19.5)	7 (16.4)	5 (51.3)	5 (51.5)	5 (30.8)	4 (28.4)	4 (43.8)	3 (42.4)	6 (12.3)	6 (9.3)
People aged 65+ years										
Cardiovascular diseases										
Ischemic heart disease	1 (1584.0)	1 (1179.0)	1 (1374.9)	1 (1085.8)	1 (1484.0)	1 (1169.0)	1 (838.9)	1 (517.2)	1 (762.3)	1 (512.1)
Stroke	3 (518.4)	2 (420.6)	3 (363.9)	2 (480.9)	3 (316.8)	2 (335.4)	3 (231.2)	2 (215.5)	2 (317.9)	2 (281.3)
Diabetes	7 (106.3)	7 (106.3)	7 (176.8)	3 (227.5)	7 (180.4)	3 (86.9)	5 (157.5)	3 (182.8)	7 (81.0)	4 (78.0)

Note. Values in parentheses are the age-specific crude mortality rates per 100,000 persons, adjusted to the 1980 standard U.S. population. Data are from Centers for Disease Control, National Center for Health Statistics, National Vital Statistics System as published in *Chronic Disease in Minority Populations* (1994) and are in the public domain. [a]Includes Hispanics. [b]Includes Hispanics of any race.

ond, regardless of age or gender, African Americans have the highest mortality rates and Asians and Pacific Islanders the lowest. For stroke, however, Native Americans and Alaska Natives, rather than Asians and Pacific Islanders, generally have the lowest mortality rate. Third, diabetes mortality is significantly higher among minorities than among Whites, with the striking exception of Asians and Pacific Islanders.

NIDDM and CVD as Causes of Morbidity

Table 2 shows age-adjusted morbidity rates for the three major CVDs (i.e., hypertension, ischemic heart disease, and stroke) and diabetes among the four major minority groups and Whites. Data were compiled from the National Health Interview Survey, 1986–1990, by the National Center for Health Statistics and are based on self-report of doctor-diagnosed conditions rather than on clinical examination (CDC, 1994). Complete national morbidity data are not available for all five ethnic groups (Whites and the four minorities). Also, reliable gender-specific estimates of ischemic heart disease and stroke morbidity were not available for Asians and Pacific Islanders and Native Americans and Alaska Natives. Estimates of diabetes mortality were also unavailable for Native American and Alaska Native men. Despite these limitations, some generalizations can be made on the basis of ethnic comparisons of the available data. First, their rank among causes of morbidity combined with their absolute prevalence rates indicate that CVD and NIDDM are significant public health problems for people in the four ethnic minority groups. Second, African Americans tend to have the highest morbidity rates and Asians and Pacific Islanders the lowest rates (when data are available); ischemic heart disease is an exception for African Americans. Third, diabetes prevalence is substantially higher in minorities than in Whites, with the exception of Asians and Pacific Islanders. In this regard, it is interesting to note that the prevalence patterns of NIDDM and IDDM in Whites and ethnic minorities are reversed. Whereas NIDDM is more prevalent in ethnic minorities than among Whites, IDDM is more prevalent in Whites than among ethnic minorities (Harris, 1991). Finally, it should be noted that the pattern of ethnic differences in CVD and NIDDM morbidity largely parallels the pattern observed for mortality.

Table 2

Rank Order and Age-Adjusted Prevalence of Cardiovascular Diseases and Diabetes for White and Minority Populations: United States, 1986–1990.

Condition	White[a]		African American		Hispanic[b]		American Indian & Alaska Native		Asian & Pacific Islander	
	Men	Women	Men	Women	Men	Women	Men	Women	Men	Women
Cardiovascular diseases										
Hypertension	1 (10.32)	1 (10.96)	1 (13.79)	1 (19.73)	1 (7.86)	1 (10.55)	1 (10.29)	1 (13.82)	1 (9.67)	1 (8.35)
Ischemic heart disease	4 (2.45)	5 (1.83)	5 (1.64)	5 (1.42)	5 (1.97)	4 (3.53)	—	—	—	—
Stroke	7 (1.14)	6 (0.98)	6 (1.54)	6 (1.20)	6 (1.27)	5 (1.10)	—	—	—	—
Diabetes	5 (3.53)	4 (2.36)	3 (4.13)	3 (4.89)	3 (3.74)	4 (3.53)	—	4 (5.04)	3 (3.37)	2 (2.38)

Notes. Values in parentheses are the age-adjusted prevalence rates of the disease in the total population (i.e., percentage of people with the disease during the survey period). Data are from Centers for Disease Control, National Center for Health Statistics, National Health Interview Survey as published in *Chronic Disease in Minority Populations* (1994) and are in the public domain. Dashes indicate that data were not presented because the relative standard error was >30%. [a]Includes Hispanics. [b]Includes Hispanics of any race.

Association Between Modifiable Health Behaviors and NIDDM and CVD in Minorities

Epidemiological studies in White populations have clearly established that lifestyle factors play a major role in the development of CVD and NIDDM. These lifestyle factors include obesity; lack of physical activity; cigarette smoking; consumption of diets low in fiber and high in fat, sodium, and cholesterol; and high consumption of alcohol (American Heart Association, 1978; Anonymous, 1993; Attvall, Fowelin, Lager, Von Schench, & Smith, 1993; Beilin & Puddey, 1992; Brownell, Bacherik, & Ayerle, 1982; Elders & Hui, 1993; Eliasson, Attvall, Taskinen, & Smith, 1994; Gordon, Castelli, Hjortland, Kannel, & Dawber, 1977; Holbrook, Barret-Connor, & Wingard, 1990; Keys, Aravanis, Blackburn, & Van Buchem, 1972; Manson et al., 1992; Ohmura et al., 1994; Paffenbarger, Hyde, Wing, & Hsieh, 1986; Shekelle et al., 1981; Shurtleff, 1974; Stampfer et al., 1988). Empirical data about the association of these lifestyle factors with CVD and NIDDM in minorities, however, are somewhat scarce and uneven across ethnic groups. In this section, we present a brief review of the data that we were able to uncover, noting gaps that occur in the research.

African Americans

Two major epidemiological studies—Coronary Atherosclerosis Risk Development in Adults and Atherosclerosis Research in Communities—have reported that standard risk factors for CVD (i.e., low high-density lipoprotein cholesterol, high total and low-density lipoprotein cholesterol, and high triglycerides) increased with levels of obesity in African Americans (Folsom et al., 1991). Both cross-sectional and epidemiological studies of adults (Adams, LaPorte, Mathews, Orchard, & Kuller, 1986; Flegal, 1982; Kumanyika & Adams-Campbell, 1991; Neser, Thomas, Semenya, Thomas, & Gillum, 1986; Van-Itallie, 1985) have also reported that obesity, measured by body mass index (weight in kilograms/height in meters squared), contributes to the higher rates of hypertension observed in African Americans compared with non-Hispanic Whites. Furthermore, obesity per se appears to be more highly correlated than body fat distribution with blood pressure in both African American adolescents and adults (Adams et al., 1986; Adams, Waashburn, Haile, & Kuller, 1987). Obesity has also been associated with increased risk of stroke in African American women (U.S. Interagency Committee on Nutrition Monitoring, 1989). Finally, both obesity and truncal distribution of body fat have been associated with increased NIDDM incidence in African Americans (Lipton, Liao, Cao, Cooper, & McGee, 1993).

Fewer data are available about the association of other lifestyle factors with CVD and NIDDM in African Americans. Evidence that exercise is helpful in controlling hypertension has been reported in clinical trials that have included African Americans (Thompson, 1985). In a cross-sectional epidemiological study, Harris (1991) reported that level of physical activity was not associated with NIDDM in African Americans; however, no prospective studies have examined this association. Smoking has been shown to increase risk of both mortality and morbidity from heart disease and stroke in African Americans (Chen, 1993). In addition, the high fat, high-sodium, low-fiber diets of African Americans compared with Whites (Block & Lanza, 1987; Flegal, 1982; Lanza, Jones, Block, & Kessler, 1987; U.S. Interagency Committee on Nutrition Monitoring, 1989) have been found to predispose African Americans to develop CVD (Dennis et al., 1985). The link between these dietary habits and prevalence of NIDDM in African Americans has yet to be established. We found no data regarding the association of alcohol with NIDDM or CVD in African Americans.

Hispanics

Much of the research on CVD and NIDDM among Hispanics has focused on Mexican Americans, with less attention given to Cuban Americans and Puerto Ricans. Some data on disease prevalence and its correlates in all three Hispanic subgroups have been published from the Hispanic Health and Nutrition Examination Survey (1982–1984; Flegal et al., 1991). Obesity, as measured by body mass index, has been associated with increased levels of cardiovascular risk factors (i.e., low high-density lipoprotein cholesterol and high triglycerides) in Mexican Americans (Haffner, Stern, Hazuda, Rosenthal, & Knapp, 1986; Welty et al., 1995). A recent study has also reported that obesity is a risk factor for embolic stroke, although less for thrombotic or hemorrhage stroke, in Mexican Americans (Gillum, 1995). In a program of blood pressure screening, education, and follow-up Bray and Edward (1991) reported that obesity is a risk factor for high blood pressure among Hispanics. However, the increased risk of hypertension associated with obesity in at least one Hispanic subgroup may be less than the risk in Whites. Mexican American participants in the San Antonio Heart Study, a large community-based epidemiological study, were more obese than non-Hispanic Whites, and the incidence of hypertension was similar in the two ethnic groups or slightly lower in Mexican Americans (Haffner, Mitchell, Stern, Hazuda, & Patterson, 1990). This paradoxical finding is consistent with findings from other prevalence studies (Samet, Coultas, Howard, Skipper, & Hanis, 1988; Sorel, Ragland, & Syme, 1991; Stern et al., 1981). Pima Indians, with whom Mexican Americans share the same genetic admixture and who are more obese than Mexican Americans, also have a low prevalence of hypertension (Welty et al., 1995). These findings suggest that there may be other lifestyle or genetic factors protecting these two ethnic groups from hypertension relative to Whites. Finally, in a recent prospective study of Mexican Americans, Monterrosa, Haffner, Stern, and Hazuda (1995) reported that obesity predicted NIDDM incidence in both men and women. However, they found this association to be stronger in women than in men.

We found fewer data for other lifestyle factors. Physical activity and alcohol consumption have been associated with both standard cardiovascular risk factors (i.e., lipids and lipoproteins; Haffner et al., 1986) and NIDDM (Monterrosa et al., 1995) in Mexican Americans. The association between smoking and cardiovascular risk factors has also been established in this ethnic group (Castro, Baezconde-Garbanati, & Beltran, 1985; Haffner et al., 1986; Lee & Markides, 1991; Mitchell, Stern, Haffner, Hazuda, & Patterson, 1990). Although an association between smoking and insulin resistance has been found in non-Hispanic Whites and Japanese (Attvall et al., 1993; Eliasson et al., 1994; Ohmura et al., 1994), no published data were located for Hispanics.

High intake of dietary fat and cholesterol have been associated with increased cardiovascular risk in Mexican Americans (Haffner, Knapp, Hazuda, Stern, & Young, 1985). In addition, high-fat, low-carbohydrate diets were associated with the onset of NIDDM and conversion of Impaired Glucose Tolerance (IGT) to NIDDM among Hispanics in the San Luis Valley Study (Marshall, Hamman, & Baxter, 1991). Stern et al. (1992) noted decreased fat consumption associated with a lower prevalence of NIDDM in Mexican men compared with Mexican American men, in spite of similar genetic admixtures. And in a recent prospective study among Mexican Americans, Monterrosa et al. (1995) reported that avoidance of saturated fat and cholesterol corresponded to decreased risk of NIDDM for women. In the same prospective study, Monterrosa et al., reported moderate alcohol intake to be associated with increased NIDDM incidence in Mexican American men but not in women.

Native Americans and Alaska Natives

More attention has been given to NIDDM than to CVD among Native Americans and Alaska Natives. The most heavily studied of the greater than 500 Indian nations in the United States are the Pima, who have the highest documented rates of NIDDM in the world (prevalence >50%). A prospective study of the Pima has shown that NIDDM incidence increases almost linearly with increasing body mass index (Knowler et al., 1991). Similarly, in their cross-sectional study Dowse et al. (1991) showed that physical activity is inversely related to glucose intolerance in Pima and that Pima who reported historically low levels of leisure physical activity had a higher rate of diabetes than those who were more active. No data were found concerning a possible link between NIDDM and smoking in Pima or other Native Americans and Alaska Natives. However, Bennett et al. (1984) did show total energy and starch intake to be associated with NIDDM in a prospective study of Pima women. No data were found concerning the association of alcohol with NIDDM among Native Americans and Alaska Natives.

The Strong Heart Study is a fairly recently initiated epidemiological investigation of NIDDM and CVD in 13 diverse Indian nations in the United States. Recently, Welty et al. (1995) reported that prevalence rates of coronary disease reported in the Strong Heart Study varied by geographical region and speculated that the regional difference in disease prevalence may be related to a corresponding difference in cigarette smoking. Welty et al. also indicated that high prevalence of obesity was correlated with low levels of high-density lipoprotein cholesterol. The contribution of alcohol consumption to CVDs has been established in Native Americans (Gibb, 1992; Gallaher, Fleming, Berger, & Sewell, 1992; Rhoades, Hammond, Welty, Handler, & Amler, 1987; Welty & Coulehan, 1993), but we found no data concerning the association of other dietary habits with CVD.

Asians and Pacific Islanders

There are few data on CVD and NIDDM in Asians and Pacific Islanders. The most frequently studied Asian and Pacific Islander subgroup
is Japanese Americans. The Honolulu Heart Study, a seminal study of
Japanese American men, has clearly documented that the standard
and lifestyle cardiovascular risk factors observed in non-Hispanic
White men also apply to Japanese American men (Stern, 1984). At
least one study has reported that, for all Asian American subgroups,
higher body mass index is a risk factor for CVD in men but not
women (Klatsky & Armstrong, 1991).

It has also been reported that Japanese living in Hawaii have higher
rates of NIDDM than Japanese living in Japan (Kawate et al., 1979),
but obesity by itself did not explain the higher NIDDM prevalence in
Japanese Americans. In a subsequent study comparing Japanese living
in Hiroshima with Japanese migrants to Hawaii, Kawate, Yamakido,
and Nishimoto (1980) found that calorie intake in the two groups was
similar, but that the Hawaiian Japanese were more sedentary, consumed more fat and simple carbohydrates, had a higher frequency of
obesity, and had approximately twice the prevalence of NIDDM.

Prevalence of Risky Health Behaviors in Minorities

Table 3 shows data on the prevalence of modifiable health behaviors,
indicated by lifestyle risk factors, associated with increased risk of
CVD and NIDDM among adults in the four minority groups and
Whites. These self-report data were collected by the CDC's Behavioral
Risk Factor Surveillance System from 1991 to 1992 (Anonymous, 1994;
CDC, 1994). Table 4 shows related data among adolescents for Whites,
African Americans, and Hispanics. These are also self-report data, col-
lected by the CDC Youth Risk Behavior Surveillance System in 1993
(Kann et al., 1993). Data were not reported for Native American and
Alaska Native or Asian and Pacific Islander adolescents. However,
growing evidence suggests that many health behaviors have their or-
igins in adolescence (Desmond, Price, Hallinan, & Smith, 1989; Desmond, Price, Lock, Smith, & Stewart, 1990; Freedman, Srinivasan, Harsha, Webber, & Berenson, 1989; Jackson, 1990; Must, Jacques, Dallal,
Bahema, & Dietz, 1992), and this is likely to hold just as true for Native

Table 3 *Prevalence of Lifestyle Risk Factors for Diabetes and Cardiovascular Diseases in Male and Female White and Minority Populations Aged 18 Years and Older: United States, 1991–1992.*

Risk factor	White[a]		African American		Hispanic[b]		American Indian & Alaska Native		Asian & Pacific Islander	
	%	SE	%	SE	%	SE	%	SE	%	SE
Men										
Sedentary lifestyle	56.2	(0.29)	62.8	(0.87)	61.5	(1.38)	50.8	(3.04)	56.6	(1.97)
Overweight	24.8	(0.81)	28.4	(0.81)	23.8	(1.17)	33.8	(2.97)	10.8	(1.12)
Cigarette smoking	24.5	(0.25)	27.4	(0.80)	22.0	(1.12)	39.9	(3.00)	19.4	(1.59)
Alcohol use:										
Chronic drinking	6.7	(0.15)	4.3	(0.36)	5.9	(0.63)	6.9	(1.42)	2.3	(0.42)
Binge drinking	23.1	(0.25)	15.7	(0.65)	27.1	(1.31)	25.9	(2.61)	12.8	(1.11)
High cholesterol	25.8	(0.31)	21.4	(0.95)	25.5	(1.54)	26.2	(3.52)	27.4	(2.19)
Women										
Sedentary lifestyle	56.4	(0.25)	67.7	(0.67)	61.9	(1.15)	64.1	(2.62)	64.7	(1.74)
Overweight	21.7	(0.21)	37.7	(0.68)	26.5	(1.05)	30.3	(2.52)	10.1	(1.03)
Cigarette smoking	21.6	(0.20)	19.4	(0.55)	14.5	(0.77)	28.7	(2.50)	9.7	(1.04)
Alcohol use:										
Chronic drinking	1.1	(0.06)	0.7	(0.11)	0.8	(0.19)	—		—	
Binge drinking	7.5	(0.14)	4.5	(0.31)	7.0	(0.61)	8.5	(1.36)	3.5	(0.57)
High cholesterol	27.0	(0.25)	25.7	(0.79)	23.5	(1.23)	28.8	(3.49)	25.8	(2.39)

Note. State aggregate data were as follows: 1991 data included 47 states and the District of Columbia; 1992 data included 48 states and the District of Columbia. Cigarette smoking = ever smoked 100 cigarettes and currently smokes regularly; Sedentary lifestyle = fewer than three 20-min sessions of leisure-time physical activity per week; Chronic drinking = 60 or more drinks of alcohol during the past month; Binge drinking = consumption of five or more alcoholic beverages on at least one occasion during the past month; Overweight = body mass index (BMI) ≥ 27.8 for men and ≥ 27.3 for women (BMI = kg/m^2); High cholesterol awareness = respondents ever told by a health professional that their cholesterol level is elevated. Data are from Centers for Disease Control, Behavioral Risk Factor Surveillance System, as published in *Chronic Disease in Minority Populations* (1994) and are in the public domain. [a]Includes Hispanic Whites. [b]Includes Hispanics of any race. Dashes indicate unstable estimates based on fewer than 50 observations.

Table 4

Prevalence (%) of Selected Risk Factors Among White, Black, and Hispanic High School Students. From the U.S. Youth Risk Behavior Survey, 1993

Risk behavior	White[a]		African American		Hispanic[b]	
	Boys	Girls	Boys	Girls	Boys	Girls
Participation in physical activity						
Vigorous activity	75.9	58.8	71.4	48.8	68.8	50.0
Stretching exercises	57.1	55.6	53.0	43.2	54.9	46.8
Strengthening exercises	62.3	44.0	58.2	33.3	57.7	41.4
Obesity						
Perceived overweight	23.9	47.5	20.8	32.2	32.0	45.4
Attempting weight loss	22.3	61.3	19.9	44.0	32.8	61.4
Cigarette use						
Lifetime	70.4	70.0	67.6	66.7	75.1	68.2
Current	32.2	35.3	16.3	14.4	30.2	27.3
Regular	28.2	38.6	9.4	9.1	19.0	18.3
Alcohol use						
Lifetime	81.0	82.4	82.0	78.1	84.9	82.2
Current	51.1	48.6	48.2	37.1	55.0	46.9
Episodic heavy drinking	35.6	29.3	25.1	13.3	39.4	27.6
Nutrient intake						
Ate 5 or more servings of fruits and vegetables	18.4	13.5	11.0	7.2	13.2	9.8
Ate no more than 2 servings of higher fat foods	56.4	77.1	54.5	63.2	66.2	79.0

Note. Obesity and nutrient intake variables were based on behavior during the day preceding the survey. Vigorous activity = Activities that caused sweating and hard breathing for at least 20 min on $\geq$ 3 of the 7 days preceding the survey, such as toe touching, knee bending, or leg stretching during $\geq$ 4 of the 7 days preceding the survey, or push-ups, sit-ups, or weight lifting during $\geq$ 4 of the 7 days preceding the survey.

Current cigarette or alcohol use = smoked cigarettes or drank alcohol on $\geq$ 1 of 30 days preceding the survey or had at least one drink on $\geq$ 20 of the 30 days preceding the survey. Regular cigarette use = smoked at least one cigarette for 30 days. Episodic heavy drinking = drank five or more drinks of alcohol on at least one occasion on $\geq$ 1 of the 30 days preceding the survey. Lifetime cigarette or alcohol use = Ever tried smoking, even one or two puffs, or ever had at least one drink of alcohol.

Fruits and vegetables = fruit, fruit juice, green salad, and cooked vegetables. Higher fat foods = Hamburgers, hot dogs, or sausages; french fries or potato chips; and cookies, doughnuts, pie, or cake.

Data are from Kann et al. (1993). [a]Does not include Hispanic Whites. [b]Does not include Black Hispanics.

Americans and Alaska Natives and Asians and Pacific Islanders as for the ethnic groups for whom data were available.

African Americans

As shown in Table 3, a sizable majority of adult African American men have a sedentary lifestyle (62.8%). Over one fourth are current smokers (27.4%) or are overweight (28.4%), and one fifth (21.4%) have high cholesterol. However, only 4.3% reported that they are chronic drinkers, and only 15.7% reported being binge drinkers. These proportions are somewhat different from those observed among adolescent African American boys. As shown in Table 4, 71.4% of African American adolescent boys reported engaging in vigorous activity, whereas, 53% and 58.2% reported engaging in stretching and strengthening exercises, respectively. Similarly, although 67.6% had tried cigarette smoking at least once, only 16.3% reported being current smokers and 9.4% regular smokers. About one fifth perceived themselves as overweight (20.8%) or reported attempting weight loss (19.9%). Most boys (54.5%) said that they eat no more than two servings of higher fat food per day, but only 11.0% eat fruits and vegetables. The proportion of those boys who have ever tried alcohol is extremely high (82%). In addition, half of African American adolescent boys said they were current drinkers (48.2%), and one quarter (25.1%) said they were episodic heavy drinkers. Thus, from adolescence to adulthood there appears to be a drift upward in the proportion of African American men who are sedentary, current smokers, or overweight and a drift downward in the proportion who are current or heavy drinkers.

Among adult African American women, fully two thirds (67.7%) had a sedentary lifestyle, and over one third (37.7%) were overweight. One fourth (25.7%) also reported having high cholesterol. One fifth (19.4%) were current smokers, but a very small proportion were chronic (0.7%) or binge (4.3%) drinkers. Among adolescent African American girls, less than one half reported engaging in vigorous physical activity (48.8%) or stretching exercises (43.2%) and only one third (33.3%) in strengthening exercises. Although 32.2% perceived themselves as overweight, close to half (44.0%) were attempting weight loss. Almost two thirds (63.2%) reported eating no more than two servings of higher fat foods in a day, yet 7.2% reportedly ate fruits and vegetables. Over three fourths of African American adolescent girls had tried alcohol, but only a little over one third (37.1%) were current drinkers and 13.3% episodic heavy drinkers. Thus, the same pattern of change in health behaviors from adolescence to adulthood observed among African American men is also observed among African American women. That is, there is a drift upward in the proportion who are sedentary, current smokers, or overweight and a drift downward in the proportion who are current or heavy drinkers.

Hispanics

Similar to African Americans, almost two thirds of adult Hispanic men (61.5%) have sedentary lifestyles. About one fourth were overweight (23.8%) or had high cholesterol (25.5%). Although only 5.9% were chronic drinkers, 27.1% reported binge drinking, and slightly more than one fifth (22.0%) were current smokers. Over two thirds of adolescent Hispanic boys (68.8%) reported that they engaged in vigorous physical activity and over one half reported doing stretching (54.9%) or strengthening (57.7%) exercises. About one third (32.0%) perceived themselves as overweight, and one third (32.8%) were attempting weight loss. Two thirds of Hispanic boys reported eating no more than two servings of higher fat foods daily, but only 13.2% reported eating fruits and vegetables. In addition, 84.9% had tried alcohol. Over half (55.0%) were current drinkers, and 39.4% reported episodic heavy drinking. About 75% had tried cigarettes at least once. Almost one third (30.2%) were current smokers, and about one fifth (19%) were regular smokers. Thus, among Hispanic men there is a noticeable drift upward in sedentary lifestyle and cigarette smoking, but a drift downward in being overweight and consuming alcohol.

Over 60% of adult Hispanic women reported having a sedentary lifestyle, and over 26.5% were overweight. Almost 25% reported having high cholesterol. However, less than 15% were current smokers, and only a small proportion reported chronic or binge drinking (0.8% and 7%, respectively). Among adolescent Hispanic girls, only 50% reported engaging in vigorous physical activity, and less than half engaged in stretching (46.8%) or strengthening (41.4%) exercises. Almost half (45.4%) perceived themselves as overweight, and more than half (61.4%) reported attempting weight loss. Over 75% said that they ate no more than two servings of higher fat foods daily, but only 9.8% ate fruits and vegetables. About two thirds had tried cigarettes, but less than 30% were current smokers and less than one fifth were regular smokers. Over 80% had used alcohol once in their lifetime, 46.9% used alcohol currently, and 27.6% reported episodic heavy drinking. Thus, among Hispanic women, there is a slight drift upward in sedentary lifestyle, but a drift downward in current smoking, overweight, and alcohol consumption.

Native Americans and Alaska Natives

Among Native American and Alaska Native adult men, only 50.8% had a sedentary lifestyle, but 33.8% were overweight and 26.2% had high cholesterol. Almost 40% were current smokers. About 7% reported chronic drinking, and 25.9% reported binge drinking. We were unable to find comparable data on Native American and Alaska Native adolescents except for those perceiving themselves as overweight and dieting (Story et al., 1994): About one fifth of boys (21%) perceived themselves as overweight and 30% had dieted at some time in their lives.

Almost two thirds of adult Native American and Alaska Native women reported having a sedentary lifestyle. About one third were overweight, and 28.8% had high cholesterol. Over one fourth were current smokers, and 8.5% reported binge drinking. The only comparable data we found for Native American and Alaska Native adolescents related to weight (Story et al., 1994): Over 40% of adolescent girls perceived themselves as overweight, and almost 50% had dieted at some time in their lives.

Asians and Pacific Islanders

Over half of adult Asian and Pacific Islander men reported having a sedentary lifestyle. However, only 10.8% were overweight. Alcohol use was low. Only 2.3% reported chronic drinking and only 12.8% binge drinking. Over one quarter had high cholesterol, but only about one fifth were current smokers. To our knowledge, no comparable data are available for Asian and Pacific Islander adolescent boys.

As with their male counterparts, a high proportion (64.7%) of adult Asian and Pacific Islander women reported a sedentary lifestyle, but only 10.1% were overweight. Cigarette smoking and alcohol consumption were low. Less than 10% were current smokers, and less than 4% reported binge drinking. No comparable data were found for Asian and Pacific Islander adolescent girls.

Summary and Comparison of Ethnic Differences in Risky Health Behaviors

Adolescents

National data on the prevalence of risky health behaviors in adolescents were available only for Whites, African Americans, and Hispanics. As with adults, these data indicated that the prevalence of adolescent risky behaviors was high across all three groups. About 25%–70% of adolescents reported that they did not engage in physical activity, depending on the type of activity and gender. Almost twice as many adolescent girls as boys reported that they did not engage in vigorous activities (41%–51% vs. 24%–31%) or strengthening exercises (56%–67% vs. 38%–42%). From 24% to 32% of boys and 32% to 48% of girls thought they were overweight on the day preceding the survey; in addition, from 20% to 33% of boys and 44% to 61% of girls reported that they were attempting weight loss. Among boys and girls, reported cigarette smoking was high. Among boys, from 68% to 75% had tried cigarettes at least once, 16% to 32% had smoked cigarettes on 1 or more days during the 30-day period prior to the survey, and 9% to 29% smoked cigarettes regularly (i.e., on 20 or more days during the 30-day period prior to the survey). Smoking prevalence was similar among girls. Reported alcohol use was also high among both genders. Among boys, 78% to 82% had tried alcohol at least once in their lifetime, 48% to 55% were current users, and 25% to 39% reported engaging in episodic heavy drinking. Prevalence rates for each type of drinking were only slightly lower among girls. Nutritional habits were fairly poor for girls and boys. From 82% to 85% of boys and 86% to 93% of girls reported that not eating adequate amounts of fruits and vegetables; in addition, 23% to 44% of boys and 21% to 37% of girls reported eating too many high-fat foods.

The rank of ethnic groups (Whites, African Americans, and Hispanics) by risk behavior prevalence varied somewhat for different behaviors. Among adolescent boys, African Americans had the highest prevalence of risky behavior for stretching exercises, attempted weight loss, and nutrient intakes, but they had the lowest prevalence for current and episodic heavy drinking as well as cigarette smoking. Hispanic boys had the highest prevalence of risky behaviors for vigorous physical activities, strengthening exercises, perceiving themselves as overweight, lifetime cigarette use, and alcohol consumption but the lowest prevalence for attempted weight loss and eating high-fat foods. White boys had the highest prevalence of current and regular cigarette smoking but the lowest prevalence of risky behavior for physical activity, perceiving themselves as overweight, lifetime use of alcohol, and eating fruits and vegetables.

Among girls, African Americans had the highest prevalence of risky behaviors for physical activity, attempted weight loss, and nutrient intakes but the lowest prevalence for cigarette smoking, being perceived as overweight, and consuming alcohol. Hispanic girls had the lowest prevalence of eating high-fat foods and were intermediate between African Americans and Whites on all other behaviors. White girls had the highest prevalence of cigarette smoking, alcohol consumption, and perceiving themselves as overweight but had the lowest prevalence of risky behaviors for physical activity and eating fruits and vegetables.

Adolescents and Adults

Although the health behavior data for adults and adolescents are not directly comparable, they are parallel. At least for Whites, African Americans, and Hispanics, it is thus possible to ask whether those ethnic groups that have the highest prevalence of risky health behaviors during adolescence also have the highest prevalence during adulthood. The answer, in large part, is *yes*, but this is more true for girls than for boys.

Both Hispanic boys and men had the highest prevalences of binge drinking. Hispanic adolescent boys also had the highest prevalence of current drinking, but White men had the highest prevalence of chronic drinking. Adolescent African American boys had the highest prevalence of risky behavior for stretching exercises, and African American men had the highest prevalence of sedentary lifestyle. However, Hispanic boys had the highest prevalence of risky behavior for vigorous physical activity and strengthening exercises. African American boys also had the highest prevalence of risky behavior for attempting weight loss, whereas African American men had the highest prevalence of obesity. However, Hispanic boys had the highest prevalence of perceived obesity. The prevalence of risky behavior for nutrient intakes was also highest among African American boys, but White men had the highest prevalence of high cholesterol. White boys had the highest prevalence of cigarette smoking, but among adult men, African Americans had the highest smoking prevalence.

African American adolescent girls had the highest prevalence of risky behaviors for physical activity, attempting weight loss, and nutrient intakes. African American women had the highest prevalence of sedentary lifestyle and perceiving themselves as overweight. Conversely, White women reported the highest prevalence of high cholesterol, and White girls had the highest prevalence of perceiving themselves as overweight. However, both White girls and White women reported the highest prevalence of cigarette smoking and the highest prevalence of current or chronic drinking.

Some of these changes from adolescence to adulthood in ethnic ranking of risky behaviors are no doubt due to the self-report nature of the data and to differences in wording and frame of reference for questions used in the adult and adolescent surveys. For example, the high ranking of adult Whites on high cholesterol may be due to their greater access to medical care and, therefore, an increased likelihood that a health professional would tell them that they have elevated cholesterol. Similarly, the physical activity questions asked of adults and adolescents were quite different, and there was no one-to-one correspondence between the nutrient intakes queried in adolescents and the high-cholesterol diagnosis queried in adults. Perceived obesity in White adolescent girls regardless of their actual weight is also known to be high, and failure to attempt weight loss may be a better predictor of adult obesity in adolescent girls as well as boys. Regardless of the relative prevalence of risky behaviors across ethnic groups, the bottom line remains that risky behaviors are high across all ethnic groups for both adults and adolescents. Because harmful lifestyle practices associated with adult CVD and NIDDM are likely to have their origins in childhood or adolescence (Andersen, Henckel, & Saltin, 1989; Kumanyika, 1987; U.S. Interagency Committee on Nutritional Monitoring, 1989), perhaps the best way to prevent these diseases in all ethnic groups is to promote the development of healthy lifestyles during adolescence.

Summary and Conclusions

Given the generally high level of risky health behaviors in minorities, both adults and adolescents, and the association between adolescent behavior and subsequent risk of CVD and NIDDM in adulthood, it is imperative that increased attention be given to health promotion among minority youth. This should include special educational strategies to raise the level of awareness among parents, teachers, and health care providers concerning the increased risk of adult CVD and NIDDM associated with negative health behaviors during adolescence. It is important that health-promotion efforts address the distinct profile of health behaviors that characterizes different minority groups. For example, the data reviewed here suggest that the most pressing need among Asian and Pacific Islanders may be to help them adopt a more physically active lifestyle, whereas obesity, alcohol consumption, and cigarette smoking are smaller problems. Among African Americans, sedentary lifestyle, obesity, and poor dietary habits are equally pressing major concerns, whereas alcohol consumption and cigarette smoking are smaller problems.

Increased research efforts are needed to document the association of health behaviors with CVD and NIDDM in all main minority groups and subgroups. For example, little research has been carried out with Asians and Pacific Islanders, and research that has been done has focused primarily on Japanese Americans. Among Hispanics, much more research has been carried out with Mexican Americans than with the other Hispanic subgroups. Increased research efforts are also needed to obtain data on health risk behavior profiles in distinct ethnic subgroups (e.g., Hispanic subgroups of Mexican Americans, Cuban Americans, Puerto Ricans, Central and South Americans, and Spanish Americans) so that health-promotion strategies can be targeted appropriately.

REFERENCES

Adams, L. L., LaPorte, R. E., Mathews, K. A., Orchard, T. J., & Kuller, L. H. (1986). Blood pressure determinants in a middle-class Black population: The University of Pittsburgh experience. *Preventive Medicine, 15,* 232–243.

Adams, L. L., Waashburn, R. A., Haile, G. T., & Kuller, L. H. (1987). Behavioral factors and blood pressure in Black college students. *Journal of Chronic Diseases, 40,* 131–136.

American Heart Association. (1978). *Diet and coronary heart disease.* Dallas, TX: Author.

Andersen, L. B., Henckel, P., & Saltin, B. (1989). Risk factors for cardiovascular disease in 16–19-year-old teenagers. *Journal of Internal Medicine, 225,* 157–163.

Anonymous. (1993). Prevalence of sedentary lifestyle—behavioral risk factor surveillance. *Morbidity and Mortality Weekly Report, 42,* 576–579.

Anonymous. (1994). Prevalence of selected risk factors for chronic disease by education level in racial/ethnic populations—United States, 1991–1992. *Mortality and Mortality Weekly Report, 43,* 894–899.

Attvall, S., Fowelin, J., Lager, I., Von Schench, H., & Smith, U. (1993). Smoking induces insulin resistance: A potential link with the insulin resistance syndrome. *Journal of Internal Medicine, 233,* 327–332.

Beilin, L. J., & Puddey, I. B. (1992). Alcohol and hypertension. *Clinical and Experimental Hypertension, Part A, Theory and Practice, 14,* 119–138.

Bennett, P. H., Knowler, W. C., Bair, H. R., Butler, W. J., Pettitt, D. J., & Reid, J. (1984). Diet and development of non-insulin-dependent diabetes mellitus: An epidemiological perspective. In G. Pozza, P. Micossi, A. L. Catapano, & R. Paoletti (Eds.), *Diet, diabetes and atherosclerosis* (pp. 109–119). New York: Raven Press.

Block, G., & Lanza, E. (1987). Dietary fiber sources in the United States by demographic group. *Journal of the National Cancer Institute, 79,* 83–91.

Bray, M. L., & Edward, L. H. (1991). Prevalence of hypertension risk factors among Hispanic Americans. *Public Health Nursing, 8,* 276–280.

Brownell, K. D., Bacherik, P. S., & Ayerle, R. S. (1982). Changes in plasma lipid and lipoprotein levels in men and women after a program of moderate exercise. *Circulation, 65*(Suppl. 3), 477–484.

Castro, F. G., Baezconde-Garbanati, L., & Beltran, H. (1985). Risk factors for coronary heart disease in Hispanic populations: A review. *Hispanic Journal of Behavioral Science, 7,* 153–175.

Centers for Disease Control and Prevention. (1994). *Chronic disease in minority populations.* Atlanta, GA: Author.

Chen, V. W. (1993). Smoking and the health gap in minorities. *Annals of Epidemiology, 3,* 159–164.

Dennis, B. H., Haynes, S. G., Anderson, J., Lui-Chi, S., Hosking, J. D., & Rifkind, B. M. (1985). Nutrient intakes among selected North American populations in the Lipid Research Clinics Prevalence Study: Composition of energy intake. *American Journal of Clinical Nutrition, 41,* 312–329.

Desmond, S. M., Price, J. H., Hallinan, C., & Smith, D. (1989). Black and White adolescents' perceptions of their weight. *Journal of School Health, 59,* 353–358.

Desmond, S. M., Price, J. H., Lock, R. S., Smith, D., & Stewart, P. W. (1990). Urban Black and White adolescents' physical fitness status and perceptions of exercise. *Journal of School Health, 60,* 220–226.

Dowse, G. K., Zimmet, P. Z., Gareboo, H., George, K., Alberti, M. M., Tuomilehto, J., Finch, C. F., Chitson, P., & Tulsidas, H. (1991). Abdominal obesity and physical activity as risk factors for NIDDM and impaired glucose tolerance in Indians, Creole and Chinese Mauritians. *Diabetes Care, 14,* 271–282.

Elders, M. J., & Hui, J. (1993). Making a difference in adolescent health. *Journal of the American Medical Association, 269*, 1425–1426.

Eliasson, B., Attvall, S., Taskinen, M. R., & Smith, U. (1994). The insulin resistance syndrome in smokers is related to smoking habits. *Arteriosclerosis and Thrombosis, 14*, 1946–1950.

Flegal, K. M. (1982). *Anthropometric evaluation of obesity in epidemiologic research on risk factors: Blood pressure and obesity in the Health Examination Survey.* Unpublished manuscript, Cornell University, Division of Nutritional Sciences.

Flegal, K. M., Ezzati, T. M., Harris, M. I., Haynes, S. G., Juarez, R. Z., Knowler, W. C., Perez-Stable, E. J., & Stern, M. P. (1991). Prevalence of diabetes in Mexican Americans, Cubans and Puerto Ricans from the Hispanic Health and Nutrition Examination Survey, 1982–1984. *Diabetes Care, 14*, 628–638.

Folsom, A. R., Burke, G. L., Byers, C. L., Hutchinson, R. G., Heiss, G., Flack, J. M., Jacobs, D. R., Jr., & Caan, B. (1991). Implications of obesity for cardiovascular disease in Blacks: The CARDIA and ARIC studies. *American Journal of Clinical Nutrition, 53*(Suppl. 6), 1604S–1611S.

Freedman, D. S., Srinivasan, S. R., Harsha, D. W., Webber, L. S., & Berenson, G. S. (1989). Relation of body fat patterning to lipid and lipoprotein concentrations in children and adolescents: The Bogalusa Heart Study. *American Journal of Clinical Nutrition, 50*, 930–939.

Gallaher, M. M., Fleming, D. W., Berger, L. R., & Sewell, C. M. (1992). Pedestrian and hypothermia deaths among Native Americans in New Mexico: Between bar and home. *Journal of the American Medical Association, 267*, 1345–1348.

Gibb, R. (1992). Alcohol-related deaths of American Indians [letter]. *Journal of the American Medical Association, 268*, 331–338.

Gillum, R. F. (1995). The epidemiology of stroke in Native Americans. *Stroke, 26*, 514–521.

Gordon, T., Castelli, W. P., Hjortland, M. D., Kannel, W. B., & Dawber, T. R. (1977). Diabetes, blood lipids, and the role of obesity in coronary heart disease risk for women: The Framingham Study. *Annals of Internal Medicine, 87*, 393–397.

Haffner, S. M., Knapp, J. A., Hazuda, H. P., Stern, M. P., & Young, E. A. (1985). Dietary intakes of macronutrients among Mexican Americans and Anglo Americans: The San Antonio Heart Study. *American Journal of Clinical Nutrition, 41*, 776–783.

Haffner, S. M., Mitchell, B. D., Stern, M. P., Hazuda, H. P., & Patterson, J. R. (1990). Decreased prevalence of hypertension in Mexican Americans. *Hypertension, 16*, 225–232.

Haffner, S. M., Stern, M. P., Hazuda, H. P., Rosenthal, M., & Knapp, J. A. (1986). The role of behavioral variables and fat patterning in explaining ethnic differences in serum lipids and lipoproteins. *American Journal of Epidemiology, 123*, 830–839.

Harris, M. I. (1991). Epidemiological correlates of NIDDM in Hispanics, Whites, and blacks in the U.S. population. *Diabetes Care, 14*, 639–648.

Holbrook, T. L., Barret–Connor, E., & Wingard, D. L. (1990). A prospective population based study of alcohol use and non-insulin-dependent diabetes mellitus. *American Journal of Epidemiology, 132,* 902–909.

Jackson, A. L. (1990). Operation Sunday School—Education caring hearts to be healthy hearts. *U.S. Public Health Reports, 105,* 85–88.

Kann, L., Warren, C. W., Harris, W. A., Collins, J. L., Douglas, K. A., Collins, M. E., Williams, B. I., Ross, J. G., & Kolbe, L. J. (1993). State and Local YRBSS Coordinators. Youth Risk Behavior Surveillance: United States, 1993. *Morbidity and Mortality Weekly Report, 44,* 1–53.

Kawate, R., Yamakido, M., & Nishimoto, Y. (1980). Migrant studies among the Japanese in Hiroshima and Hawaii. In W. K. Waldhaust (Ed.), *Diabetes, 1979: Proceedings of the 10th Congress of the International Diabetes Federation* (pp. 526–531). Princeton, NJ: Excerpta Medica.

Kawate, R., Yamakido, M., Nishimoto, Y., Bennet, P. H., Hamman, R. F., & Knowler, W. C. (1979). Diabetes mellitus and its vascular complications in Japanese migrants on the island of Hawaii. *Diabetes Care, 2,* 161–170.

Keys, A., Aravanis, C., Blackburn, H., & Van Buchem, F. S. (1972). Probability of middle-aged men developing coronary heart disease in five years. *Circulation, 45,* 815–828.

Klatsky, A. L., & Armstrong, M. A. (1991). Cardiovascular risk factors among Asian Americans living in northern California. *American Journal of Public Health, 81,* 1423–1428.

Knowler, W. C., Pettitt, D. J., Saad, M. F., Charles, M. A., Nelson, R. G., Howard, B. V., Bogardus, C., & Bennet, P. H. (1991). Obesity in the Pima Indians: Its magnitude and relationship with diabetes. *American Journal of Clinical Nutrition, 53,* 1543S–1551S.

Kumanyika, S. (1987). Obesity in Black women. *Epidemiological Review, 327,* 31–50.

Kumanyika, S., & Adams-Campbell, L. L. (1991). Obesity, diet and psychosocial factors contributing to cardiovascular disease in Blacks. *Cardiovascular Clinics, 21,* 47–73.

Lanza, E., Jones, D. Y., Block, G., & Kessler, L. (1987). Dietary fiber intake in the U.S. population. *American Journal of Clinical Nutrition, 46,* 790–797.

Lee, D. J., & Markides, K. S. (1991). Health behaviors, risk factors, and health indicators associated with cigarette use in Mexican Americans: Results from the Hispanic HANES. *American Journal of Public Health, 81,* 859–864.

Lipton, R. B., Liao, Y., Cao, G., Cooper, R. S., & McGee, D. (1993). Determinants of incident non-insulin-dependent diabetes mellitus among Blacks and Whites in a national sample. The NHANES I Epidemiologic Follow-Up Study. *American Journal of Epidemiology, 138,* 826–839.

Manson, J. E., Tosteson, H., Satterfield, S., Hebert, P., O'Connor, G. T., Buring, J. E., & Hennekens, C. H. (1992). The primary prevention of myocardial infarction. *New England Journal of Medicine, 326,* 1406–1416.

Marshall, J. A., Hamman, R. F., & Baxter, J. (1991). High-fat, low-carbohydrate diet and the etiology of non-insulin dependent diabetes mellitus: The San Luis Valley Diabetes Study. *American Journal of Epidemiology, 134,* 590–603.

Mitchell, B. D., Stern, M. P., Haffner, S. M., Hazuda, H. P., & Patterson, J. K. (1990). Risk factors for cardiovascular mortality in Mexican Americans and non-Hispanic Whites. *American Journal of Epidemiology, 131,* 423–433.

Monterrosa, A., Haffner, S. M., Stern, M. P., & Hazuda, H. P. (1995). Sex differences in lifestyle factors predictive of NIDDM in Mexican Americans. *Diabetes Care, 18,* 448–456.

Must, A., Jacques, P. F., Dallal, G. E., Bahema, C. J., & Dietz, W. H. (1992). Long-term morbidity and mortality of overweight adolescents. *New England Journal of Medicine, 327,* 1350–1355.

Neser, W. B., Thomas, J., Semenya, K., Thomas, D. J., & Gillum, R. F. (1986). Obesity and hypertension in a longitudinal study of Black physicians: The Meharry Cohort Study. *Journal of Chronic Diseases, 39,* 105–113.

Ohmura, T., Ueda, K., Kiyohara, Y., Kato, I., Iwamoto, H., Nakayama, K., Nomiyama, K., Ohmori, S., Yoshitake, T., Shinkawa, A., Hasuo, Y., & Fujishama, M. (1994). The association of the insulin resistance syndrome with impaired glucose tolerance and NIDDM in the Japanese general population: The Hisayama Study. *Diabetologia, 37,* 897–904.

Paffenbarger, R. S. J., Hyde, R. T., Wing, A. L., & Hsieh, C. C. (1986). Physical activity, all-cause mortality, and longevity of college alumni. *New England Journal of Medicine, 314,* 605–613.

Rhoades, E. R., Hammond, J., Welty, T. K., Handler, A. O., & Amler, R. W. (1987). The Indian burden of illness and future health interventions. *U.S. Public Health Reports, 102,* 361–368.

Samet, J. M., Coultas, D. B., Howard, C. A., Skipper, B. J., & Hanis, C. L. (1988). Diabetes, gallbladder disease, obesity and hypertension among Hispanics in New Mexico. *American Journal of Epidemiology, 128,* 1302–1311.

Shekelle, R. B., Shryook, A. M., Paul, O., Lepper, M., Stamler, J., Liu, S., & Raynor, W. J. J. (1981). Diet, serum cholesterol, and death from coronary heart disease. The Western Electric Study. *New England Journal of Medicine, 304,* 65–70.

Shurtleff, D. (1974). Some characteristics related to the incidence of cardiovascular disease and death: Framingham Study, 18-year follow-up. W. B. Kannel and T. Gordon (Eds.), *The Framingham Study* (Publication No. DHEW NIH 74-599). Washington, DC: U.S. Government Printing Office.

Sorel, J. E., Ragland, D. R., & Syme, S. L. (1991). Blood pressure in Mexican Americans, Whites and Blacks: The Second National Health and Nutrition Examination Survey. *American Journal of Epidemiology, 134,* 370–378.

Stampfer, J. M., Colditz, G. A., Willet, W. C., Manson, J. E., Arky, R. A., Hennekens, C. H., & Speizer, F. E. (1988). A prospective study of moderate alcohol drinking and risk of diabetes in women. *American Journal of Epidemiology, 128,* 549–558.

Stern, M. P. (1984). Honolulu Heart Study: Review of epidemiologic data and design. *Progress in Clinical & Biological Research, 147,* 93–104.

Stern, M. P., Gaskill, S. P., Allen, S. R., Garza, V., Gonzales, J. L., & Waldrop, R. H. (1981). Cardiovascular risk factors in Mexican Americans in Laredo,

Texas: II. Prevalence and control of hypertension. *American Journal of Epidemiology, 113*, 556–562.

Stern, M. P., Gonzales, C., Mitchell, B. D., Villalpando, E., Haffner, S. M., & Hazuda, H. P. (1992). Genetic and environmental determinants of Type II diabetes in Mexico City and San Antonio. *Diabetes, 41*, 484–492.

Story, M., Hauck, F. R., Broussard, B. A., White, L. L., Resnick, M. D., & Blum, R. W. (1994). Weight perception and weight control practices in American Indian and Alaska Native adolescents. *Archives of Pediatric Adolescent Medicine, 148*, 567–571.

Thompson, G. E. (1985). Non-pharmacologic therapy of hypertension in Blacks. In W. D. Hall, E. Saunders, & N. B. Shulman (Eds.), *Hypertension in Blacks: Epidemiology, pathophysiology and treatment* (pp. 159–181). Chicago: Year Book Medical Publishers.

U.S. Interagency Committee on Nutrition Monitoring, U.S. Public Health Service and U.S. Department of Agriculture. (1989). *Nutrition monitoring in the United States: The directory of Federal nutrition monitoring activities* (Pub. No. 89-1255). Rockville, MD: U.S. Department of Health and Human Services.

Van-Itallie, T. B. (1985). Health implications of overweight and obesity in the United States. *Annals of Internal Medicine, 103*(Pt. 2), 983–988.

Welty, T. K., & Coulehan, J. L. (1993). Cardiovascular disease among American Indians and Alaska Natives. *Diabetes Care, 16*(Suppl. 1), 277–283.

Welty, T. K., Lee, E. T., Yeh, J., Cowan, L. D., Go, O., Fabsitz, R. R., LeNa, Oopik, A. J., Robbins, D. C., & Howard, B. V. (1995). Cardiovascular disease risk factors among American Indians: The Strong Heart Study. *American Journal of Epidemiology, 142*, 269–287.

III

Interventions for Minority Adolescent Populations

INTRODUCTION

Interventions for Minority Adolescent Populations

This part presents a unique look at clinical perspectives on health promotion in minority populations. Chapters in previous parts of the book have examined conceptual, cultural, and developmental issues related to health promotion in minority adolescents and addressed specific behavioral health risk factors associated with adolescence. This part comprises four chapters that discuss clinical approaches for enhancing adolescent health behaviors, with a particular focus on culturally sensitive interventions. The interventions described in these chapters have a theoretical underpinning, and they have been empirically evaluated. It is increasingly necessary for clinicians to provide evidence substantiating the efficacy of their interventions with adolescents. Chapter authors in this part provide not only ample evidence for treatment efficacy with minority populations but also valuable descriptions of health-promotion strategies that can be used in different settings and across multiple contexts.

Health psychologists are employed in a wide range of settings, including (but certainly not limited to) private practice, university settings, academic health centers, community health centers, and public schools. The chapters in this part provide clinically useful strategies for health promotion among minority adolescents with a particular emphasis on the diverse settings in which health psychologists work. In chapter 9, Resnicow, Braithwaite, and Kuo examine the role of interpersonal approaches for promoting health among minority adolescents. Using social–cognitive theory as the conceptual framework for health behavior change, the authors highlight important considerations in the development of culturally sensitive strategies for increasing personal efficacy and motivating behavioral effort among adolescents. In chapter 10, Brondino and colleagues provide an excellent description of the specific elements of multisystemic therapy with minority youth. Drawing on family systems theory, the multisystemic approach to promoting adolescent health incorporates into treatment those contextual influences and diverse systems in which the minority adolescent is embedded. The need to conceptualize adolescent health behavior within broader socioecological contexts is further highlighted in chapter 11, by Forgey, Schinke, and Cole. This chapter provides an example of how school-based substance abuse prevention programs can be effectively used with culturally diverse groups of adolescents. Finally, in chapter 12, Yung and Hammond urge psychologists to consider the relative importance of community-based health-promotion programming for adolescents. A thoughtful and careful review of the advantages and limitations of community-based services for minority adolescents is presented. Collectively, the chapters in this part provide a wide range of clinical approaches to adolescent health promotion in minority populations and highlight culturally relevant issues of conceptualization, implementation, and evaluation of these services.

James R. Rodrigue

Chapter 9

Interpersonal Interventions for Minority Adolescents

Ken Resnicow, Ronald L. Braithwaite, and JoAnne Kuo

Social–cognitive theory (SCT; previously called *social learning theory*) has been used to explain and modify a diverse set of health behaviors, including smoking, diet, exercise, sexual habits, and disease self-management (Bandura, 1986, in press; Baranowski, 1989–1990; Calfas, Sallis, & Nader, 1991; Ellickson & Bell, 1990; Kirby et al., 1994; Levy et al., 1995; Sallis, Hovell, Hofstetter, & Barrington, 1992; Strecher, DeVellis, Becker, & Rosenstock, 1986; Walter et al., 1993). In this chapter, we use SCT as a reference framework for developing culturally sensitive interventions for minority youth. We begin by providing a brief overview of SCT and how it conceptualizes health behavior change in minority adolescents. We then present several examples of individual- and environmental-level factors that differ among minority and White Americans and discuss how these differences can be integrated within culturally sensitive SCT interventions.

We conclude the chapter with recommendations for future research. Although the discussion focuses primarily on African Americans and Black–White differences, examples are also presented for other minority groups. Because there has been ambiguity, inconsistency, and disparity in conceptualization of the terms *race* and *ethnicity* (Fish, 1995; Lewontin, 1982), we use the combined term *racial–ethnic group* throughout the chapter. In additional, we use the terms *African American* and *Black* as well as *Hispanic* and *Latino* interchangeably throughout.

Social Cognitive Theory (SCT): An Overview

At the core of SCT is the triadic model comprising person, behavior, and environment (see Figure 1). The dynamic interaction of these three factors, referred to as *reciprocal determinism*, forms the basis of SCT (Bandura, 1986, in press). To illustrate, individual, person-level factors such as outcome expectations and self-efficacy may increase the likelihood of an individual executing a behavior; conversely, the behavior of individuals can shift group norms among others within the shared social environment, which in turn may influence their personal motivation (e.g., outcome expectations) and subsequent behavior. Environmental factors can also enable or impede behavior (e.g., availability of exercise facilities or a high cigarette tax, respectively), serving either to enhance or suppress individual motivation. Given this chapter's theme of interpersonal interventions, we focus our discussion on person-level factors; environmental factors are only nominally addressed. Within the person domain, SCT delineates several determinants of behavior change: self-efficacy, outcome expectations, skills, and goals. We review each of these below.

Self-Efficacy

Self-efficacy is broadly defined as the confidence in one's ability to execute a specific behavior or set of behaviors. Self-efficacy has been associated with numerous health behaviors, including condom use, diet, substance use, exercise, and weight loss (Bandura, 1995; Clark, Abrams, Niaura, Eaton, & Rossi, 1991; J. B. Jemmott, Jemmott, Spears, Hewitt, & Cruz-Collins, 1992; Sheeska, Woolcott, & MacKinnon, 1993; Strecher et al., 1986). Two fundamental assumptions regarding self-

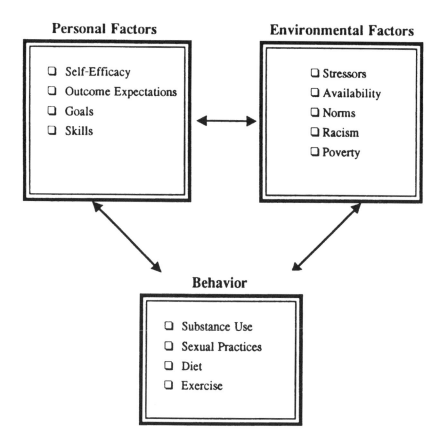

Figure 1. A representation of social–cognitive theory as it applies to interventions with minority adolescents. The dynamic interaction of the three factors—referred to as *reciprocal determinism*—forms the basis of social–cognitive theory.

efficacy are critical to understanding its central role in SCT. First, efficacy is seen as a cause of behavior, not (as operant learning theorists may contend) simply the result of it (see Hawkins, 1992, for a competing explanation of the causal role of self-efficacy). Second, self-efficacy is task-specific, as distinguished from more global personality attributes such as self-esteem, self-concept, and locus of control (i.e., externality). Individuals are not self-efficacious in general but, rather, their sense of efficacy is tied to specific behaviors or tasks. Though self-efficacy is conceptualized as task-specific, when tasks are similar in their cognitive and behavioral demands, as well as the context in which they occur, crossover or generalizability of self-efficacy can occur. A gradient of efficacy can be plotted, with levels of self-efficacy generally decreasing as the complexity or difficulty of the task increases. Thus, an adolescent may be highly self-efficacious with regard to asking a long-time partner to use a condom, but less efficacious with a new partner (Maibach & Murphy, 1995).

Efficacy can develop through four sources: performance mastery experience, vicarious observation, verbal persuasion, and physiologic and psychologic states. *Performance mastery experiences* are considered the most influential source, producing the strongest and most enduring efficacy effects. Performance success raises efficacy beliefs, whereas failure lowers them. Thus, individuals who are convinced (either through their own appraisal or the assessment of others) they performed well on a task, independent of actual performance, develop stronger efficacy beliefs and are more likely to continue efforts than individuals performing well but perceiving their performance as unsuccessful. This suggests a need to provide minority adolescents with strong efficacy beliefs, despite seemingly daunting environmental constraints. *Vicarious observation* involves seeing (or visualizing) individuals under comparable demand parameters successfully perform the target behavior. This can include vicarious observation of simulated performance in clinical settings or instructional media or "in vivo" observation of peers and family members. Absence of positive role models can then be recast as an absence of positive observational learning situations and, therefore, a problem of low personal efficacy rather than low self-esteem. *Verbal persuasion*—encouraging an individual to attempt a behavior change and assuring them that they have the skills necessary to do so—can be an effective motivational strategy, although encouragement must be matched to the behavioral and cognitive capacity of the individual. Determining "how high to aim," requires considerable understanding of an individual's talents, interests, motivation, and baseline efficacy. Finally, *physiologic* and *psychologic* states such as excessive arousal, anxiety, and depression can diminish efficacy and discourage continued efforts, whereas positive states such as stimulation, euphoria, and physical enjoyment can encourage future effort. Pressuring an adolescent to attempt a new behavior or modify an existing one when he or she is not prepared or sufficiently motivated to do so can create dysphoric levels of anxiety, arousal, anger, or resentment that, even with successful performance, can result in diminished motivation to continue efforts.

Efficacy operates through four processes: choice behavior, effort expenditure and persistence, thought patterns, and emotional reactions. The first two processes are reflected in the behavioral domain, whereas the second two are largely cognitive in nature. Individuals with high self-efficacy are more likely to attempt performing a behavior (i.e., exercise choice) and more likely to continue their efforts in the face of initial setbacks or frustration (i.e., expenditure and persistence). On the cognitive level, highly self-efficacious individuals tend to visualize and dwell on their successes more than their failures (i.e., thought patterns) and to process positive affective aspects of their performance more than the negative (i.e., emotional reactions).

Outcome Expectations

Outcome expectations include the perceived positive and negative results of a behavior, that is, its pros and cons. Initial and continued behavioral efforts are more likely when perceived benefits outweigh the perceived costs (Prochaska et al., 1994). SCT delineates three categories of outcome effects: physical, social, and self-evaluative. *Physical effects* include anticipated positive and negative sensory experiences (pleasure or pain) as well as assumed short- and long-term health consequences resulting from a behavior. This may include achievement of positive physical effects (e.g., losing weight) or avoidance of negative effects (e.g., reducing risk of heart disease). It is within this domain that health knowledge operates. Knowledge regarding what behaviors improve or impair health as well as what resources and options are at one's disposal are necessary, though insufficient precursors, of outcome expectations. *Social effects* include approval from friends and family, recognition, monetary reward, and improved status as well as such inhibiting factors as disapproval, rejection, censure, or ostracization. Social effects are particularly influential among adolescents, who largely determine their identities through peer relationships and normative comparison. Studies on substance use and sexual habits have demonstrated that perceptions regarding peer behaviors and group norms are strongly associated with individual health behaviors (Botvin et al., 1992; Walter et al., 1993; Wulfert & Wan, 1993). *Self-evaluation* includes the positive and negative internal reactions resulting from behavior. Although related to perceived social effects (insofar as personal values are largely derived from peer standards and social mores), self-evaluative expectations refer more to the perceived intrapersonal or intrapsychic consequences of behavior (i.e., how a person will feel about himself or herself morally and emotionally as a result of engaging in a behavior, beyond the external, social contingencies). During adolescence, moral development is largely under construction and contingent more on external than internal reference (Kohlberg, Levine, & Hewer, 1983). As a result, self-evaluative effects are seen as less influential than social effects at this developmental time. Nonetheless, as we discuss below, higher levels of religiosity among African Americans suggests a possible role of self-evaluative expectations in adolescent interventions (e.g., use of moral and spiritual appeals; Barnes, Farrell, & Banerjee, 1994; Taylor & Chatters, 1991).

Modifying outcome expectations is an important component of many health-promotion programs targeting adolescents. For example, substance use programs often include information regarding the positive and negative physical health effects of tobacco, marijuana, and alcohol use. Given the "present" orientation of most adolescents, saliency of health information for this population is enhanced by focusing on immediate rather than delayed consequences of behavior. For example, substance use prevention programs that place greater emphasis on concurrent or short-term physical effects, such as impaired stamina and athletic performance, appear more effective than those emphasizing long-term health effects such as cancer, cirrhosis, or heart disease (Glynn, Boyd, & Gruman, 1990).

Modifying perceived social effects may have an even greater impact on adolescent behavior than improving knowledge of physical consequences. Social effects include perceptions of how engaging in a behavior will alter social status. For example, decisions regarding substance use are influenced by how the individual perceives that these behaviors will affect his or her social image. On the basis of the observation that many adolescents overestimate the prevalence and, therefore, the normalcy of substance use, researchers have developed programs aimed at correcting erroneous perceptions regarding prevalence and acceptability, and initial results of these interventions appear promising (Hansen & Graham, 1991; Sussman et al., 1993). Though most normative influences programs have focused on substance use behaviors, this approach appears applicable to influencing other health habits, such as sexual behavior and diet (Baranowski, 1989–1990; L. S. Jemmott & Jemmott, 1992).

Goals

Setting discrete, realistically ambitious goals and then attaining them can significantly increase performance motivation. Attainment of goals that are too easily achieved produces little motivation, whereas setting unrealistic goals, though initially motivating, can eventually take its toll, resulting in low-efficacy states, if not helplessness and depression. The relation between attainability and motivation may differ for short- and long-term goals. Ambitious long-term goals can be useful, if the short-term goals needed to achieve them are divided into realistic, hierarchical steps and are sequentially attained. Rather than hinging all sense of success on glamorous future goals, individuals can be taught to gain satisfaction from progressive mastery of "mini-goals," using short-term successes as stepping stones toward their ultimate ambition.

According to SCT, personal goals mediate motivation in three ways. First, anticipated self-satisfaction from achieving performance standards can stimulate initial efforts and continued persistence. Second, successful performance and goal attainment can enhance personal efficacy, motivating heightened efforts and progression to more complex tasks and hierarchical goal achievement. The third type of influence involves adjustment of standards in response to performance attainment. Individuals who readjust their goals upward after successful performance are more likely to continue efforts, whereas those satisfied with simply attaining the same standard again invest little subsequent effort. Whereas upward readjustment of goals can help maintain motivation, during this process it is also important to enjoy the success attained. Failure to do so can result in the "Type A treadmill" of escalating accomplishment and drive, without the accompanying sense of efficacy and personal satisfaction (Friedman & Rosenman, 1974).

The relationship between expectations, goals, and motivation can be somewhat complex. In the face of initial failure, some individuals become demoralized and others persist. Motivation is best maintained by a strong sense of efficacy not only to succeed, but to withstand failure. Applying this principle to adolescents, it may be important not only to provide them with motivation to attempt new behaviors but also to prepare them to regroup and try again if initial efforts are not entirely successful. This strategy—encouraging realistic expectations for success and preempting defeatist interpretations of failure—is an essential element of relapse prevention (Brownell, Marlatt, Lichtenstein, & Wilson, 1986; Marlatt & Gordon, 1985). The challenge, again, lies in providing realistic expectations without injecting a self-fulfilling prophecy of failure.

Skills

For some behaviors, high self-efficacy and motivation (i.e., strong positive outcome expectations) are insufficient to produce successful behavior change; task-specific skills are often needed. During the 1980s, researchers developed numerous skills-based substance use prevention programs aimed at increasing general and substance-use specific skills, such as assertiveness and peer resistance (e.g., Botvin, Dusenbury, Baker, James-Ortiz, & Kerner, 1989; McCaul & Glasgow, 1985; Schinke, Gilchrist, & Snow, 1985). Although initial results were encouraging, many of these skills-based programs included multiple intervention strategies, such as modifying outcome expectations and increasing personal efficacy, and the effectiveness of skills training has recently been questioned (Resnicow, Cherry, & Cross, 1993). Several studies that tested the independent effects of skills training have found this approach to be largely ineffective (Elder, Sallis, Woodruff, & Wildey, 1993; Hansen & Graham, 1991; Sussman et al., 1993). Instead, these studies indicated that modifying normative beliefs and social outcome expectations—adolescents' assumptions regarding the prevalence and acceptability of substance use—appears to be the "active ingredient" of many so-called "skills-training" programs. Despite the questionable effectiveness of skills training in substance use prevention, this approach may be important in other behavioral domains, such as sexuality, nutrition, and exercise (Baranowski, 1989–1990; St. Lawrence, Jefferson, Alleyne, & Brasfield, 1995; Warzak, Grow, Poler, & Walburn, 1995).

The Interaction of Self-Efficacy, Outcome Expectations, Skills, and Goals

Given the central role of self-efficacy in SCT, it is important to understand how it interacts with other personal and environmental determinants of behavior. Individuals with high self-efficacy are more likely to attempt a behavior if they have strong positive outcome expectancies and possess the skills necessary to accomplish the task. Possessing requisite skills is also likely to increase opportunities to attain mastery experiences, which increases efficacy and spurs continued behavioral effort. In addition, if realistic goals are set, performance is more likely to be perceived as successful, and efficacy beliefs will be strengthened. If unattainable goals are set, performance may be perceived as failure, which will decrease efficacy and discourage persistence. On the environmental level, excessive levels of family stress, chaotic living conditions, lack of positive peer and adult models, and insufficient access to preventive services can suppress positive outcome expectations and initial effort, as well as the likelihood of experiencing positive mastery experiences—all of which can decrease efficacy and persistence.

SCT and Minority Adolescents

Is SCT an appropriate intervention model for African American and other minority adolescents? The answer is perhaps determined more by philosophical and political orientation than empirical evidence. Some Afrocentric scholars, for example, contend that theoretical and empirical models developed from a Eurocentric perspective fail a priori to adequately incorporate the social, psychological, cultural, historical, and genetic characteristics of African Americans (Akbar, 1984; Asante, 1987). For example, SCT includes several individual-based components, such as self-efficacy, personal goals, self-evaluative expectations, self-management, and assertiveness skills (Bandura, 1995; Baranowski, 1989–1990), that are rooted in Eurocentric, predominantly male values of competitiveness, materialism, personal achievement, impulse control, and self-determinism (Nobles, Goddard, Cavil, & George, 1993). Such individual-centered models, it has been argued, are too mechanistic and fail to adequately account for environmental determinants such as stress, racism, and poverty; high availability of guns and drugs; and low availability of recreational, educational, and health facilities that, for many African Americans, may be more influential than individual motivation (Airhihenbuwa, 1992; Cochran & Mays, 1993). Moreover, Eurocentric models generally situate White as the norm for what constitutes appropriate, acceptable, and desired as well as what are considered risk and resiliency factors. Such ethnocentric contrasts often impose a deficit model on African Americans and other nonmajority groups, whose performance may not measure up to White standards or whose cultures may operate by different principles (Akbar, 1984; Nobles et al., 1993).

The Afrocentric view asserts, to some degree, that individual and social learning principles may operate differently in African Americans, not only in degree but in kind. For example, assumptions regarding an individual-centered, linear, rational model of behavior change may not be appropriate for African or other non-Western cultures (Akbar, 1984; Asante, 1987; Nobles et al., 1993). A "one-size-fits-all" application of SCT, even with culturally sensitive adaptation, is seen as less effective than developing a uniquely African-centered paradigm (Cochran & Mays, 1993; Nobles et al., 1993). The Afrocentric paradigm does not assert racial superiority or that all Eurocentric science and thought are inherently invalid, only that these models should not be imposed on people—be they African American, Latino, or Asian Pacific Islander—from whom they did not emanate and for whom they may not be well suited.

A contrasting approach assumes that the fundamental determinants of behavior operate similarly in all populations and that psychological and behavioral models, such as SCT, can, despite their Eurocentric origins, be successfully adapted for a range of sociodemographic, racial, and ethnic populations. It is this view that guides our discussion for the remainder of this chapter. Adaptation, however, requires an integrative understanding of the unique personal and environmental characteristics of the target population and an ability to translate this knowledge into culturally sensitive messages and behavior change strategies. In recognition of the potential bias of Eurocentricism, the adaptation process requires researchers to first examine ethnocentric (and possibly racist) assumptions inherent in their models and then attempt to incorporate alternative conceptualizations of human experience. In the next section, using SCT as the organizing framework, we provide examples of how personal and environmental characteristics unique to African Americans and other minority groups can be incorporated into culturally sensitive interventions.

Prior to our discussion, several caveats are in order. First, for many of the examples presented, it is not clear to what degree the racial–ethnic differences exist independent of socioeconomic factors. Many putative racial–ethnic differences in social, psychological, behavioral, and medical phenomena disappear after inequities in education, income, and opportunity are controlled for, for example, differences in cancer rates and locus of control (Banks, 1988; Baquet, Horm, Gibbs, & Greenwald, 1991; Krieger, Rowley, Herman, Avery, & Phillips, 1993). Racial differences in other phenomena—such as obesity, smoking, blood pressure reactivity, preterm delivery rates, cognitive learning styles, and stress coping skills—however, appear to persist independent of socioeconomic status (SES; i.e., across racial–ethnic groups within the same SES class; Banks, 1988; Krieger et al., 1993; Shea et al., 1991; Ulbrich, Warheit, & Zimmerman, 1989). However, the persistence of these phenomena after adjustment for socioeconomic variables does not prove that these differences are genetic or even independent of SES. Adjustment for SES variables—most commonly education, income, and occupation—often fails to capture subtle social and psychological differences in how these variables may operate differently in African American and other minority communities. For example, the economic return of education is lower for African Americans than Whites; after education is controlled for, African Americans still earn less and have lower status jobs (Krieger et al., 1993), and the African American poor have fewer assets and more debts than the White poor. Many middle and upper SES African Americans are the first in their families to achieve upward mobility. They are more likely to live with lower SES family members and friends and to live in mixed-SES neighborhoods as well as participate in mixed-SES activities and organizations (Banks, 1988; Krieger et al., 1993). Generational economic status is a potentially important component of SES that is rarely measured. In summary, determining whether racial–ethnic differences are artifacts of inequities in education and income or are bona fide cultural, ethnic, or even genetic characteristics cannot be accomplished with covariate adjustment or stratification of statistics.

Our second caveat is that the studies we cite varied considerably in their scientific rigor. They include moderate to severe methodological limitations, such as small numbers of participants and convenience samples. Generalizing findings from these studies to the larger African American population or other minority groups should be tempered by these considerations. Despite these limitations, the examples provided may have heuristic utility for program planners and evaluators.

Example 1: Attitudes Toward Obesity and Standards of Physical Beauty

African Americans. Several studies have found that African Americans possess different standards than Whites regarding what constitutes an ideal body image and "how overweight is overweight" (Kumanyika, Morssink, & Agurs, 1992; Kumanyika, Wilson, & Guilford-Davenport, 1993). African American women report a higher ideal body weight and are more likely to be satisfied with their weight, even when they are statistically overweight, than White women. African American women and men appear to prefer fuller body types than Whites. The obsession with thinness, exemplified by the credo "you can never be too rich or too thin," may reflect Eurocentric values that do not resonate in the African American community. These differences appear to occur independent of education and are evident among adolescent as well as elderly African Americans. That these differences exist across generations suggests that this standard may have relatively deep roots in African American culture (Kumanyika et al., 1992, 1993).

How these cultural differences developed is a matter of debate. Obesity is largely uncommon among native Africans, and low prevalence in Africa may somehow contribute to the relative higher tolerance among African Americans. Conversely, because more African American women are obese, comparison to the African American norm may result in a higher expected norm than comparison with Whites (Kumanyika et al., 1992, 1993). Another explanation offered is the earlier transition of African Americans into roles as mother or grandmother, after which the importance placed on physical beauty may diminish. Finally, being large may have secondary social benefit. In urban settings, physical size may be used to convey a sense of strength or invulnerability, a "shield" against a potentially hostile environment. It also may, as in preindustrial Europe, be seen as a sign of wealth and success.

Ironically, this cultural standard represents a double-edged sword. On the one hand, it probably decreases the likelihood of developing such eating disorders as anorexia and bulimia, which are driven largely by White American values regarding thinness, femininity, and shame. In fact, African Americans have a significantly lower incidence of eating disorders than Whites (American Psychiatric Association, 1994). On the other hand, tolerance for fuller body types may encourage development of obesity and discourage motivation to seek or comply with necessary treatment. African Americans, particularly women, have a significantly higher prevalence of obesity than Whites, independent of education (Centers for Disease Control and Prevention [CDC], 1994; Shea et al., 1991).

With regard to SCT, these differences are examples of race-specific social outcome expectations, and interventions designed to prevent or treat obesity among African American adolescents need to work within these social norms. In practice, one option for program developers and clinicians would be to place greater emphasis on the health consequences of being overweight rather than its social consequences. Alternatively, strategies to alter perceptions regarding its social acceptability (i.e., decrease the perceived acceptability and attractiveness of being overweight) may also be effective. This, however, raises a potential ethical and public health dilemma. Increasing social sanctions against overweight people may increase pathological concern over body image, and the consequent morbidity (e.g., eating disorders) may cancel some of the public health benefits that resulted from decreasing obesity prevalence.

Application to other racial and ethnic groups. Among females, prevalence of obesity is higher among Hispanics than among Whites (CDC, 1994; Resnicow, Futterman, & Vaughan, 1993). Though there are little published data regarding body image among Hispanics, there is at least indirect evidence of higher tolerance, if not preference, for a larger body type among Hispanics, particularly those of Puerto Rican and Dominican descent (Stern, Pugh, Gaskill, & Hazuda, 1982). Conversely, the prevalence of obesity is lower among Asian Americans, and the tolerance or preference for a larger body type is likely less applicable to this group (CDC, 1994).

Example 2: Attitudes Toward Individualism Versus Communalism

African Americans. Contemporary health-promotion interventions place significant emphasis on individual responsibility for behavior change (e.g., self-efficacy, personal goals, self-evaluative expectations, self-management, and assertiveness skills; Bandura, 1986). These elements of behavior change theory are rooted in Eurocentric, predominantly male values of competitiveness, materialism, personal achievement, impulse control, and self-determinism (Akbar, 1984; Asante,

1987; Nobles et al., 1993). In contrast, Afrocentric values place greater emphasis on community, interpersonal relations, expressiveness, and spiritualism (e.g., "It takes an entire village to raise a child"; Nobles et al., 1993). Although the degree that African Americans, particularly adolescents, possess or aspire to these Afrocentric values and the degree that communality differs by race have not been adequately assessed, this unique psychological and philosophical orientation has several implications for program planners.

In the SCT framework, these differences suggest that self-efficacy, self-evaluative outcomes, and individual-based goals may be less effective behavior change strategies among African Americans and, therefore, should be de-emphasized in culturally sensitive SCT interventions. Instead, greater emphasis could be placed on social outcome expectations related to communal benefits: interpersonal rather than intrapersonal motivation and collective rather than personal goals. Appropriate messages for African American adolescents developed from this perspective might include "Do it for yourself, your family, and your people," "We need more healthy brothers for the struggle," or "Do it with a friend." These messages could be applied, with modification, to multiple health behaviors, including substance use, exercise, diet, and sexual practices. To some degree, the positive health behaviors prevalent among Nation of Islam followers (decreased alcohol, tobacco, and drug use and abstention from pork) can be attributed to the high value placed on community responsibility, spirituality, and discipline.

Application to other racial and ethnic groups. Hispanic culture has also been characterized as having a strong sense of collectivism (*colectivismo*), which includes high levels of personal interdependence, conformity, and sacrifice for the communal good (Schinke, Moncher, Palleja, Zayas, & Schilling, 1988; U.S. Department of Health and Human Services [U.S. DHHS], 1995). Hispanic youth appear less self-centered than other Americans (Szalay, Canino, & Vilov, 1993). Emphasis, then, on communal versus self-centered motivation for behavior may also be appropriate for this population.

Example 3: Religiosity

African Americans. Several studies of adults and adolescents have found higher levels of religiosity among African Americans than Whites (Levin, Taylor, & Chatters, 1994; Taylor & Chatters, 1991). African Americans are more likely to attend church, they place a higher value on religion, and they are more likely to use religion as a coping strategy. The salience of religion in African American life is supported by the finding that religiosity is a stronger predictor of life satisfaction for African Americans than Whites, whereas among African American adolescents, religion appears more protective of substance use than for Whites (Thomas, Bethlehem, & Holmes, 1992). In addition, the church serves different functions in African American and White communities. Beyond spiritual sustenance, African American churches also provide a forum for social discourse and political activism; in particular, African American churches were major contributors to the civil rights movement. Many African American churches also provide social and medical services, such as health screenings, voter registration campaigns, and food programs for the disadvantaged (Thomas et al., 1992; U.S. DHHS, 1989).

With regard to SCT, religiosity relates to social and self-evaluative outcome expectations. Linking health messages to religious or spiritual themes or using religious leaders as messengers or models may be appropriate strategies for African Americans. This can involve manipulation of social effects, such as linking health behaviors to specific biblical commandments or using the norms of the faith community as a source of positive or negative sanctions. In addition, self-evaluative expectations, for example, that emphasize personal feelings of spiritual or religious pride or shame can be used to encourage positive health behaviors. Increased involvement in religion may also be associated with an increased responsiveness to fear messages among African Americans. African Americans may be more receptive to fear messages regarding health, particularly when these are tied to religious themes. Research is needed to determine the effectiveness of fear messages among African Americans and to discern the degree to which responsiveness to such messages is related to religiosity.

Application to other racial and ethnic groups. Hispanic youth may also have higher levels of religiosity than majority youth, and so culturally sensitive interventions for this population should also consider religion as a possible motivational factor in health behavior decisions (Neff & Hoppe, 1992; U.S. DHHS, 1995).

Example 4: Peer Influence

African Americans. It is largely accepted that adolescent health behavior is influenced by peer attitudes and behaviors (Newcomb &

Bentler, 1989; Stein, Newcomb, & Bentler, 1987). Peers can influence health habits directly (e.g., by offering, purchasing, or otherwise making available cigarettes, alcohol, or other drugs) or indirectly (e.g., by affecting group norms and social outcome expectations). In the substance use literature, peer influences are generally measured as either the number or proportion of friends who smoke, drink, or use drugs or perceptions of peer attitudes toward these substances and individuals who use them. Several studies have reported significant racial and ethnic differences in both direct and indirect peer influence, with peers generally having weaker effects on substance use behaviors among African Americans than among Whites (Landrine, Richardson, Klonoff, & Flay, 1994; Sussman, Dent, Flay, Hansen, & Johnson, 1987; Vega, Zimmerman, Warheit, Apospori, & Gil, 1993). However, these findings have been somewhat inconsistent (Catalano et al., 1993; Farrell, Danish, & Howard, 1992).

From an SCT perspective, differential effects of peers can be cast in the person or environment domains. On the personal level, peer influences affect social outcome expectations and thereby affect individual motivation. On the environmental level, peer influences contribute to social norms, which can affect social expectations by increasing opportunities for use, either through direct appeals or increasing availability. Regardless of which box peer influence is placed in the figure of the SCT model, these data suggest that substance use interventions, and possibly other interventions for African Americans, should place less emphasis on altering group norms and resisting peer pressure and greater emphasis on such other factors as parental smoking and family interaction (Landrine et al., 1994; Vega et al., 1993). Specifically, this could entail developing activities that address why parents smoke as well as strategies to encourage parents who smoke (or use other substances) to quit. Interventions could also be developed that better engage African American family and community members to participate in local substance use prevention and broader health-promotion programs. Little research specifically examining the relative effectiveness of parental versus peer influences among African Americans has been reported.

Application to other racial and ethnic groups. There is evidence that the predictors of substance use differ among Hispanics and Asians relative to Whites, yet the effects of peer influence appear similar between these groups (Sussman et al., 1987; Vega et al., 1993), although in one study peer influence had a greater impact on smoking patterns for Asian youth compared with African American, White, or Hispanic youth (Koepke, Flay, & Johnson, 1990). There is also some evidence that Hispanic and Asian youth have stronger family ties than other groups. Tapping these inherent support systems may increase the effectiveness of health-promotion programs among these populations (Koepke et al., 1990; Schinke et al., 1988; U.S. DHHS, 1995).

Example 5: Stressful Life Events

African Americans. A substantial body of evidence has established that stressful life events can have an impact on human physiology (Delongis, Coyne, Dakof, Folkman, & Lazarus, 1982; Herbert & Cohen, 1993; Kiecolt-Glaser & Glaser, 1987; Selye, 1978) and health behavior (Brownell et al., 1986; Marlatt & Gordon, 1985; Wills, Vaccaro, & McNamara, 1992). Compared with Whites, African Americans experience a greater number of negative stressful events. They experience different types of stressors and use different types of coping strategies in response to stress (Airhihenbuwa & Cole, 1988; Fitzpatrick & Boldizar, 1993; Garrison, Schoenbach, Schluchter, Kaplan, & Berton, 1987). They also derive social support—a buffer against stress—from different sources (Thomas et al., 1992). Specifically, African American adolescents are more likely than their White counterparts to be victims or witnesses to violence, to experience the death of a parent or sibling, to be involved in the criminal justice system, and to have parents whose income has recently decreased (Fitzpatrick & Boldizar, 1993; Garrison et al., 1987). African American youth also rate the impact of stressful events differently than do White adolescents (Newcomb, Huba, & Bentler, 1986). Another important source of stress for African Americans is the overt and covert effects of racism, which can increase feelings of anger, hostility, and helplessness, each of which have been associated with negative health outcomes (Scherwitz et al., 1992; Siegler, Peterson, Barefoot, & Williams, 1992). There are also data to suggest that African Americans are more likely to use drugs to anesthetize dysphoric states resulting from poverty, oppression, and lack of opportunity (Dawkins, 1988).

In terms of intervention, African American youth may require more and different stress coping skills that are tailored to the specific stressors they experience. Appropriate interventions might include relaxation exercises, yoga, meditation, martial arts, or cognitive coping strategies such as thought stopping, imagery, and reframing (Braith-

waite, 1985; Schinke et al., 1988). Another means of buffering the del-
eterious effects of stress is to increase the amount of social support
available to African American and other minority youth, by engaging
family members, adult mentors, community members, religious leaders, or mental health professionals (Schinke et al, 1988; U.S. DHHS,
1995). Either approach—providing stress-management skills or social
support—can help individuals regain a sense of equilibrium, control,
and hope that is essential for continued learning and personal growth.

Application to other racial and ethnic groups. Urban Hispanic
youth face many of the same stressors as their African American counterparts, such as noise, overcrowding, unemployment, racial discrimination, school failure, substandard housing, and safety concerns
(Schinke et al., 1988). There is also evidence that Hispanic and Asian
youth face unique stressors, and the effects of specific stressors may
differ between these groups (Schinke et al., 1988; Szalay et al., 1993).
One stressor of particular interest is acculturation. Acculturation is the
process by which immigrants assimilate the culture of their host country. Substance use as well as other health risks appear to increase after
immigration, particularly among those unable to master English or
navigate in American society (Neff & Hoppe, 1992; Szalay et al., 1993).
There is evidence that increasing biculturality, appreciation, and identification with both native and host cultures may decrease substance
use and other problem behaviors (Schinke et al., 1988). As noted earlier for African Americans, increasing ethnic and racial pride, instilling
traditional values, and engaging family and community as sources of
social support may be effective intervention strategies for minority
immigrant youth. SCT has been used as a framework for developing
such interventions (Schinke et al., 1988).

Future Research Priorities

Examination of Afrocentric Approaches to Behavior Change

Afrocentricity denotes both a philosophical and a sociopolitical construct. With regard to the philosophical sense of the term, Afrocentricity has been defined as an orientation that places African ideals at
the center of any analysis that involves African culture and behavior
(Asante, 1987) as well as a conceptual framework that centers on the

history, culture, and philosophy of African people (Baldwin, 1987; Baldwin, Brown, & Rackley, 1990). It is seen as a way of knowing, defined by distinctive use of language, time, and reasoning along with a unique appreciation of nature, mythology, spirituality, and community (Akbar, 1984; Asante, 1987; Morgan, 1991).

As a sociopolitical construct, Afrocentricity refers to the role of racial identity in personality development (Akbar, 1984; Cross, 1991; Harris, 1992). Two dimensions of Afrocentricity addressed by most theorists are (a) awareness of and pride in African and Black heritage and (b) recognition of and opposition to racism (Baldwin et al., 1990). These constructs have also been referred to as "pro-Black" and "anti-White" attitudes (Baldwin, Duncan, & Bell, 1987; Parham & Helms, 1985). Although the philosophical definition of Afrocentricity provides a basis for understanding what being African American "is," the sociopolitical interpretation provides prescriptive guidelines for how African Americans "should be." In this regard, many Afrocentric leaders believe that increasing Afrocentricism can be therapeutic for many members of the African American community. Examples of Afrocentric interventions include incorporation of rites of passage and celebration of Kwaanza as well as study of the Nguzo Saba (the seven spiritual principles of Kwanzaa), African history, and African culture within substance use, school dropout, and violence prevention programs.

Although, as a sociopolitical construct, Afrocentricity has in cross-sectional research been positively associated with a wide range of personality traits and behaviors—including self-actualization, anxiety, hostility, juvenile crime, substance use, depression, and self-esteem—little controlled research examining the therapeutic effects of Afrocentric interventions has been conducted (Cross, 1991; Parham & Helms, 1985; Terrell, Taylor, & Terrell, 1980). Many interventions that include Afrocentric components also include secular, non-Afrocentric strategies. As a result, it is often difficult to disentangle the specific effects of Afrocentric approaches when they are delivered as part of comprehensive, multicomponent interventions. Therefore, studies examining the effectiveness of Afrocentric versus more secular approaches appear warranted. The effects of increasing cultural awareness and ethnic pride among Hispanic and Asian youth similarly merit investigation (Schinke et al., 1988).

Appreciating Heterogeneity Within Ethnic Groups

Cultural sensitivity includes an appreciation for the variation within social groups, not only between groups. Thus, African Americans as well as other racial groups cannot be considered a homogeneous entity with a single mind-set. As described by Cross (1991), there is great variation in the degree that African Americans define themselves by their race and in how racial identity influences overall personal identity. Some place great significance on their African heritage, others define themselves in relation to Whites, and still others do not define themselves by their race at all. Hence, there exists no single definition of what it means to "be Black." Moreover, racial identity is only one dimension on which African Americans vary; within the African American community there is also extensive variation in religiosity, education, income, political beliefs, dietary habits, musical preference, and so on. Interestingly, even on the genetic level, there is evidence that differences are greater within members of an ethnic group than between different ethnic groups. Thus, any two African Americans will be more dissimilar on a chromosomal level than any pair of White and African American individuals (Lewontin, 1982).

Culturally sensitive programs also assume heterogeneity within the target population. Although, for example, many African American youth may respond positively to Afrocentric messages (e.g., linking their dietary practices to Black history or Africa), many others may not. Similarly, an intervention for Hispanic youth might include messages incorporating healthy foods from their indigenous cultural or family homeland, but youth interested in assimilating into American culture may be repelled by such appeals. Thus, although identifying culturally unique determinants is an important step in developing interventions for minority populations, program planners should notassume that these factors will be applicable or meaningful to all members of their target population. Public health professionals need to better understand the diversity within groups and, to the degree possible, tailor programs according to the needs and diversity of the population being served.

Distinguishing Myth From Fact

In this chapter, we have discussed how and why cultural and racial differences should be incorporated into health-promotion interventions for minority adolescents. It is perhaps equally important to examine inaccurate and invalid assumptions regarding racial differences in order to delineate those factors that should specifically not be considered. For example, there is a belief among some that minority youth exhibit lower impulse control and more aggressive behavior and that interventions for this group should perhaps include more punitive measures or other strategies to help control "unruly" youth. There are little data to support this assertion, and to the degree that these differences do exist, they may exist only in well-defined subpopulations, and factors such as nutritional habits and stressful living conditions are more likely etiological explanations than race per se (Krieger et al., 1993). Similarly, there is a belief, based in part on the doll studies conducted in the 1940s by Clark and Clark, that African American youth have lower self-esteem than Whites. Analysis of more than 160 self-concept studies as well as several recent scholarly reviews on this topic (see Cross, 1991), however, question this assertion. Finally, significant controversy was roused with the recent publication of Herrnstein and Murray's (1994) *The Bell Curve*, which discusses racial differences in intelligence and aptitude test scores, achievement, and social class. That the distribution of scores on standardized tests may differ between racial and ethnic groups is in itself an important empirical observation that requires elucidation. However, attributing these differences to genetic rather than to environmental, social, historical, and cultural factors begins to suggest inherent racial superiority and negates the vast social, economic, and political inequities that may contribute to these statistical differences (Fraser, 1995). Moreover, such biological explanations inherently discourage remedial programs aimed at mitigating the underlying social inequities that are certainly at least part of the cause. Instead of assuming that African American youth (or adults) are less intelligent, have lower self-esteem, or are more impulsive, program developers need to understand and incorporate different learning styles, language patterns, and other social and psychological characteristics that can influence how and why information is processed and used. In summary, it is important to discern legitimate racial and ethnic differences from myth, stereotype, and fallacy. Failure to do so may result not only in culturally insensitive interventions but also in interventions that may cause more harm than good.

Conclusion

There is a consensus that health interventions should be customized to match the social, psychological, cultural, environmental, and economic characteristics of the target population (Catalano et al., 1993; Schinke et al., 1988). In this chapter, we have provided a framework for adapting one model of health behavior change, SCT, for use with minority adolescents. Successful adaptation of SCT or other models of behavior change (e.g., stages of change, health belief model, and the theory of planned action) for special populations requires a two-stage process. First, program planners should describe the major individual-level determinants (i.e., self-efficacy, outcome expectations, normative beliefs, goal setting, and skills) and environmental factors (e.g., availability and cost of foods in the local neighborhoods) that influence the targeted behavior in the population. This might entail examining the published literature as well as collecting new qualitative data (through focus groups or individual interviews) or quantitative data (e.g., baseline surveys) to determine which factors should be targeted by the intervention and how. The specific cognitive and behavioral skills required to achieve the desired outcome must be delineated, and culturally sensitive strategies for increasing personal efficacy and motivating behavioral effort can then be developed. Cultural sensitivity should be addressed on two levels: surface and deep structure. *Surface structure* includes using familiar images (e.g., members from the target population), settings, language, foods, etc., in print and video materials. *Deep structure* refers to the culturally syntonic representation of psychological, spiritual, and historical issues related to the target behavior. It is the latter level of sensitivity that is more difficult to attain. For a dietary intervention, deep structure might include appeals to adopt improved nutritional habits for the "sake of the community" or, perhaps, linking messages to religious or historical themes. Culturally sensitive programs also assume heterogeneity within the target population. Thus, although identifying culturally unique determinants is an important step in developing interventions for minority populations, program planners should not assume that these factors will be applicable or meaningful to all members of their target population.

A core premise of this chapter is that the fundamental determinants of behavior are essentially similar across populations and that models of health behavior change can be successfully adapted for minority populations. Unique characteristics of minority populations can be incorporated within extant models by recognizing the strengths and weaknesses of a target group, appropriately emphasizing or de-emphasizing intervention elements based on the unique behavioral determinants of the population, and designing salient messages and materials. Alternatively, depending on the magnitude of adaptation, it could be argued that these modified models become different not only in degree but in kind. This suggests a potential need for developing new paradigms for understanding and modifying health behavior—whether unique to each racial and ethnic subpopulation or a general model applicable to any demographic, ethnic, and racial minority. We therefore encourage controlled studies that test the efficacy of "generic" versus "ethnocentric" models of health behavior change. Such research requires that causal elements be well defined and that putative differences between models be based on sound theoretical distinctions.

REFERENCES

Airhihenbuwa, C. O. (1992). Health promotion and disease prevention strategies for African Americans: A conceptual model. In R. L. Braithwaite & S. E. Taylor (Eds.), *Health issues in the Black community* (pp. 267–277). San Francisco: Jossey-Bass.

Airhihenbuwa, C. O., & Cole, G. E. (1988). Results of a pilot study of the relationships of psychosocial measures among Black adolescent students. *The Western Journal of Black Studies, 12*, 204–209.

Akbar, N. (1984). Afrocentric social sciences for human liberation. *Journal of Black Studies, 14*, 395–414.

American Psychiatric Association. (1994). *Diagnostic and statistical manual of mental disorders* (4th ed.). Washington, DC: Author.

Asante, M. K. (1987). *The Afrocentric idea.* Philadelphia: Temple University Press.

Baldwin, J. A. (1987). African psychology and Black personality testing. *The Negro Educational Review, 38*(2–3), 56–66.

Baldwin, J. A., Brown, R., & Rackley, R. (1990). Some socio-behavioral correlates of African self-consciousness in African-American college students. *Journal of Black Psychology, 17*, 1–17.

Baldwin, J. A., Duncan, J. A., & Bell, Y. R. (1987). Assessment of African self-consciousness among Black students from two college environments. *Journal of Black Psychology, 13*, 27–41.

Bandura, A. (1986). *Social foundations of thought and action: A social cognitive theory*. Englewood Cliffs, NJ: Prentice Hall.

Bandura, A. (in press). *Self-efficacy: The exercise of control*. New York: Freeman.

Banks, J. A. (1988). Ethnicity, class, cognitive and motivational styles: Research and teaching implications. *Journal of Negro Education, 57*, 452–467.

Baquet, C. R., Horm, J. W., Gibbs, T., & Greenwald, P. (1991). Socieconomic factors and cancer incidence among Blacks and Whites. *Journal of National Cancer Institute, 83*, 551–556.

Baranowski, T. (1989–1990). Reciprocal determinism at the stages of behavior change: An integration of community, personal and behavioral perspectives. *International Quarterly of Community Health Education, 10*, 297–327.

Barnes, G. M., Farrell, M. P., & Banerjee, S. (1994). Family influences on alcohol abuse and other problem behaviors among Black and White adolescents in a general population sample. *Journal of Research on Adolescence, 4*, 183–201.

Botvin, G. J., Dusenbury, L., Baker, E., James-Ortiz, S., Botvin, E. M., & Kerner, J. (1992). Smoking prevention among urban minority youth: Assessing effects on outcome and mediating variables. *Health Psychology, 11*, 290–299.

Botvin, G. J., Dusenbury, L., Baker, E., James-Ortiz, S., & Kerner, J. (1989). A skills-training approach to smoking prevention among Hispanic youth. *Journal of Behavioral Medicine, 12*, 279–295.

Braithwaite, R. (1985). *Stress management manual*. Norfolk, VA: Norfolk Area Health Education Center.

Brownell, K. D., Marlatt, G. A., Lichtenstein, E., & Wilson, G. T. (1986). Understanding and preventing relapse. *American Psychologist, 7*, 765–782.

Calfas, K. J., Sallis, J. F., & Nader, P. R. (1991). The development of scales to measure knowledge and preference for diet and physical activity behavior in 4- to 8-year-old children. *Journal of Developmental and Behavioral Pediatrics, 12*, 185–190.

Catalano, R. F., Hawkins, J. D., Krenz, C., Gillmore, M., Morrison, D., Wells, E., & Abbott, R. (1993). Using research to guide culturally appropriate drug abuse prevention. *Journal of Consulting and Clinical Psychology, 61*, 804–811.

Centers for Disease Control and Prevention. (1994). Prevalence of selected risk factors for chronic disease by education level in racial/ethnic populations. *Morbidity and Mortality Weekly Report, 43*, 894–899.

Clark, K. B., & Clark, M. P. (1947). Racial identification and preference in Negro children. In T. M. Newcomb & E. L. Hartley (Eds.), *Readings in social psychology*. New York: Holt, Rinehart & Winston.

Clark, M. M., Abrams, D. B., Niaura, R. S., Eaton, C. A., & Rossi, J. S. (1991). Self-efficacy in weight management. *Journal of Consulting and Clinical Psychology, 59*, 739–744.

Cochran, S. D., & Mays, V. M. (1993). Applying social psychological models to predicting HIV-related sexual risk behaviors among African Americans. *Journal of Black Psychology, 19*, 142–154.

Cross, W. E. (1991). *Shades of Black: Diversity in African American identity*. Philadelphia: Temple University Press.

Dawkins, M. P. (1988). Alcoholism prevention and Black youth. *Journal of Drug Issues, 18*, 15–20.

DeLongis, A., Coyne, J. C., Dakof, G., Folkman, S., & Lazarus, R. S. (1982). Relationship of daily hassles, uplifts, and major life events to health status. *Health Psychology, 1*, 119–136.

Elder, J. P., Sallis, J. F., Woodruff, S. I., & Wildey, M. B. (1993). Tobacco-refusal skills and tobacco use among high risk adolescents. *Journal of Behavioral Medicine, 16*, 629–642.

Ellickson, P. L., & Bell, R. M. (1990). Drug prevention in junior high: A multi-site longitudinal test. *Science, 247*, 1299–1305.

Farrell, A. D., Danish, S. J., & Howard, C. W. (1992). Risk factors for drug use in urban adolescents: Identification and cross-validation. *American Journal of Community Psychology, 20*, 263–286.

Fish, J. M. (1995). Why psychologists should learn some anthropology. *American Psychologist, 50*, 44–45.

Fitzpatrick, K. M., & Boldizar, J. P. (1993). The prevalence and consequences of exposure to violence among African-American youth. *Journal of the American Academy of Child and Adolescent Psychiatry, 32*, 424–430.

Fraser, S. (Ed.). (1995). The bell curve wars: Race, intelligence, and the future of America. New York: Harper Collins.

Friedman, M., & Rosenman, H. (1974). Type A behavior and your heart. New York: Knopf.

Garrison, C. R., Schoenbach, V. J., Schluchter, I., Kaplan, M. D., & Berton, H. (1987). Life events in early adolescence. *Journal of the American Academy of Child and Adolescent Psychiatry, 26*, 865–872.

Glynn, T. J., Boyd, G. M., & Gruman, J. C. (1990). Essential elements of self-help/minimal intervention strategies for smoking cessation. *Health Education Quarterly, 17*, 329–345.

Hansen, W. B., & Graham, J. W. (1991). Preventing alcohol, marijuana, and cigarette use among adolescents: Peer pressure resistance training versus establishing conservative norms. *Preventive Medicine, 20*, 414–430.

Harris, N. (1992). A philosophical basis for an Afrocentric orientation. *Western Journal of Black Studies, 16*, 154–159.

Hawkins, R. M. (1992). Self-efficacy: A predictor but not a cause of behavior. *Journal of Behavior Therapy and Experimental Psychiatry, 23*, 251–256.

Herbert, T. B., & Cohen, S. (1993). Stress and immunity in humans: A meta-analytic review. *Psychosomatic Medicine, 55*, 364–379.

Herrnstein, R. J., & Murray, C. (1994). *The bell curve: Intelligence and class structure in American life.* New York: Free Press.

Jemmott, J. B., Jemmott, L. S., Spears, H., Hewitt, N., & Cruz-Collins, M. (1992). Self-efficacy, hedonistic expectancies, and condom-use intentions among inner-city Black adolescent women: A social cognitive approach to AIDS risk behavior. *Journal of Adolescent Health, 13*, 512–519.

Jemmott, L. S., & Jemmott, J. B. (1992). Increasing condom-use intentions among sexually active Black adolescent women. *Nursing Research, 41*, 273–279.

Kiecolt-Glaser, J. K., & Glaser, R. (1987). Psychosocial moderators of immune function. *Annals of Behavioral Medicine, 9*, 16-20.

Kirby, D., Short, L., Collins, J., Rugg, D., Kolbe, L., Howard, M., Miller, B., Sonenstein, F., & Zabin, L. S. (1994). School-based programs to reduce sexual risk behaviors: A review of effectiveness. *Public Health Reports, 109,* 339–360.

Koepke, D., Flay, B., & Johnson, C. A. (1990). Health behaviors in minority families: The case of cigarette smoking. *Family and Community Health, 13,* 35–43.

Kohlberg, L., Levine, C., & Hewer, A. (1983). Moral stages: A current formulation and a response to critics. *Contributions to Human Development, 10,* 174.

Krieger, N., Rowley, D. L, Herman, A. A., Avery, B., & Phillips, M. T. (1993). Racism, sexism, and social class, implications for studies for health, disease, and well-being. *American Journal of Preventive Medicine, 9,* 82–122.

Kumanyika, S. K., Morssink, C., & Agurs, T. (1992). Models for dietary and weight change in African-American women: Identifying cultural components. *Ethnicity and Disease, 2,* 166–175.

Kumanyika, S. K., Wilson, J. F., & Guilford-Davenport, M. (1993). Weight-related attitudes and behaviors of Black women. *Journal of the American Dietetic Association, 93,* 416–422.

Landrine, H., Richardson, J. L., Klonoff, E. A., & Flay, B. (1994). Cultural diversity in the predictors of adolescent cigarette smoking: The relative influence of peers. *Journal of Behavioral Medicine, 17,* 331–346.

Levin, S. J., Taylor, R. J., & Chatters, L. M. (1994). Race and gender differences in religiosity among older adults: Findings from four national surveys. *Journal of Gerontology, 49*(Suppl. 3), S137–S145.

Levy, S. R., Perhats, C., Weeks, K., Handler, A. S., Zhu, C., & Flay, B. R. (1995). Impact of a school-based AIDS prevention program on risk and protective behavior for newly sexually active students. *Journal of School Health, 65,* 145–151.

Lewontin, R. (1982). *Human diversity.* New York: Freeman.

Maibach, E., & Murphy, D. A. (1995). Self-efficacy in health promotion research and practice: Conceptualization and measurement. *Health Education Research, 10,* 37–50.

Marlatt, G. A., & Gordon, J. R. (1985). *Relapse prevention maintenance strategies in addictive behavior change.* New York: Guilford Press.

McCaul, K. D., & Glasgow, R. E. (1985). Preventing adolescent smoking: What have we learned about treatment construct validity? *Health Psychology, 4,* 361–387.

Morgan, G. D. (1991). Afrocentricity in social science. *Western Journal of Black Studies, 15,* 197–206.

Neff, J. A., & Hoppe, S. K. (1992). Acculturation and drinking patterns among U.S. Anglos, Blacks, and Mexican Americans. *Alcohol and Alcoholism, 27,* 293–308.

Newcomb, M. D., & Bentler, P. M. (1989). Substance use and abuse among children and teenagers. *American Psychologist, 44,* 242–248.

Newcomb, M. D., Huba, G. J., & Bentler, P. M. (1986). Desirability of various life change events among adolescents: Effects of exposure, sex, age, and ethnicity. *Journal of Research in Personality, 20,* 207–227.

Nobles, W. W., Goddard, L. L., Cavil, W. E., & George, P. Y. (1993). An African-centered model of prevention for African-American youth at high risk. In Lawford L. Goddard (Ed.), *An African-centered model of prevention for African-American youth at high risk* (U.S. DHHS/CSAP Tech. Rep. No. 6, DHHS Publication No. SMA 93-2015, pp. 115–129). Rockville, MD: Public Health Service/SAMHSA.

Parham, T. A., & Helms, J. E. (1985). Relation of racial identity attitudes to self-actualization and affective states of Black students. *Journal of Counseling Psychology, 32*, 431–440.

Prochaska, J. O., Velicer, W. F., Rossi, J. S., Goldstein, M. G., Marcus, B. H., Rakowski, W., Fiore, C., Harlow, L. L., Redding, C. A., Rosenbloom, D., & Rossi, S. R. (1994). Stages of change and decisional balance for 12 problem behaviors. *Health Psychology, 13*, 39–46.

Resnicow, K., Cherry, J., & Cross, D. (1993). Ten unanswered questions regarding comprehensive school health promotion. *Journal of School Health, 63*, 171–175.

Resnicow, K., Futterman, R., & Vaughan, R. (1993). Body mass index as a predictor of systolic blood pressure in a multiracial sample of U.S. schoolchildren. *Ethnicity and Disease, 3*, 351–361.

Sallis, J. F., Hovell, M. F., Hofstetter, C. R., & Barrington, E. (1992). Explanation of vigorous physical activity during two years using social learning variables. *Social Science and Medicine, 34*, 25–32.

Scherwitz, L. W., Perkins, L. L., Chesney, M. A., Hughes, G. H., Sidney, S., & Manolio, T. A. (1992). Hostility and health behaviors in young adults: The CARDIA Study. *American Journal of Epidemiology, 136*, 136–145.

Schinke, S. P., Gilchrist, L., & Snow, W. H. (1985). Skills intervention to prevent cigarette smoking among adolescents. *American Journal of Public Health, 75*, 665–667.

Schinke, S. P., Moncher, M. S., Palleja, J., Zayas, L. H., & Schilling, R. F. (1988). Hispanic youth, substance abuse, and stress: Implications for prevention research. *International Journal of the Addictions, 23*, 809–826.

Selye, H. (1978). *The stress of life.* New York: McGraw-Hill.

Shea, S., Stein, A., Basch, C., Lantigua, R., Maylahn, C., Strogatz, D., & Novick, L. (1991). Independent associations of educational attainment and ethnicity with behavioral risk factors for cardiovascular disease. *American Journal of Epidemiology, 134*, 567–582.

Sheeska, J. D., Woolcott, D. M., & MacKinnon, N. J. (1993). Social and cognitive theory as a framework to explain intentions to practice healthy eating behaviors. *Journal of Applied Social Psychology, 23*, 1547–1573.

Siegler, I. C., Peterson, B. L., Barefoot, J. C., & Williams, R. B. (1992). Hostility during late adolescence predicts coronary risk factors at mid-life. *American Journal of Epidemiology, 136*, 146–154.

St. Lawrence, J. S., Jefferson, K. W., Alleyne, E., & Brasfield, T. L. (1995). Comparison of education versus behavioral skills training interventions in lowering sexual HIV-risk behavior of substance-dependent adolescents. *Journal of Consulting and Clinical Psychology, 63*, 154–157.

Stein, J. A., Newcomb, M. D., & Bentler, P. M. (1987). An 8-year study of multiple influences on drug use and drug use consequences. *Journal of Personality and Social Psychology, 53*, 1094–1105.

Stern, M. P., Pugh, J. A., Gaskill, S. P., & Hazuda, H. P. (1982). Knowledge, attitudes, and behavior related to obesity and dieting in Mexican Americans and Anglos: The San Antonio Heart Study. *American Journal of Epidemiology, 115*, 917–928.

Strecher, V. J., DeVellis, B. M., Becker, M. H., & Rosenstock, I. M. (1986). The role of self-efficacy in achieving health behavior change. *Health Education Quarterly, 13*, 73–92.

Sussman, S., Dent, C. W., Flay, B. R., Hansen, W. B., & Johnson, C. A. (1987). Psychosocial predictors of cigarette smoking onset by White, Black, Hispanic, and Asian adolescents in southern California. *Morbidity and Mortality Weekly, 36*, 11S–16S.

Sussman, S., Dent, C. W., Stacy, A. W., Sun, P., Craig S., Simon, T. R., Burton, D., & Flay, B. R. (1993). Project Towards No Tobacco Use: One-year behavior outcomes. *American Journal of Public Health, 83*, 1245–1250.

Szalay, L. B., Canino, G., & Vilov, S. K. (1993). Vulnerabilities and cultural change: Drug use among Puerto Rican adolescents in the United States. *International Journal of the Addictions, 28*, 327–354.

Taylor, L. M., & Chatters, R. J. (1991). Religious life. In James Jackson (Ed.), *Life in Black America* (pp. 105–123). Newbury Park, CA: Sage.

Terrell, F., Taylor, J., & Terrell, S. (1980). Self-concept of juveniles who commit Black on Black crimes. *Corrective and Social Psychiatry, 26*, 107–109.

Thomas, M. E., Bethlehem, L. U., & Holmes, B. J. (1992). Determinants of satisfaction for Blacks and Whites. *Sociological Quarterly, 33*, 459–472.

Ulbrich, P. M., Warheit, G. J., & Zimmerman, R. S. (1989). Race, socioeconomic status, and psychological distress: An examination of differential vulnerability. *Journal of Health and Social Behavior, 30*, 131–146.

U.S. Department of Health and Human Services and National Institutes of Health. (1989). *Churches as an avenue to high blood pressure control* (NIH Publication No. 89–2725). Washington, DC: Author.

U.S. Department of Health and Human Services and U. S. Public Health Service. (1995). *CSAP implementation guide: Hispanic/Latino natural support systems* (DHHS Publication No. 95–3033). Rockville, MD: Public Health Service/SAMHSA.

Vega, W. A., Zimmerman, R. S., Warheit, G. J., Apospori, E., & Gil, A. G. (1993). Risk factors for early adolescent drug use in four ethnic and racial groups. *American Journal of Public Health, 83*, 185–189.

Walter, H. J., Vaughan, R. D., Gladis, M. M., Ragin, D. F., Kasen, S., & Cohall, A. T. (1993). Factors associated with AIDS-related behavioral intentions among high school students in an AIDS epicenter. *Health Education Quarterly, 20*, 409–420.

Warzak, W. J., Grow, C. R., Poler, M. M., & Walburn, J. N. (1995). Enhancing refusal skills: Identifying contexts that place adolescents at risk for unwanted sexual activity. *Journal of Developmental and Behavioral Pediatrics, 16*, 98–100.

Wills, T. A., Vaccaro, D., & McNamara, G. (1992). The role of life events, family support, and competence in adolescent substance use: A test of vulnerability and protective factors. *American Journal of Community Psychology, 20*, 349–374.

Wulfert, E., & Wan, C. K. (1993). Condom use: A self-efficacy model. *Health Psychology, 12*, 346–353.

10

Multisystemic Therapy and the Ethnic Minority Client: Culturally Responsive and Clinically Effective

Michael J. Brondino, Scott W. Henggeler, Melisa D. Rowland, Susan G. Pickrel, Phillippe B. Cunningham, and Sonja K. Schoenwald

R acial and ethnic minority groups constitute an increasing proportion of the American population. Indeed, projections estimate that one third of the U.S. population by the Year 2000 and more than one half by the Year 2010 will be composed of racial and ethnic minority group members (D. W. Sue, Arredondo & McDavis, 1992; Whitfield, 1994). Over the same period of time, ethnic minority mental health needs are expected to increase at rates faster than those of the U.S. White majority (Benjamin, 1993). In light of these demographic trends, the development of services that are responsive to the needs of the

Preparation of this chapter was supported by the National Institute on Drug Abuse (Grant DA08029), the National Institute of Mental Health (Grant MH51852), and the Office of Juvenile Justice and Delinquency Prevention (Grant 16542).

various racial and ethnic groups should be a goal of all social service systems.

In the area of mental health, evidence suggests that services have not been sufficiently responsive to the needs of ethnic minority clients. When compared with the White majority, ethnic minority group populations are less likely to use mental health services (Atkinson & Gim, 1989; S. Sue & Morishima, 1982), more likely to drop out of treatment prematurely (S. Sue, 1977; Vernon & Roberts, 1982), and less likely to openly discuss their problems with therapists (Atkinson & Gim, 1989). Such underutilization of mental health services has persisted despite the increased rates at which ethnic minority groups are exposed to stressors arising from cultural and intergenerational conflicts and prejudicial and discriminatory practices in comparison with the cultural majority (Atkinson & Gim, 1989; Gibbs & Huang, 1990; Padilla, Wagatsuma, & Lindholm, 1985).

Several explanations have been offered to account for the low rates of ethnic minority involvement in psychotherapy. One common explanation is that minority clients' values are in conflict with the process of traditional psychotherapy. Many minority individuals associate stigma and shame with mental health service use or hold beliefs about mental illness that bring them to seek medical or spiritual care rather than mental health care for their problems (Flaskerud, 1986; Franklin, 1992; Ruiz, 1990). On the other hand, traditional mental health services have been criticized for insufficiently addressing cultural factors important to the clients and for their inaccessibility because of inconvenient appointment times and locations (Atkinson & Gim, 1989; Flaskerud, 1986; Ho, 1992; S. Sue & Zane, 1987). Such difficulties are exacerbated by the fact that the majority of therapists come from White cultural groups and have been trained to provide psychotherapy using procedures largely developed among this dominant culture (D. W. Sue, 1981). Given the expanding role of ethnic minorities in society and the problems that minority groups experience in relation to traditional therapies, alternative therapies capable of addressing the needs of cultural minorities need to be developed, validated, and disseminated across systems of care.

Among the attempts to address the deficiencies in traditional mental health services is a model of treatment known as *multisystemic therapy* (MST; Henggeler & Borduin, 1990). We will discuss in depth the definition and use of MST later in the chapter. MST has demonstrated considerable success in engaging and retaining African American and

White families in treatment. More important, findings from clinical trials also show that MST has been equally effective with these cultural groups in obtaining favorable clinical outcomes. Such success is attributable, in part, to the manner in which MST addresses key issues believed to contribute to minority underutilization of mental health services. To illustrate this thesis, we briefly discuss several issues in therapy with minority group clients as well as provide recommendations for resolving these issues. The focus of our discussion is African Americans, because MST clinical trials have primarily included this minority group. However, MST may be a valuable approach to treatment with clients from a variety of ethnic minority backgrounds, and efforts are underway to demonstrate its applicability in other ethnic minority populations (e.g., see Thomas' [1994] study with a predominantly Hispanic sample in Galveston, Texas).

Issues in Therapy with Minority Clients

In the provision of mental health services to cultural minorities, problems may arise for several reasons. Among these are (a) therapist misinterpretation of culturally determined client social behaviors when such behaviors are viewed outside of their cultural context, (b) the client's preferences for counselor characteristics, (c) unique characteristics of minority family structure, (d) socioecological pressures on and social isolation of the client, (e) the provision of services that insufficiently address minority family needs, and (f) the client's mistrust of the people and systems providing services. Although this is only a partial listing, these issues represent formidable barriers to successful outcome in therapy with ethnic minority clients.

Therapist Misinterpretation of Client Behavior

To design effective interventions, therapists must appreciate how behaviors arise from their cultural substratum (Cross, Bazron, Dennis, & Isaacs, 1989; P. Wade & Bernstein, 1991). A failure to do so may result in misunderstandings about the meaning or relevance of a behavior and, consequently, the provision of inappropriate treatments. Carter (1974), for example, described an African American client whose behaviors in a clinical interview seemed to reflect paranoia. Such interpersonal suspiciousness, however, may actually reflect a normative response to interacting with White authority figures rather than any serious underlying psychopathology. Others have noted that the same indexes of mental illness in African Americans and Whites can result in different psychiatric diagnoses: African Americans are more often diagnosed as suffering from schizophrenia and Whites as having affective disorders (Adebimpe, 1981; Snowden & Cheung, 1990). Moreover, such differences in diagnostic outcomes can occur outside of any overt prejudicial beliefs or discriminatory practices of a therapist or system of care, and instead, may be attributable to such factors as social conventions regarding the physical distance between patient and clinician (Adebimpe, 1981). Unless these social conventions are understood by therapists and the minority client's behaviors are viewed within their cultural context, it is likely that mistakes in diagnosis and treatment will continue. The key to developing the capacity to distinguish between clinical psychopathology and differences in social convention most likely pertains to two processes. First, therapists must become as familiar as possible with the social conventions of the ethnic minorities that they serve. Second, clinical problems should always be examined with regard to their functionality, which may or may not be linked to social conventions. That is, in developing an understanding of the factors determining and maintaining a particular clinical problem, the therapist must consider cultural variables along with other aspects of the client's social environment.

Client Preferences for Counselor Characteristics

The impact of social distance extends beyond therapists' interpretations of clients' behavior to clients' preference for therapists with characteristics similar to their own. Several studies have found that clients prefer counselors who are racially or ethnically similar to themselves. For example, counselors of similar cultural backgrounds were rated more highly by clients than ethnically dissimilar counselors on the characteristics of trustworthiness, expertness, attractiveness, and the client's willingness to see the therapist (Ponce & Atkinson, 1989; Terrell & Terrell, 1984). Overall, this research suggests that matching clients to therapists on racial and ethnic dimensions may increase the willingness of members of minority groups to use mental health services and increase minority retention (Terrell & Terrell, 1984).

Several factors, however, may offset the potentially detrimental effects of racial and ethnic or cultural dissimilarity. Atkinson, Furlong, and Poston (1986), for example, found that African American clients preferred therapists who, in order of importance, (a) had a higher education, (b) held attitudes and values similar to their own, (c) were older in age than the client, (d) had a similar personality, and (e) were of the same ethnicity. Similar results have been reported among Native Americans (Bennett & BigFoot-Sipes, 1991). The ameliorating effect of perceived attitudinal similarity on ethnic and racial dissimilarity has been replicated in a number of studies involving a variety of minority groups including: (a) Mexican American college students (Atkinson, Ponce, & Martinez, 1984), (b) Chicano students (Furlong, Atkinson, & Casas, 1979), and (c) African American adolescents (Porche & Banikotes, 1982). Across these studies, attitudinal similarity was more strongly associated with positive personal impressions (increased attractiveness, expertise, and trust) than was simple ethnic similarity. Likewise, cultural dissimilarity effects may be moderated by the degree of the client's acculturation. Highly acculturated ethnic minority people show less preference for therapists of the same cultural background (Sanchez & Atkinson, 1983), increased recognition of the possible value of mental health services, and increased tolerance of the stigma attached to seeking such services (Atkinson & Gim, 1989). The demonstration of such moderating effects offers hope for service systems in which the therapists are drawn predominantly from the majority culture. In contrast with attempts to match therapists to clients on racial and ethnic dimensions, which may be difficult to implement because of the demographic characteristics of most mental health agency personnel pools, moderators may be more amenable to change by service systems. For example, practices involving (a) the disclosure of educational and continuing educational statuses of therapists, (b) the appropriate use of self-disclosure or the discussion of attitudinal and value systems during therapy, and (c) the inclusion of respected and more acculturated members of the minority community in therapeutic alliance building could be adopted by service systems to offset the effects of ethnic and racial dissimilarity.

Minority Family Structure

Because of cultural, historical, racial, and socioeconomic factors, family structure varies considerably across cultural groups. Filipino families, for example, typically function around egalitarian rather than patrilineal principles (Agbayani-Siewert, 1994), whereas family decision making and authority in Asian Indian families are centered with the husband and his mother (Hines, Garcia-Preto, McGoldrick, Almeida, & Weltman, 1992). African American families may be matriarchal, egalitarian, patriarchal, or intergenerational in structure (i.e., extended families spanning several generations and living in close geographical proximity to each other; J. C. Wade, 1994). Much, for example, has been written about the African American extended family, which is likely to include blood relations as well as people who have been informally adopted into the family (Boyd-Franklin, 1989; Hines et al., 1992).

Structural differences may also be found in the degree of role flexibility and boundary permeability in minority families. For example, African American families may be characterized by a high degree of role or boundary flexibility. Boyd-Franklin (1989) noted that role flexibility can be a strength as a survival mechanism but can also result in boundary confusion or situations in which one family member becomes overburdened from assuming too many roles. In African American families, boundary confusion is often intergenerationally based, centering around grandmothers who raise their children and grandchildren as their own. In comparison, the intergenerational relations in Irish families are often handled by the mother (Hines et al., 1992).

Because the structural form of a family is multidetermined, mental health problems associated with family structure can present a considerable challenge to therapists and may not be as changeable as therapeutic goals require (Boyd-Franklin, 1989). Boyd-Franklin, for example, provided an example of a woman who became a mother at an early age but continued to live with her mother in the same household in which the (now) grandmother was raising both the mother and grandchild as her children. In such a case, it can be extremely difficult to empower the mother sufficiently to take over the role of parent to the child because of her continuing dependence on her own mother, possible hesitancy of the grandmother to relinquish her maternal role, and possible resistance of the child.

Socioecological Pressures and Social Isolation

Socioecological pressures resulting from poverty, unemployment, prejudice, and discrimination have been linked to differences in family structure, parenting style, and child socialization techniques within and between ethnic minority populations (Fagan & Wexler, 1987;

Steinberg, Mounts, Lamborn, & Dornbusch, 1991). J. C. Wade (1994), for example, noted that between 1880 and 1925, African American households were typically headed by males and had two parents. During the 1960s, a drastic shift toward single-parent families began to take place, so that by 1980, 45.8% of African American homes were headed by single parents. According to Wade the increase in single-parent homes is partly attributable to U.S. society's emphasis on judging men by their ability to provide for their families in conjunction with societal discriminatory practices that limit the employment opportunities of African American men. Together, these social forces can engender feelings of low self-worth, with the result that many men find it difficult to associate with their families, and their role in socializing children decreases (J. C. Wade, 1994).

Social isolation is another problem faced by many families from ethnic minority groups. Agbayani-Siewart (1994), for example, noted that Filipino values stress interdependence and cooperation among family members and that these values are often lost in the emigration or acculturation process, which results in a loss of social support from the extended family. This loss may lead to conflict within the family because extended family members no longer act to buffer life stressors. Problems associated with social isolation have also been described for African American single mothers (Lindblad-Goldberg & Dukes, 1985; Loury, 1987), although extended family networks may offset any negative impact of stressors (Gray-Ray & Ray, 1990; Lindblad-Goldberg & Dukes, 1985). Thus, the possible importance of the extended family and informal support networks in addressing socioecological issues should not be overlooked when dominant-culture therapists work with ethnic minority clients. Incorporating these significant others in therapy can increase a therapist's effectiveness (Luckey, 1994).

Services That Do Not Meet Minority Family Needs

Traditional services may not address immediate family priorities for many reasons. Among these reasons are (a) inappropriate treatment resulting from misdiagnosis, as discussed previously; (b) the failure to address basic living needs such as health care, education, employment, and housing, which are often of greater concern to the clients than the goals therapists set for family functioning; and (c) strict adherence to clinical ideologies that have little bearing on the real-world functioning of ethnic minority families. Regarding basic living needs, if a service agency does not provide the needed case-management functions to address housing, vocational, and other needs, then mental health efforts may be wasted. Moreover, the failure to provide needed services can reinforce a client's beliefs in the inability of the service system to help with their problems in living, which may further impede the therapeutic process. Regarding agency ideological barriers to appropriate care, agency rules concerning confidentiality and "therapeutic boundaries" may prevent the therapist from enlisting the help of the client's informal support network, which may also decrease the possibility of obtaining a favorable clinical outcome.

Client's Lack of Confidence in People and Systems Providing Services

In response to discriminatory practices, issues of power, trust, and control have become central to the lives of many African Americans (J. C. Wade, 1994). The lack of cooperation that arises in therapy between White therapists and African American clients can sometimes be attributed to these factors as well as to one of the following: (a) prior experience with unresponsive institutions that are perceived as prying into the client's personal life; (b) the fact that traditional sources of help are nested in the client's family, friends, and church; (c) fear of having family secrets exposed; and (d) being remanded to therapy under threat or pressure (Boyd-Franklin, 1989). To enhance cooperation and achieve the goals of therapy, the establishment of a trusting client–therapist relationship is critical. However, as noted above, many potential barriers can attenuate the development of such a relationship. Next, we present possible solutions to the factors that impede mental health care use and favorable outcomes for ethnic minority individuals.

Prescriptions

One of the principle recommendations to address the aforementioned ethnic minority issues has been to increase the number of ethnic minority and bilingual counselors—essentially, to better match clients and therapists on ethnic characteristics (Flaskerud, 1986). Although increasing the percentage of ethnic minority mental health providers is an important long-term goal, matching clients to therapists is not a viable immediate solution in many communities. More useful are alternative recommendations for enhancing the cultural competence of existing mental health professionals (Hardy & Laszloffy, 1992; Pinderhughes, 1989) and for changing models of service delivery to improve accessibility of services (Berg & Miller, 1992; Henggeler, 1994). Unlike matching, changes in training and service delivery models can be implemented across varied systems of care and used by therapists of all racial and ethnic origins.

Cultural Competence

The current impetus for creating culturally competent systems of care has developed partly in response to the report by Knitzer (1982) entitled *Unclaimed Children*. Knitzer described many of the deficiencies in the service systems for children and adolescents and cited the failure of the federal government to provide leadership in addressing these deficiencies. In response to this report and through the work of several advocacy groups, the Child and Adolescent Service System Program (CASSP) was founded at the National Institute of Mental Health. CASSP's purpose was to help states develop competent systems of care for youth with severe emotional disturbances. The efforts of CASSP led to the publication of a monograph by Stroul and Friedman (1986) that outlined a series of core principles believed to serve as the foundation for effective systems of care. One of the core principles is that systems be culturally competent.

Although the idea of cultural competence was quickly espoused by social service agencies, few attempts were made initially to define the term sufficiently or to develop specific guidelines for training and professional standards that could be implemented across systems of care. Over the past decade, however, several efforts have been made to address these deficiencies (cf. Cross et al., 1989; Ho, 1992; D. W. Sue et al., 1992). Some have suggested the use of specific techniques in therapy with certain cultural groups. Ponce and Atkinson (1989), for example, found a directive style to be preferred by Mexican American college students. Shipp (1983) suggested using a group counseling format for African Americans. Some (e.g., Niles, 1993; Todisco & Salomone, 1991) have proposed guidelines to reduce or eliminate a lack of knowledge, bias, and awareness in counselors providing cross-cultural services. Still others (e.g., Boynton, 1987; Pedersen, 1981) have devised models of cross-cultural counseling or have suggested such system-level changes as the relocation of service centers in the community, the introduction of flexible hours, the use of brief therapy, the use of family members in therapy, and the involvement of clergy to increase cultural competence (Flaskerud, 1986).

In one of the most comprehensive attempts to address the issue of cultural competence to date, the Professional Standards Committee of the Association for Multicultural Counseling and Development developed guidelines that encompass a set of 31 competencies of therapists (D. W. Sue et al., 1992). These competencies include, for example, (a) an awareness of the therapist's own personal culturally based values and biases, (b) an awareness of the client's worldview, (c) the need to develop a broader range of skills, such as learning the client's language; and (d) a willingness to use additional resources compatible with cultural beliefs, such as consulting with traditional healers (D. W. Sue et al., 1992).

Although one can agree in principle, with many of these recommendations, shortcomings in their application should be acknowledged. Recommendations for applying particular methods of therapy with specific cultural groups have been criticized for ignoring individual differences among and within ethnic minority groups (e.g., Niles, 1993; S. Sue & Zane, 1987). A primary concern with recommending particular treatments for particular cultural groups is that therapists will use the advocated techniques in a boiler-plate fashion, without regard for the level of acculturation or other unique characteristics of the family (S. Sue, 1983). Educational programs designed to increase therapists' knowledge of cultures are unlikely to be effective in and of themselves because, as noted by S. Sue and Zane (1987), cultural knowledge is distal to the outcomes desired in therapy. To be useful, knowledge must be operationalized and then applied in conjunction with key intervening processes (e.g., development of client–therapist trust) if desired goals are to be achieved. The primary problem with most of the recommendations regarding cultural competence is that they are insufficiently operationalized in terms of training and criteria by which to judge the proficiency of their application. In addition, little empirical evidence supports the use of specific therapeutic techniques in relationship to the principles listed.

In summary, for several reasons pertaining to characteristics of minority families, therapists, and service systems, mental health services have often fit poorly with the needs of minority families. Although several groups of investigators are attempting to address key issues in the field of cultural competence, researchers are far from achieving "the answer," and much work remains. Nevertheless, some progress toward the development of family-based services that are culturally competent and clinically effective has been demonstrated for MST (Henggeler & Borduin, 1990). As described next, MST has shown favorable clinical outcomes for youth presenting serious clinical problems and their families. More important, such outcomes have not varied with the race of the family. That is, MST has been equally effective with African American families and White families. After describing the outcomes from several recent clinical trials, we discuss the basis of MST's cultural competence.

Outcome Studies Involving MST

The effectiveness of MST in addressing minority issues is evidenced by several completed and ongoing clinical trials, all of which have included relatively high percentages of minority families. In three of these studies, Borduin et al. (1995), Henggeler, Melton, and Smith (1992), and Henggeler, Pickrel, and Brondino (1996) demonstrated that favorable outcomes were not moderated by race. Brief descriptions of those pertinent studies are provided next.

Simpsonville, South Carolina

The Simpsonville project included 84 violent and chronic juvenile offenders who were at imminent risk for out-of-home placement because of their serious criminal activity (Henggeler et al., 1992). The youth averaged 3.5 arrests and 9.5 weeks of previous placement in correctional facilities. Their average age was 15.2 years; 56% were African American, 77% were male, the average Hollingshead (1975) social class score was 25 (i.e., at a level for semiskilled workers), and 26% lived with neither biological parent. Youth were randomly assigned to receive MST ($n = 43$) or usual services provided by the Department of Juvenile Justice ($n = 41$). Of the families assigned to MST, 86% completed treatment. At posttreatment, the MST youth reported greater reductions in criminal activity than did youth receiving usual services, with the effect being maintained through a 59-week follow-up, at which time MST youth averaged 0.87 rearrests versus

1.52 for the usual-services group and 5.8 weeks of incarceration versus 16.2 for the usual-services group. Data from a 2.4-year follow-up (Henggeler, Melton, Smith, Schoenwald, & Hanley, 1993) supported the continued effectiveness of MST for reducing criminal activity. Families that received MST also reported increased family cohesion and decreased aggression in their adolescent's peer relations. In contrast, family cohesion decreased and adolescent aggression with peers remained the same for adolescents who received usual services. Finally, data analyses indicated that the clinical changes were not associated with participants' race, age, social class, gender, or arrest and incarceration histories.

Columbia, Missouri

Borduin et al. (1995) compared the effectiveness of MST versus individual therapy (IT) in treating 200 12- to 17-year-old juvenile offenders and their families from Columbia, Missouri. The adolescents in the study averaged four previous arrests ($SD = 1.3$), and 61% had been incarcerated prior to their entry in the study. The adolescents averaged 14.7 years of age ($SD = 1.6$); 67% were male, 67% White, and 32.2% African American. Approximately 65% of the families were of low socioeconomic status (Hollingshead, 1975). At posttest, the families that received MST, compared with IT counterparts, showed greater increases in adaptability, cohesion, and supportiveness; decreased conflict-hostility during family discussions; and greater decreases in parental psychiatric symptomatology. MST effects on criminal behavior were maintained through a 4-year follow-up, and youth in the MST condition were found to be arrested less often, to be arrested for less serious offenses, and to have significantly lower rates of violent offenses and substance-related arrests (Henggeler et al., 1991) than IT youth. More important, 73.7% of the adolescents and families in the MST condition completed the full course of therapy. Again, favorable clinical outcomes were not mediated by participant demographic characteristics, including race.

Orangeburg and Spartanburg, South Carolina

The purpose of this 3-year multisite study was to evaluate the diffusability of MST across two rural mental health sites. In a preliminary examination of outcomes (Scherer, Brondino, Henggeler, Melton, &

Hanley, 1994), participating adolescents ranged in age from 11.7 to 17.3 years (M = 15.12 years); 82% were male, 78% were African American, and 22% were White. For 77% of the families, a single female was head of the household. Approximately 73% of the youth had been in at least one out-of-home placement, and 63% had committed a crime against another person. Findings indicated significant decreases in adolescent socialized aggression; decreases in parent symptomology, including depression; increases in parental monitoring; and improvements in family functioning for youth and families in the MST conditions. Participants receiving usual services deteriorated or did not change on these indicators. As in the earlier studies, outcomes did not differ across racial, urban versus rural, or socioeconomic categories. Comprehensive analyses on the full sample are currently under way and are expected to be complete by late 1996.

Charleston, South Carolina

The effectiveness of MST versus usual community services in the treatment of substance abusing or dependent delinquents is being examined in a 5-year study (Pickrel & Henggeler, 1996). Participants are 120 youth referred by the South Carolina Department of Juvenile Justice who had a *DSM-III-R* diagnosis of substance abuse or dependence. Researchers have examined dropout rates for this sample (Henggeler, Pickrel, Brondino, & Crouch, 1996) of which 47.5% of families were African American. Although substance abusing individuals make up a population that traditionally has low rates of retention in treatment (Stark, 1992), in the Pickrel and Henggeler study, only 1 of 60 families in the MST condition left treatment prematurely, and that family received 28 hrs of therapy over a period of 6 weeks. In addition, analyses of key ultimate and instrumental outcomes incorporating race as a moderator variable resulted in nonsignificant main and interaction effects for race across all dependent measures (Henggeler, Pickrel, & Brondino, 1996). Thus, irrespective of racial status, MST was extremely effective for engaging families in treatment and had similar outcomes.

Summary

Together, the research presented above supports our thesis that MST has shown considerable success in engaging and retaining participants while achieving positive outcomes in an increasing number of clinical trials. More important, these findings have been completed in different geographic locations with diverse populations, and the effects have been independent of participants' racial or ethnic and socioeconomic statuses. Next, we explore the clinical effectiveness of MST with minority families, which stems in part from the capacity of MST to successfully address the aforementioned issues that have been identified as important for providing mental health services for minority families.

Multisystemic Therapy and Minority Issues

Based on Bronfenbrenner's (1979) theory of social ecology, MST is a family-based treatment approach in which serious clinical problems are conceptualized as being multidetermined with the role of the individual, family, and extrafamilial systems playing important functions in the development and maintenance of such problems. Systemic as well as nonsystemic (individual) interventions are used, and special emphasis is placed on ensuring that strategies are developmentally appropriate for youth. All intervention strategies used throughout treatment are empirically derived and monitored for outcome.

For a model of service delivery, published clinical trials of MST have used the family preservation approach. In this approach, therapists provide MST work with families in their natural environment; that is, most meetings occur in the home, school, neighborhood, or community. The MST therapist is a generalist, who provides multiple therapeutic services (individual, family, marital therapy, and school consultation) as well as case management when indicated. Counselors are accessible 24 hr a day and 7 days a week and carry a caseload of four to six clients. Contact with the family occurs frequently (daily, if indicated) and treatment lasts 3 to 4 months.

With its social–ecological treatment approach and family preservation model of service delivery, MST by its very nature addresses key issues believed to contribute to ethnic minority underutilization of mental health services. To illustrate, we describe the clinical process of delivering MST and discuss how this process addresses the key treatment issues mentioned earlier that arise when working with minorities.

The Initial Assessment

Two ethnic minority issues directly targeted by the initial MST assessment are the concerns that services often do not meet ethnic minority family needs and that ethnic minority family structures are often misunderstood and not considered during therapy. The MST counselor helps to ensure that services are targeted to family need by emphasizing the role of the family in generating goals and by working with caregivers to ensure that basic living needs such as health care, education, and housing are met. MST assessments occur primarily in the home at times that are convenient for family members. Initially, the therapist meets with all individuals that live with the client or play a substantial caregiver role. The therapist's first goal is to affirm the parent's authority while obtaining each member's perspective about the presenting problems. The second goal is to assess the strengths and weaknesses of the individual, the family system, and the extrafamilial systems (peer, school, and support networks) to gain a better understanding of the fit of the identified problems with this broader systemic context. Finally, the therapist helps the family members develop a clear operational definition of the behaviors or problems that they would like to solve (Henggeler & Borduin, 1990). In this way, the natural setting and systemic focus of MST promote the development of interventions that include and use all pertinent individuals in the environment, thereby minimizing the chance that important resources in the family will go unnoticed.

Treatment Planning and Delivery

The possible misinterpretation of minority client behavior is directly addressed by the MST treatment planning and delivery process. As noted above, the therapist must appreciate the multidetermined nature of a client's behavior, including how it arises from the cultural substratum (Cross et al., 1989; P. Wade & Bernstein, 1991). Misinterpretation of this behavior and the resulting misunderstanding of its significance may lead to the provision of inappropriate and ineffective interventions. When assessing the fit between the identified problems and their broader systemic context, the MST therapist is trained to consider the role that culture plays in contributing both to the problem and to possible solutions. Regular supervision, input from other therapists, and continuous evaluation of the efficacy of interventions from multiple perspectives (client, family, therapist, teacher, and team supervisor) serve to reduce the misinterpretation of client behavior. Reducing misinterpretation of behavior enables accurate reconceptualizations of problems and modification of interventions when treatment goals are not being attained.

A second treatment issue addressed by MST in the process of treatment planning and delivery is the impact of social–ecological pressures and social isolation on the efficacy of interventions with ethnic minority clients. In MST, the importance of the extended family and informal support network is emphasized, and individuals in the natural environment are often used to assist family members in obtaining and maintaining therapeutic goals. Thus, at the close of the initial assessment, the therapist and family reach a consensus regarding the nature of the problems. The therapist's first treatment task is to provide interventions that are logically associated with these problems and that build on the strengths of individuals, family, and extrafamilial systems. Therapists are encouraged to develop treatment strategies that are present focused and action oriented, targeting specific and well-defined problems. Support systems are assessed early in the treatment process and extensive effort goes toward the development of networks, if these are insufficient. The ultimate goal of the interventions is the promotion of treatment generalization and long-term maintenance of therapeutic change. Thus, treatment strategies emphasize the development of skills that are to be used in the natural environment, and therapists work with family members to increase their capacity to develop and implement appropriate solutions to problems that enhance the family's link with natural community supports (e.g., extended family, neighbors, and the church).

Therapist Characteristics

The ethnic minority client's perceived lack of confidence in people and systems providing services suggests that treatments need to be more accessible and sensitive to the cultural needs of the individual (Berg & Miller, 1992; Hardy & Laszloffy, 1992; Henggeler, 1994). Although MST therapists are usually master's-level professionals from a variety of training backgrounds (e.g., social work, counseling, psychology, and education), we believe that it is the personal and interpersonal qualities of the therapists that are key to the delivery and efficacy of treatment. Some of the qualities emphasized in the selection of an MST therapist are social and interpersonal flexibility, self-confidence, intelligence, real-world experience, commitment to the families, and capacity to identify individual and family strengths. Thus, therapists who have experience with a range of human problems and who are sensitive to important cultural and ethnic issues are selected for the program. In addition, the MST therapist is trained to honor the racial, ethnic, cultural, and socioeconomic diversity of each family and to be flexible in adjusting their interpersonal styles to changing treatment needs. The family, therapist, and supervisor work together to design interventions that meet the needs of the family and fit with the counselor's characteristics, but the responsibility for therapeutic change ultimately rests with the therapist and treatment team (Henggeler et al., 1994). By holding the therapist and treatment program responsible for engaging and retaining the client in therapy as well as for clinical outcome, interventions are more likely to be readily accessible and to promote client confidence in therapists.

MST clients are not matched with therapists on a racial or ethnic basis, but treatment teams are composed of a cultural mix similar to the population being treated. Thus, supervision occurs regularly in a group format that provides multiple ethnic perspectives. This multi-ethnic group format, along with the counselor's strength-based focus and supportive stance, helps to promote an alliance with clients from diverse cultural backgrounds. If ethnic dissimilarities are a therapeutic issue, then they are addressed through the same process as with other family–therapist dissimilarities (e.g., family complaints that a therapist is too young, too old, does not have children, or is male vs. female).

Conclusion

Traditional mental health services have often fit poorly with the needs of minority families for reasons pertaining to characteristics of the families, therapists, and service systems. Criticisms of traditional services have ranged from the inconvenience of appointment times and locations and a failure to address basic family needs to the provision of services according to values that conflict with those of ethnic minority clients. These deficiencies are compounded by a predominance of therapists from the White majority culture, problems stemming from ethnic minority family structure in interaction with the larger societal context, social–ecological pressures on families, and client preferences for therapists. Together, these characteristics act to reduce ethnic minority involvement in therapy. Attempts by service systems to address these problems have often been piecemeal, involving such practices as matching clients to therapists or making available more bilingual therapists. More recently, an emphasis has been placed on increasing a service system's overall level of cultural competence. Although this is laudable in principle, insufficient operationalization of recommendations for cultural competence training and evaluation impedes the viability of this approach in the immediate future. Alternatively, as documented from outcomes of clinical trials of MST with African American and White families, it is possible to address identified failings of mental health systems by building cultural competence into the specification of treatment and service delivery models. Moreover, we contend that the proof of cultural competence is best demonstrated in positive client and family outcomes.

REFERENCES

Adebimpe, V. R. (1981). Overview: White norms and psychiatric diagnosis of Black patients. *American Journal of Psychiatry, 138*, 279–285.

Agbayani-Siewert, P. (1994). Filipino American culture and family: Guidelines for practitioners. *Families in Society, 75*, 429–438.

Atkinson, D. R., Furlong, M. J., & Poston, W. C. (1986). Afro-American preferences for counselor characteristics. *Journal of Counseling Psychology, 33*, 326–330.

Atkinson, D. R., & Gim, R. H. (1989). Asian-American cultural identity and attitudes toward mental health services. *Journal of Counseling Psychology, 36*, 209–212.

Atkinson, D. R., Ponce, F. Q., & Martinez, F. M. (1984). Effects of ethnic, sex, and attitude similarity on counselor credibility. *Journal of Counseling Psychology, 31*, 588–590.

Benjamin, M. P. (1993). *Child and adolescent service system program minority initiative research monograph.* Washington, DC: Georgetown University Child Development Center.

Bennett, S. K., & BigFoot-Sipes, D. S. (1991). American Indian and White college student preferences for counselor characteristics. *Journal of Counseling Psychology, 38*, 440–445.

Berg, I. K., & Miller, S. D. (1992). Working with Asian American clients: One person at a time. *Families in Society, 73,* 356–363.

Borduin, C. M., Mann, B. J., Cone, L. T., Henggeler, S. W., Fucci, B. R., Blaske, D. M., & Williams, R. A. (1995). Multisystemic treatment of serious juvenile offenders: Long-term prevention of criminality and violence. *Journal of Consulting and Clinical Psychology, 63,* 569–578.

Boyd-Franklin, N. (1989). *Black families in therapy: A multisystems approach.* New York: Guilford Press.

Boynton, G. (1987). Cross-cultural family therapy: The ESCAPE model. *American Journal of Family Therapy, 15,* 123–130.

Bronfenbrenner, U. (1979). *The ecology of human development: Experiments by nature and design.* Cambridge, MA: Harvard University Press.

Carter, J. H. (1974). Recognizing psychiatric symptoms in Black Americans. *Geriatrics, 29,* 95–99.

Cross, T. L., Bazron, B. J., Dennis, K. W., & Isaacs, M. R. (1989). *Towards a culturally competent system of care* (Vol. 1). Washington, DC: Georgetown University Child Development Center.

Fagan, J., & Wexler, S. (1987). Family origins of violent delinquents. *Criminology, 25,* 643–669.

Flaskerud, J. H. (1986). The effects of culture-compatible intervention on the utilization of mental health services by minority clients. *Community Mental Health Journal, 22,* 127–141.

Franklin, A. J. (1992). Therapy with African American men. *Families in Society, 73,* 350–355.

Furlong, M. J., Atkinson, D. R., & Casas, J. M. (1979). Effects of counselor ethnicity and attitudinal similarity on Chicano students' perceptions of counselor credibility and attractiveness. *Hispanic Journal of Behavioral Science, 1,* 41–43.

Gibbs, J. T., & Huang, L. N. (1990). *Children of color: Psychological intervention with minority youth.* San Francisco, CA: Jossey-Bass.

Gray-Ray, P., & Ray, M. C. (1990). Juvenile delinquency in the Black community. *Youth and Society, 22,* 67–84.

Hardy, K. V., & Laszloffy, T. A. (1992). Training racially sensitive family therapists: Context, content, and contact. *Families in Society, 73,* 364–370.

Henggeler, S. W. (1994). A consensus: Conclusions of the APA task force report on innovative models of mental health services for children, adolescents, and their families. *Journal of Clinical Child Psychology, 23*(Suppl.), 3–6.

Henggeler, S. W., & Borduin, C. M. (1990). *Family therapy and beyond: A multisystemic approach to treating behavior problems of children and adolescents.* Pacific Grove, CA: Brooks/Cole.

Henggeler, S. W., Borduin, C. M., Melton, G. B., Mann, B. J., Smith, L., Hall, J. A., Cone, L., & Fucci, B. R. (1991). Effects of multisystemic therapy on drug use and abuse in serious juvenile offenders: A progress report from two outcome studies. *Family Dynamics of Addiction Quarterly, 1,* 40–51.

Henggeler, S. W., Melton, G. B., & Smith, L. A. (1992). Family preservation using multisystemic therapy: An effective alternative to incarcerating serious juvenile offenders. *Journal of Consulting and Clinical Psychology, 60,* 953–961.

Henggeler, S. W., Melton, G. B., Smith, L. A., Schoenwald, S. K., & Hanley, J. H. (1993). Family preservation using multisystemic treatment: Long-term follow-up to a clinical trial with serious juvenile offenders. *Journal of Child and Family Studies, 2,* 283–293.

Henggeler, S. W. Pickrel, S. G., and Brondino, M. J. (1996). *Multisystemic treatment of substance abusing and dependent delinquents: Outcomes for drug use, criminality, and out-of-home placement at posttreatment and 6-month follow-up.* Manuscript submitted for publication.

Henggeler, S. W., Pickrel, S. G., Brondino, M. J., & Crouch, J. L. (1996). Eliminating (almost) treatment dropout of substance abusing or dependent delinquents through home-based multisystemic therapy. *American Journal of Psychiatry, 153,* 427–428.

Henggeler, S. W., Schoenwald, S. K., Pickrel, S. G., Brondino, M. J., Borduin, C. M., & Hall, J. A. (1994). *Treatment manual for family preservation using multisystemic therapy.* Columbia: South Carolina Health and Human Services Finance Commission.

Hines, P. M., Garcia-Preto, N., McGoldrick, M., Almeida, R., & Weltman, S. (1992). Intergenerational relationships across cultures. *Families in Society, 73,* 323–338.

Ho, M. K. (1992). *Minority children and adolescents in therapy.* Newbury Park, CA: Sage.

Hollingshead, A. B. (1975). *Four factor index of social status.* Unpublished manuscript, Yale University, Department of Sociology, New Haven.

Knitzer, J. (1982). *Unclaimed children.* Washington, DC: Children's Defense Fund.

Lindblad-Goldberg, M., & Dukes, J. L. (1985). Social support in Black, low income, single parent families: Normative and dysfunctional families. *American Journal of Orthopsychiatry, 58,* 104–120.

Loury, G. C. (1987). The family as context for delinquency prevention: Demographic trends and political realities. In J. Q. Wilson & G. C. Loury (Eds.), *From children to citizens, Vol. 3. Families, schools, and delinquency prevention* (pp. 3–26). New York: Springer-Verlag.

Luckey, I. (1994). African American elders: The support network of generational kin. *Families in Society, 75,* 82–89.

Niles, F. S. (1993). Issues in multicultural counselor education. *Journal of Multicultural Counseling and Development, 21,* 14–21.

Padilla, A., Wagatsuma, Y., & Lindholm, K. (1985). Acculturation and personality as predictors of stress in Japanese and Japanese Americans. *Journal of Social Psychology, 125,* 295–305.

Pedersen, P. (1981). Triad counseling. In R. Corsini (Ed.), *Handbook of innovative psychotherapies* (pp. 840–854). New York: Wiley.

Pickrel, S. G., & Henggeler, S. W. (1996). Multisystemic therapy for adolescent substance abuse and dependence. *Child and Adolescent Psychiatric Clinics of North America, 5*(1), 201–211.

Pinderhughes, E. (1989). *Understanding race, ethnicity, and power*. New York: Free Press.

Ponce, F. Q., & Atkinson, D. R. (1989). Mexican-American acculturation, counselor ethnicity, counseling style, and perceived counselor credibility. *Journal of Counseling Psychology, 36*, 203–208.

Porche, L. M., & Banikotes, P. G. (1982). Racial and attitudinal factors affecting the perceptions of counselors by Black adolescents. *Journal of Counseling Psychology, 29*, 169–174.

Ruiz, D. S. (1990). *Handbook of mental health and mental disorder among Black Americans*. New York: Greenwood Press.

Sanchez, A. R., & Atkinson, D. R. (1983). Mexican-American cultural commitment, preference for counselor ethnicity, and willingness to use counseling. *Journal of Counseling Psychology, 30*, 215–220.

Scherer, D. G., Brondino, M. J., Henggeler, S. W., Melton, G. B., & Hanley, J. H. (1994). Multisystemic family preservation therapy: Preliminary findings from a study of rural and minority serious adolescent offenders. *Journal of Emotional and Behavioral Disorders, 2*, 198–206.

Shipp, P. L. (1983). Counseling Blacks: A group approach. *Personnel and Guidance Journal, 62*, 108–111.

Snowden, L. R., & Cheung, F. K. (1990). Use of inpatient mental health services by members of ethnic minority groups. *American Psychologist, 45*, 347–355.

Stark, M. J. (1992). Dropping out of substance abuse treatment: A clinically oriented interview. *Clinical Psychology Review, 12*, 93–116.

Steinberg, L., Mounts, N. S., Lamborn, S. D., & Dornbusch, S. M. (1991). Authoritative parenting and adolescent adjustment across varied ecological niches. *Journal of Research on Adolescence, 1*, 19–36.

Stroul, B. E., & Friedman, R. M. (1986). *A system of care for children and youth with severe emotional disturbances*. Washington, DC: Georgetown University Child Development Center.

Sue, D. W. (1981). *Counseling the culturally different: Theory and practice*. New York: Wiley.

Sue, D. W., Arredondo, P. A., & McDavis, R. J. (1992). Multicultural counseling competencies and standards: A call to the profession. *Journal of Multicultural Counseling and Development, 20*, 64–88.

Sue, S. (1977). Community mental health services to minority groups: Some optimism, some pessimism. *American Psychologist, 32*, 616–624.

Sue, S. (1983). Ethnic minority issues in psychology: A reexamination. *American Psychologist, 38*, 583–592.

Sue, S., & Morishima, J. K. (1982). *The mental health of Asian Americans*. San Francisco: Jossey-Bass.

Sue, S., & Zane, N. (1987). The role of culture and cultural techniques in psychotherapy. *American Psychologist, 42*, 37–45.

Terrell, F., & Terrell, S. (1984). Race of counselor, client sex, cultural mistrust level, and premature termination from counseling among Black clients. *Journal of Counseling Psychology, 31*, 371–375.

Thomas, C. R. (1994). *Island youth programs*. Unpublished manuscript, University of Texas Medical Branch, Galveston.

Todisco, M., & Salomone, P. R. (1991). Facilitating effective cross-cultural relationships: The White counselor and the Black client. *Journal of Multicultural Counseling and Development, 19,* 146–157.

Vernon, S. W., & Roberts, R. E. (1982). Prevalence of treated and untreated
psychiatric disorders in three ethnic groups. *Social Science and Medicine,
16,* 1575–1582.

Wade, J. C. (1994). African American fathers and sons: Social, historical, and
psychological considerations. *Families in Society, 75,* 561–570.

Wade, P., & Bernstein, B. L. (1991). Culture sensitivity training, and counselor's
race: Effects on Black female clients' perceptions and attrition. *Journal of
Counseling Psychology, 38,* 9–15.

Whitfield, D. (1994). Toward an integrated approach to improving multicultural counselor education. *Journal of Multicultural Counseling and Development, 22,* 239–252.

School-Based Interventions to Prevent Substance Use Among Inner-City Minority Adolescents

Mary Ann Forgey, Steven Schinke, and Kristin Cole

Because the use of tobacco, alcohol, and drugs is physically harmful, physiologically addictive, and psychologically and socially detrimental, efforts to prevent the use of these substances among young people are forcefully advocated and widely practiced. Numerous substance use prevention approaches have evolved over the years. Typically, these interventions are targeted primarily at majority culture youth and take place in schools. School settings provide researchers with efficient access to large numbers of adolescents. Yet few school-based prevention approaches have proven effective in reducing substance use among adolescents, and even fewer have been tested with youth of minority cultures.

In this chapter, we discuss and illustrate issues in conducting school-based, culturally sensitive substance abuse prevention research with minority youth on the basis of our own research experiences.

251

Although our study targeted African American and Hispanic youth, the principles and skills drawn from its development process can be applied to work with other ethnic and racial groups. We begin by considering the history of school-based substance abuse prevention programs. Next, we present our substance abuse intervention study among inner-city minority youth. Finally, we discuss the implications of our findings for inner-city minority youth.

Past Approaches to Substance Abuse Prevention

The most common approach to school-based substance use prevention over the past few decades has been to simply provide adolescents with factual information about tobacco, alcohol, and drug use. This approach, known as information education, dwells on the nature, pharmacology, and adverse consequences of substance use, with the assumption that, once individuals are aware of the health hazards of using tobacco, alcohol, and drugs, they will develop antidrug attitudes and make the rational and logical decision not to use drugs. Empirical evidence of the ineffectiveness of such traditional approaches to tobacco, alcohol, and drug use prevention is extensive (e.g., see Berberian, Gross, Lovejoy, & Paparella, 1976; Kinder, Pape, & Walfish, 1980; Richards, 1969; Schaps, Di Bartolo, Moskowitz, Palley, & Churgin, 1981; Schaps, Moskowitz, Malvin, & Schaeffer, 1986; Swisher & Hoffman, 1975). In fact, there has even been some evidence that information education may lead to increased usage (Mason, 1973; Swisher, Crawford, Goldstein, & Yura, 1971).

In the mid-1970s, researchers began to recognize the need to provide guidance, as well as information, to help adolescents. This realization progressively shifted focus away from an informational approach and toward an emphasis on personal and social growth. The underlying assumption of this approach is that adolescents use drugs because they have low self-esteem and inappropriate values (Swisher, 1979). Such affective education programs typically include experiential classroom activities intended to increase self-esteem, communication skills, values clarification, and decision making.

Affective education approaches have, in some instances, been able to demonstrate an impact on one or more of the correlates of substance use, but they have not been successful in changing behavior. Studies on the efficacy of Here's Looking at You, a widely used affective education program, have shown an increase in knowledge about alcohol but no positive impact on drinking behavior (e.g., see Kim, 1988). In evaluating a similar approach, the Me–Me program (conducted with students in Grades 2 through 6), Kearney and Hines (1980) found that—despite an increase in self-esteem, decision making, knowledge about drugs, and a positive change in attitudes toward drug use—no behavioral effects were evident.

The affective programs mentioned above were not developed in a culturally sensitive context. Some minority investigators have argued that prevention strategies with minority youth need to incorporate the traditions and rituals of the targeted ethnic or racial populations into the content and process of prevention programs (Tucker, 1985). Emphasizing cultural pride, according to these investigators, is critical to building self-esteem among minority group adolescents (Tucker, 1985). In particular, Knox (1985) has recommended exploring sources of hope, strength, and spirituality in the African American community when attempting to prevent substance abuse among African American youth.

Emerging Approaches to Substance Use Prevention

Emerging approaches to the prevention of tobacco, alcohol, and drug use among youth draw from psychosocial theories that identify those elements of the individual's social environment that affect his or her behavior. These interventions differ from affective education because they emphasize behavioral rehearsal. On the basis of a slowly growing understanding of the psychological, social, and environmental factors that contribute to drug use, these approaches have been the most promising so far (Botvin, 1986). Two theories that have influenced the growing recognition of the importance of sociocultural environment to preventive interventions are social–cognitive theory (Bandura, 1986) and problem behavior theory (Jessor & Jessor, 1977).

Social–cognitive theory views learning as a reciprocal interaction between an individual's environment, cognitive processes, and behavior. According to this theory, substance abuse is learned through a process of modeling and reinforcement and is mediated by such intrapersonal factors as thoughts, attitudes, and expectations. As adolescents develop self-concepts and begin to mimic adult behavior, they are particularly keen observers of role models other than their parents, such as peers, older siblings, or high-profile media celebrities. If adolescents perceive high-status role models to be using substances, then they are likely to consider smoking, drinking, or drug use as a means of achieving such social status themselves.

General susceptibility to social influences (Bandura, 1986), and, in particular, social influences promoting substance use (Demone, 1973; Jessor, Collins, & Jessor, 1972; Wechsler & Thum, 1973), have been related to low self-esteem, low self-satisfaction, low self-confidence, a greater need for social approval, diminished sense of personal control, low assertiveness, and an impatience to assume adult roles or appear grown up. On the basis of this theoretical formulation and existing empirical evidence, researchers have hypothesized that resistance to social influences could be promoted by fostering the development of specific thoughts, attitudes, and expectations that counter any positive association with drugs, as well as skills for coping positively with life situations and for dealing with offers to use drugs (Schinke, Botvin, & Orlandi, 1991).

Problem behavior theory begins by defining a "problem behavior" as one that is considered inappropriate within the context of a particular value system and that typically elicits a social response designed to control it, whether informal (e.g., getting grounded) or formal and substantial (e.g., getting arrested). Many problem behaviors are age graded; that is, they are permissible for members of an older age group but are viewed as problems for younger individuals (e.g., smoking, drinking, and sexual involvement). For these behaviors, age norms may serve as defining characteristics.

Problem behavior theory recognizes the social function of problem behavior in the lives of many adolescents and argues that an important reason adolescents engage in problem behaviors is that these behaviors help the adolescent achieve personal goals (e.g., acceptance from a particular peer group). Problem behaviors might also serve as a way of coping with failure (real or anticipated), boredom, social anxiety, unhappiness, rejection, social isolation, low self-esteem, or a lack of self-efficacy.

According to problem behavior theory, vulnerability to engage in substance use is greater for adolescents who have fewer effective coping strategies in their repertoire, have fewer skills for handling social situations, and have greater anxiety about social situations. For these adolescents, discomfort in interpersonal situations is great, motivating them to take some action in an effort to alleviate that discomfort. Unless adolescents are given alternative ways of achieving personal and social goals, coping with anxiety, and establishing effective interpersonal relationships, they may be unwilling to give up substance use.

Psychosocial approaches to preventing drug abuse, like their antecedents, use school-based interventions targeted at adolescents, and they include some of the techniques found most promising in affective education. The primary content difference in psychosocial approaches is that the messages delivered to the students are based on social–cognitive theory (Bandura, 1986) and problem behavior theory (Jessor & Jessor, 1977). The primary methodological difference in psychosocial approaches has been recognition of the need for special instructor training and intervention delivery procedures.

Some psychosocial approaches place a primary emphasis on increasing students' awareness of the social influences promoting tobacco and alcohol use (i.e., psychological inoculation) and teaching specific techniques for resisting such pressures. Others emphasize the development of social competence by teaching general personal and social coping skills. These skills-based approaches take a somewhat broader perspective on the problem of substance use by attempting to target several of its most significant underlying determinants.

The prevention of substance abuse through the provision of personal and social skills training is an approach based on both social–cognitive theory and problem behavior theory (Botvin, Baker, Dusenbury, Tortu, & Botvin, 1990; Botvin, Baker, Filazzola, & Botvin, 1990; Gilchrist & Schinke, 1983; Pentz, 1983; Schinke & Blythe, 1981; Schinke & Gilchrist, 1984). Of the several tests of this approach, the most impressive results have been for smoking prevention. Studies have demonstrated that generic skills approaches to smoking prevention can produce reductions in experimental smoking ranging from 42% to 75%. Schinke and Gilchrist (1983) found a 79% reduction in the prevalence of experimental smoking after intervention. Other studies (Botvin & Eng, 1982; Botvin, Renick, & Baker, 1983) have demonstrated reductions ranging from 56% to 67% in the proportion of pretest nonsmokers becoming regular smokers at the 1-year follow-up. In another study, Botvin, Dusenbury, Baker, and James-Ortiz (1989) reported an 87% reduction in the initiation of regular smoking for students who participated in a prevention program.

Studies focused on preventing drug abuse with personal and social skills training have also shown positive results (e.g., see Botvin, Baker, Renick, Filazzola, & Botvin, 1984; Gilchrist, Schinke, Trimble, & Cvetkovich, 1987; Pentz et al., 1989; Schinke, Bebel, Orlandi, & Botvin, 1988). Alcohol use, however, has proven less preventable with this approach (Ellickson & Bell, 1990; Hansen, Malotte & Fielding, 1988).

Warranting further study is the relative effectiveness of different delivery strategies of personal and social skills training for various target populations. Thus far, the majority of programs based on the social influence and social skills model have been implemented with majority culture youth, although some programs have focused on Native American youth (Gilchrist et al., 1987; Schinke, Orlandi, et al., 1988) and others with predominantly African American and Hispanic students (Ellickson & Bell, 1990; Hansen, Johnson, Flay, Graham, & Sobel, 1988). Of those programs implemented with minority youth, few have been designed to address culturally specific risk factors. In the remainder of this chapter, we report on our efforts to develop and test a culturally tailored, school-based strategy for drug abuse prevention for inner-city minority youth.

Intervention Development

On the basis of findings from empirical research and representative focus groups, we developed a school-based, culturally tailored intervention to prevent substance abuse among inner-city minority youth (Forgey, 1994)—the Culturally Tailored Intervention, or CTI—and compared its effectiveness to a personal and social skills training intervention called Life Skills Training (LST; Botvin, Baker, Renick, Filazzola, & Botvin, 1984). Both the CTI and the LST approach are grounded in the theoretical assumptions of social–cognitive theory and problem behavior theory. Both methods thus involve teaching domain-specific and generic social skills to enable adolescents to resist substance use and teaching personal and social skills to increase adolescents' overall social competence and promote the development of interpersonal characteristics associated with decreased substance-use risk. Specific skills delivered by both interventions include decision making, communication, resistance (to both personal and media influences), stress management, self-esteem building, and help seeking. Furthermore, both interventions use cognitive–behavioral techniques of demonstration, behavioral rehearsal, feedback, reinforcement, and homework assignments.

Although the skills content of the CTI approach mirrors that of LST, the CTI differs from LST in its focus on addressing specific risk factors for African American and Hispanic youth. Specifically, the CTI uses a professional storyteller to relate mythic, culturally relevant stories; a contemporary rap video; and peer leaders to deliver certain sections of the curriculum.

The multicultural mythic stories in the CTI curriculum are drawn from ancient African, Spanish, and Greek cultures. Students witness a dramatization of the story and later, during skills sessions, review those parts of the story that highlight a particular skill. Skills illustrated in the mythic stories are subsequently related to students' contemporary circumstances in skills sessions. By seeing the positive consequences of using skills first, in the story structure, students see the application and meaning of the skill, which in turn enhances their observational learning process (Bandura, 1986). The multicultural ancient stories ground the skills lessons in a meaningful context for the target population. Such a context was meant to increase students' self-esteem, race-consciousness, cultural pride, and understanding of other cultures—all factors that are associated with minority risk for substance abuse (Gary & Berry, 1985; Kleiman & Lukoff, 1978; Szapocznik & Kurtines, 1980; Tucker, 1985).

The CTI also includes stories of historical and contemporary African American and Hispanic heroes and heroines. These biographies have been adapted to highlight how each hero or heroine used skills to overcome obstacles. Many of the obstacles in the biographies (e.g., poverty, discrimination, and family dissolution) are similar to those faced by inner-city African American and Hispanic adolescents today. The biographies in the CTI also address the sense of hopelessness that plagues so many inner-city adolescents. Each biography serves as an example of positive options to substance use and drug culture involvement. Because the stories also relate how each hero or heroine achieved his or her goals along conventional pathways, the risk factor of alienation from social institutions is concurrently addressed (Kaplan, Martin, Johnston, & Robbins, 1986). There is a lack of evidence for the use of culturally specific biographies in substance abuse prevention, but such stories have been proven effective for treating anxiety symptoms in Hispanic children (Constantino, Malgady, & Rogler, 1990).

A contemporary rap video is also used in the CTI. The video portrays two female and two male characters and the situations they encounter growing up in the inner city. As they negotiate situations, the characters model skills from the CTI curriculum. Students view distinct episodes of the video during class sessions, with each segment teaching a different skill.

To enhance the cultural sensitivity of the rap videotape, we recruited peer leaders and school personnel to help develop its script. The purpose in using a videotape was to demonstrate intervention skills in an engaging and meaningful style, and, as Bandura (1986) has noted, positive identification with characters and the contextual relevance of the modeling incident are important components of successful observational learning. An example of a contextually relevant modeling incident in the CTI videotape is a scene involving drug dealing. According to the peer leaders involved in script development, such a scene was more relevant to youth than a drug-using situation. These perceptions were echoed in a U.S. General Accounting Office (1990) drug education survey, in which students criticized the drug education they received because it did not address the subject of drug selling, a problem they said was as prevalent as drug use itself. The CTI rap videotape reflects inner-city African American and Hispanic risk factors by teaching skills within the context of an environment that offers easy access to drugs and strong peer influences. Other videotape segments teach skills to increase positive peer and adult support.

Empirical evidence supports the use of videotapes to enhance students' attentional, retentional, and conceptualization processes (Elias, 1983; Greenfield & Beagles-Roos, 1988; Harwood & Weissberg, 1987; Newcomb & Collins, 1979). Particularly with students who are less academically skilled—and thus, at higher risk for substance abuse (Barnes & Welte, 1986; Jessor, Chase, & Donavan, 1980)—the use of videotape with its attention-focusing capabilities (instant playback, visual focusing, and explicit verbal labeling) appears well suited for teaching skills.

Peer leaders were included in the CTI to model skills through role-playing and to assist adult leaders. Researchers have identified peer influence as one of the strongest risk factors for majority and minority culture substance abuse among youth (Beauvais, 1992; Oetting & Beauvais, 1987). Others (e.g., Botvin, Baker, Dusenbury, et al., 1990; Comstock & Cobbey, 1979; Murray, Johnson, Luepker, & Mittlemark, 1984; Tobler, 1986) have documented the effectiveness of using peer leaders in substance use prevention. Finally, a life story component in the CTI gives students an opportunity to record how each skill relates to their own lives. The use of a life story as a positive coping technique in dealing with adverse life events also has clinical support (see Borden, 1989, 1992).

In addition to having a different delivery strategy, the CTI approach differs from the LST approach because it does not include a knowledge component. A knowledge component was consciously omitted from the CTI because previous research (Berberian et al., 1976; Kinder et al., 1980; Swisher et al., 1971) has questioned its usefulness. Against the backdrop of theoretical and empirical support for a culturally tailored prevention intervention, we planned and executed an empirical test of the CTI with a sample of inner-city minority youth, described next.

Empirical Evaluation of the CTI

Sample

We recruited six schools from the New York City public school system for study participation. Of the 757 seventh-grade students who participated in our study, 639 (84%) provided complete data at both pre- and posttest. The mean age of students in the sample was 12.7 years. The sample was evenly split by gender. Approximately half (49%) of the students were African American; the remainder of the sample was 37% Hispanic, 5% White, and 1% Asian.

Research Design

Participating schools were randomly assigned to one of the three study conditions: CTI, LST, and test-only control. Next, informed and consenting seventh-grade students completed pretest measurements. After the students in the first two conditions received their respective interventions, all students completed posttest measurements. Measurements consisted of a 149-item self-report questionnaire and a breathalyzer test. Booster sessions were delivered 6 and 12 months after initial intervention to those in the treatment conditions.

Measures

Selecting sound measurement instruments is frequently a problem when one is working with minority communities. Most measures that exist for study phenomena have been developed for general population studies and are not sensitive to ethnic or racial populations. Instruments measuring risk factors for substance abuse, for example, typically do not include items assessing cultural pride and race consciousness—both factors associated with minority youth substance abuse (Gary & Berry, 1985; Tucker, 1985). Options for resolving these issues include using a widely accepted measure that does not have normative data for the target group; adjusting a widely accepted measure that used normative data; and developing new measures to respond to some of the culturally specific risk factors relevant to the target population. The choice of which option or combination of options to use often depends on time limitations and financial resources of the study.

In our own research experience, we have formatively and psychometrically tested outcome measurement instruments for use in quantifying the effects of substance abuse prevention programs with minority adolescents. Formative testing with focus groups of target subjects refines and adds precision to each measurement instrument and scale. Yet, focus-group data can be marred by participants' biases. Investigators can also prejudice focus-group data by asking participants leading questions. To help guard against such biases, researchers should conduct multiple sessions with a random selection of community participants.

Once focus-group data have informed changes to the format, ordering, and language of each item, one should psychometrically test the measures. Psychometric tests determine the reliability of each instrument and scale through test–retest and split–half procedures. Whenever feasible, we cross-validate our measures' scores with data from parallel instruments. For example, data from a new or adapted measure can be compared with findings from extant measures on the same variables.

In this study of the CTI and LST approaches to substance use prevention, participants completed a 149-item self-report questionnaire in 1 hour at pretest and posttest. Questionnaire items measured reported substance use behavior and intentions to use substances in the next year. Also included in the self-report questionnaire were items concerning the perceived prevalence of smoking, drinking, and marijuana use by peers and the perceived attitudes of significant others toward the respondents' use of these substances. Other questions measured cognitive, attitudinal, skills, and psychological variables associated with substance use. Included in the psychological variables was a measure of hopelessness. This variable was incorporated in an effort to capture the impact of the interventions on the risk factors related to low expectations for the future and alienation from social institutions (Kaplan, Martin, & Robbins, 1982; Kaplan, Martin, Johnston, & Robbins, 1986; Wilson, 1987). We used the Hopelessness Scale for Children (Kazdin, French, Unis, Esveldt-Dawson, & Sherick, 1983) to measure this variable. Because of time limitations and financial constraints, we did not develop measures to study the effects of other culturally specific mediating variables.

Results

The results of our empirical evaluation demonstrated that both the CTI and LST approaches were useful for high-risk minority youth. At posttest, these findings emerged primarily with respect to behavioral intention to drink or use drugs in the future. Disproving our hypotheses, both approaches were equally effective in decreasing risk for drinking beer or wine at posttest. Both prevention programs influenced several mediating variables in a direction consistent with avoidance of drug use.

Differences in the effectiveness of the two interventions did emerge at the 2-year follow-up. By this time, students in both prevention approaches still drank alcohol less often; were drunk less often; and had lower intentions to drink beer, wine, or liquor in the future relative to students in the control condition. However, participants in the CTI condition drank less and intended to drink less than did those from the LST and control conditions.

In other research into the effectiveness of substance use prevention, alcohol has proven the most difficult substance to affect (Ellickson & Bell, 1990; Hansen, Malotte, & Fielding, 1988). According to a National Survey for High School Seniors (NSHSS), alcohol had the highest usage rate at all grade levels surveyed (8th, 10th, 12th grades; National Institute on Drug Abuse, 1993). Given the young age of participants in our study and their low prevalence rates at pretest, lowering intentions to use alcohol is the best outcome measure of prevention effects for this age group. Thus, the 2-year finding that CTI participants drank less and intended to drink less in the future than participants in the LST condition is evidence for the greater effectiveness of the CTI for preventing substance abuse. Maintenance of intervention outcomes—indeed, improving them over the course of 2 years—is strong evidence for the merits of the CTI.

Although multivariate analysis did not support our hypothesis that CTI participants would have higher levels of self-esteem, self-efficacy, and hopefulness at posttest, univariate analysis revealed differential effects on the variable of hopefulness. The CTI participants showed significant increases in levels of hopefulness compared with LST participants at posttest; LST participants actually decreased in levels of hopefulness at posttest.

One explanation for the increased levels of hopefulness in CTI participants is that the CTI specifically addressed hope within the context of the students' own cultural realities, through the ancient and contemporary stories. Characters in these stories practiced intervention skills and experienced positive outcomes as a result. Perhaps viewing and hearing these stories increased students' beliefs that their lives could be improved by using these same skills. Recent research conducted on the stages of change has indicated the importance of addressing such motivational issues prior to introducing the skills needed to implement a change (Miller & Rollick, 1991).

Because we did not measure such variables as cultural pride, racial consciousness, and understanding of other cultures, it remains unclear what impact the CTI had on these variables and what mediating effect they may have had on outcomes.

Conclusion

We have dealt with tailoring research into school-based substance abuse prevention to the needs of minority adolescents. In much of the chapter, we have reviewed past school-based programs and emerging approaches to school-based substance use prevention. We subsequently discussed ways to enhance the cultural sensitivity of existing school-based programs to prevent substance use among minority groups. Despite our emphasis on substance abuse prevention research among African American and Hispanic youth in particular, the processes and principles we have described in tailoring the intervention to respond to these groups' cultural and environmental risk factors can be applied to research with other ethnic and racial groups as well.

Conclusions from our empirical investigation with CTI and LST were limited by a lack of data measuring specific cultural risk factors for substance abuse that were addressed in the CTI. Although study measures were normed for the target population, financial and time constraints prohibited us from developing measures to assess these culturally specific variables. Thus, the measurement instrument was not capable of discerning what impact these mediating variables might have had on outcome results. Future substance abuse prevention research aimed at culturally specific populations needs not only to norm widely accepted measures for the target group but also to concentrate on developing measures specifically related to the risk factors associated with the target group. Our study conclusions were further limited by the relatively young age of study participants (seventh graders). It remains unclear whether study outcomes would apply to older, substance-using adolescents.

Despite the limitations of our study, it is apparent that conducting culturally sensitive research has several benefits. Specifically, it can be more relevant, meaningful, and important than research that pays only cursory attention to cultural nuances. Researchers who sensitively and accurately assess cultural variables can have greater confidence that study outcomes resulted from the intervention itself. Conversely, researchers whose methods ignore or minimize cultural issues may reach erroneous conclusions. Although the development and testing of culturally sensitive interventions are particularly time-consuming because of a lack of previous research efforts, the rewards of such research are great.

REFERENCES

Bandura, A. (1986). *Social foundations of thought and action: A social cognitive theory.* Englewood Cliffs, NJ: Prentice-Hall.

Barnes, G. M., & Welte, J. W. (1986). Patterns and predictors of alcohol use among 7-12th grade students in New York state. *Journal of Studies on Alcohol, 47,* 3–61.

Beauvais, F. (1992). An integrated model for prevention and treatment of drug abuse among American Indian youth. *Journal of Addictive Diseases, 11,* 63–80.

Berberian, R. M., Gross, C., Lovejoy, J., & Paparella, S. (1976). The effectiveness of drug education programs: A critical review. *Health Education Monographs, 4,* 377–398.

Borden, W. (1989). Life review as a therapeutic frame in the treatment of young adults with AIDS. *Health and Social Work,* 253–259.

Borden, W. (1992). Narrative perspectives in psychosocial intervention following adverse life events. *Social Work, 37,* 135–141.

Botvin, G. J. (1986). Substance abuse prevention research: Recent developments and future direction. *Journal of School Health, 56,* 368–386.

Botvin, G. J., Baker, E., Dusenbury, L., Tortu, S., & Botvin, E. M. (1990). Preventing adolescent drug abuse through a multi-modal cognitive–behavioral approach: Results of a three year study. *Journal of Consulting and Clinical Psychology, 58,* 437–446.

Botvin, G. J., Baker, E., Filazzola, A. D., & Botvin, E. M. (1990). A cognitive–behavioral approach to substance abuse: One-year follow-up. *Addictive Behaviors, 15,* 47–63.

Botvin, G. J., Baker, E., Renick, N. L., Filazzola, A. D., & Botvin, E. M. (1984). A cognitive–behavioral approach to substance abuse prevention. *Addictive Behaviors, 9,* 137–147.

Botvin, G. J., Dusenbury, L. Baker, E., & James-Ortiz, S. (1989). A skills training approach to smoking prevention among Hispanic youth. *Journal of Behavioral Medicine, 12,* 279–296.

Botvin, G. J., & Eng, A. (1982). The efficacy of a multi-component approach to the prevention of cigarette smoking. *Preventive Medicine, 11,* 199–211.

Botvin, G. J., Renick, N., & Baker, E. (1983). The effects of scheduling format and booster sessions on a broad spectrum psychosocial approach to smoking prevention. *Journal of Behavioral Medicine, 6,* 358–379.

Comstock, G., & Cobbey, R. E. (1979). Television and the children of ethnic minorities. *Journal of Communication, 29,* 104–115.

Constantino, G., Malgady, R. G., & Rogler, L. H. (1990). Culturally sensitive psychotherapy for Puerto Rican children and adolescents: A program of treatment outcome research. *Journal of Consulting and Clinical Psychology, 58,* 704–712.

Demone, H. W. (1973). The nonuse and abuse of alcohol by the male adolescent. In M. Chafetz (Ed.), *Proceedings of the Second Annual Alcoholism Conference* (DHEW Publication No. HSM 73-9083, pp. 24–32). Washington, DC: U.S. Government Printing Office.

Elias, M. J. (1983). Improving coping skills of emotionally disturbed boys through television-based social problem solving. *American Journal of Orthopsychiatry, 53,* 61–72.

Ellickson, P. L., & Bell, R. M. (1990). Drug prevention in junior high. *Science, 247,* 1299–1305.

Forgey, M. A. (1994). Substance abuse prevention approaches for inner-city African-American and Hispanic youth. *Dissertation Abstracts International, 55*(6), 29–34. (University Microfilms No. 9427069)

Gary, L. E., & Berry, G. L. (1985). Predicting attitudes toward substance use in a Black community: Implications for prevention. *Community Mental Health Journal, 21*, 42–51.

Gilchrist, L. D., & Schinke, S. P. (1983). Self-control skills for smoking prevention. In P. F. Engstrom & P. Anderson (Eds.), *Advances on cancer control* (pp. 125–130). New York, NY: Alan R. Liss.

Gilchrist, L. D., Schinke, S. P., Trimble, J. E., & Cvetkovich, G. (1987). Skills enhancement to prevent substance abuse among American Indian adolescents. *International Journal of the Addictions, 22*, 869–879.

Greenfield, P., & Beagles-Roos, J. (1988). Radio vs. television: Their cognitive impact on children of different socioeconomic and ethnic groups. *Journal of Communication, 38*, 71–92.

Hansen, W. B., Johnson, C. A., Flay, B. R., Graham, J. W., & Sobel, J. L. (1988). Affective and social influences approaches to the prevention of multiple substance abuse among seventh grade students: Results from project SMART. *Prevention Medicine, 17*, 135–154.

Hansen, W. B., Malotte, C., & Fielding, J. (1988). Evaluation of a tobacco and alcohol abuse prevention curriculum for adolescents. *Health Education Quarterly, 15*, 93–114.

Harwood, R. L., & Weissberg, R. P. (1987). The potential of video in the promotion of social competence in children and adolescents. *Journal of Early Adolescence, 7*, 345–363.

Jessor, R., Chase, H. A., & Donavan, J. E. (1980). Psychosocial correlates of marijuana use and problem drinking in a Natural Sample of adolescents. *American Journal of Public Health, 70*, 604–614.

Jessor, R., Collins, M. I., & Jessor, S. L. (1972). On becoming a drinker: Social–psychological aspects of adolescent transition. *Annals of the New York Academy of Sciences, 197*, 199–213.

Jessor, R., & Jessor, S. L. (1977). *Problem behavior and psychosocial development: A longitudinal study of youth.* San Diego, CA: Academic Press.

Kaplan, H. B., Martin, S. S., Johnston, R. J. & Robbins, C. A. (1986). Escalation of marijuana use: Application of a general theory of deviant behavior. *Journal of Health and Social Behavior, 27*, 44–61.

Kaplan, H. B., Martin, S. S., & Robbins, C. A. (1982). Applications of a general theory of deviant behavior: Self-derogation and adolescent drug use. *Journal of Health and Social Behavior, 23*, 274–294.

Kazdin, A. E., French, H. H., Unis, A. S., Esveldt-Dawson, K, & Sherick, R. B. (1983). Hopelessness, depression and suicide intent among psychiatrically disturbed children. *Journal of Consulting and Clinical Psychology, 51*, 504–510.

Kearney, A. L., & Hines, M. H. (1980). Evaluation of the effectiveness of a drug prevention education program. *Journal of Drug Education, 10*, 127–134.

Kim, S. (1988). *A short- and long-term evaluation of Here's Looking at You alcohol education program.* Paper submitted for publication.

Kinder, B., Pape, N., & Walfish, S. (1980). Drug and alcohol education programs: A review of outcome studies. *International Journal of the Addictions, 15*, 1035–1054.

Kleiman, P. H., & Kukoff, I. F. (1978). Ethnic differences in factors related to drug use. *Journal of Health and Social Behavior, 19,* 190–199.

Knox, D. H. (1985). Spirituality: A tool in the assessment and treatment of Black alcoholics and their families. *Alcholism Treatment Quarterly, 2,* 31–44.

Mason, M. L. (1973). Drug education effects. *Dissertation Abstracts, 34*(4-B), 418.

Miller, W. R., & Rollick, S. (1991). *Motivational interviewing: Preparing people to change addictive behaviors.* New York: Guilford Press.

Murray, D. M., Johnson, C. A., Luepker, R. V., & Mittlemark, M. B. (1984). The prevention of cigarette smoking in children: A comparison of four strategies. *Journal of Applied Social Psychology, 14,* 274–288.

National Institute on Drug Abuse. (1993). *National survey results on drug abuse from the Monitoring the Future study, 1975-1992: Vol. 1, secondary school students.* Rockville, MD: Author.

Newcomb, A. F., & Collins, W. A. (1979). Children's comprehension of family role portrayals in televised dramas: Effects of socioeconomic status, ethnicity, and age. *Developmental Psychology, 15,* 417–423.

Oetting, E., & Beauvais, F. (1987). Peer cluster theory, socialization characteristics and adolescent drug use: A path analysis. *Journal of Counseling Psychology, 34,* 205–213.

Pentz, M. A. (1983). Prevention of adolescent substance abuse through social skill development. In T. J. Glynn, C. G. Leukefeld, & J. P. Ludford (Eds.), *Preventing adolescent drug abuse: Intervention strategies* (NIDA Research Monograph No. 47, pp. 195–232). Washington, DC: U.S. Government Printing Office.

Pentz, M. A., Dwyer, J., Mackinnon, D., Flay, B. R., Hansen, W. B., Yu, E., Wang, M. S., & Johnson, C. A. (1989). A multi-community trial for primary prevention of adolescent drug abuse effects on drug use prevalence. *Journal of the American Medical Association, 261,* 3259–3266.

Richards, L. G. (1969, August–September). *Government programs and psychological principals in drug abuse education.* Paper presented at the 77th Annual Convention of American Psychological Association, Washington, DC.

Schaps, E., Di Bartolo, R., Moskowitz, J., Palley, C. S., & Churgin, S. (1981). A review of 127 drug abuse prevention program evaluations. *Journal of Drug Issues, 12,* 17–43.

Schaps, E., Moskowitz, J. M., Malvin, J., & Schaeffer, G. (1986). Evaluation of seven school-based prevention programs: A final report of the Napa Valley Project. *International Journal of the Addictions, 21,* 1081–1112.

Schinke, S. P., Bebel, M. Y., Orlandi, M. A., & Botvin, G. J. (1988). Prevention strategies for vulnerable pupils: School social work practices to prevent substance abuse. *Urban Education, 22,* 510–519.

Schinke, S. P., & Blythe, B. J. (1981). Cognitive–behavioral prevention of children's smoking. *Child Behavior Therapy, 3,* 25–42.

Schinke, S. P., Botvin, G. J., & Orlandi, M. A. (1991). *Substance abuse in children and adolescents: Evaluation and intervention.* Newbury Park, CA: Sage.

Schinke, S. P., & Gilchrist, L. D. (1983). Primary prevention of tobacco smoking. *Journal of School Health, 53,* 416–419.

Schinke, S. P., & Gilchrist, L. D. (1984). Preventing cigarette smoking with youth. *Journal of Primary Prevention, 5*, 48–56.

Schinke, S. P., Orlandi, M. A., Botvin, G. J., Gilchrist, L. D., Trimble, J. E., & Locklear, V. S. (1988). Preventing substance abuse among American Indian adolescents: A bicultural competence skills approach. *Journal of Counseling Psychology, 35*, 87–90.

Swisher, J. D. (1979). Prevention issues. In R. I. Dupont, A. Goldstein, & J. O'Donnell (Eds.), *Handbook on drug abuse* (pp. 49–62). Washington, DC: U.S. Government Printing Office.

Swisher, J. D., Crawford, J. L., Goldstein, R., & Yura, M. (1971). Drug education: Pushing or preventing? *Peabody Journal of Education, 49*, 68–75.

Swisher, J. D., & Hoffman, A. (1975). Information: The irrelevant variable in drug education. In B. W. Corder, R. A. Smith, & J. D. Swisher (Eds.), *Drug abuse prevention: Perspectives and approaches for educators* (pp. 49–62). Dubuque, IA: William C. Brown.

Szapocznik, J., & Kurtines, W. (1980). Acculturation, biculturalism and adjustment among Cuban Americans. In A. M. Padilla (Ed.), *Acculturation: Theory, models, and some new findings*. Boulder, CO: American Association for the Advancement of Science.

Tobler, N. S. (1986). Meta-analysis of 143 adolescent drug prevention programs: Quantitative outcome results of program participants compared to a control or comparison group. *Journal of Drug Issues, 16*, 537–567.

Tucker, M. B. (1985). U.S. ethnic minorities and drug abuse: An assessment of the science and practice. *International Journal of the Addictions, 20*, 1021–1047.

U.S. General Accounting Office. (1990). *Drug education: School-based programs seen as useful but impact unknown* (GAO/HRD 91-27; Report to the Chairman, Committee on Governmental Affairs, U.S. Senate). Washington, DC: U.S. Government Printing Office.

Wechsler, H., & Thum, D. (1973). Alcohol and drug use among teenagers: A questionnaire study. In M. Chafetz (Ed.), *Proceedings of the Second Annual Alcoholism Conference* (DHEW Publication No. HSM 73-9083, pp. 33–46). Washington, DC: U.S. Government Printing Office.

Wilson, W. J. (1987). *The truly disadvantaged: The inner-city, the underclass and social policy*. Chicago: Chicago University Press.

Community-Based Interventions

Betty R. Yung and W. Rodney Hammond

Community-based health-promotion programs have real potential for helping ethnic minority adolescents to acquire, maintain, or increase positive health practices and to reduce those behaviors that compromise their well-being. However, creating, carrying out, and evaluating the effectiveness of such programs presents a formidable challenge. Some of the difficult issues faced by providers of community-based health-promotion services include access and appeal to young ethnic minority consumers, cultural compatibility of the prevention approach, pragmatic concerns about limited or unstable funding, and design issues such as selecting assessment methods that are culturally appropriate and acceptable in both the target and the scientific communities.

We begin this chapter by describing a rationale for providing health-promotion services for ethnic minority adolescents in community-based settings and then review selected programs directed at a variety of health concerns. The review of programs is not intended to be exhaustive, and although we have chosen primarily to describe programs that reported outcome results, it is not our intention to provide a detailed methodological critique of research design. Instead, we hope to give the reader a flavor for the range of approaches, the nature, and the findings of representative programs, as well as for barriers encountered in the conceptualization, implementation, and evaluation of these prevention services. Throughout, we focus special attention on the issue of cultural sensitivity as a key characteristic of many of the successful initiatives. We also emphasize the need for rigorous, long-term studies of the behavioral outcomes of health-promotion programs for ethnic minority adolescents.

Rationale for Community-Based Health-Promotion Programming

Most health-promotion and risk-reduction programs for adolescents are provided in school settings (Guerra, Tolan, & Hammond, 1994). This is a logical and feasible choice because it reduces barriers of cost and transportation and provides access to a large, already assembled population (Hammond & Yung, 1991). However, there are concerns about the limitations of school-based programs in reaching and making a behavioral impact on the health practices of ethnic minority adolescents, particularly those with the highest needs.

Access

Frequent absenteeism and school dropout limit the exposure of all high-risk adolescents to school-based health-promotion programs (Orlandi, 1986). These factors are more likely to affect certain ethnic minority youth groups because of higher school dropout rates among Hispanic, African American, and Native American youth. Dropout rates for Hispanic and African American youth have been estimated to range from 35% to 50% in some inner-city neighborhoods (Chavez, Oetting, & Swaim, 1994; Soriano, 1994; U.S. Department of Education,

1992). Similar rates have been calculated for Native American youth (Shafer, 1995).

Dropout youth are much more likely to be engaged in health-risky behavior, such as alcohol or drug abuse, carrying weapons, drug sales, violence, and other unsafe activities (Sheley, 1994). Although some studies (e.g., Boles, Casas, Furlong, Gonzalez, & Morrison, 1994; Chavez, Edwards, & Oetting, 1989; Chavez et al., 1994) have found that there were few ethnic differences in health-compromising behavior among school dropouts, they have concluded that there is greater overall health risk for ethnic minority dropouts simply because their population is proportionally larger and because all young people within this subgroup appear to have heightened risk for negative health behaviors. Among the most deviant of the dropout population, the extent of health-risk behavior is not fully known. Runaway and homeless youth, young prostitutes, and drug sellers and users are rarely included in health survey research because of difficulties in locating them or in convincing them to participate (Chavez et al., 1989). School-based programs are not well positioned for the labor-intensive effort required to find, engage, and retain the most vulnerable among the hard-to-reach, out-of-school youth (Brooks-Gunn, Boyer, & Hein, 1988).

Cultural Relevance

It is not clear that schools are able to easily mount health-promotion programs that respond to the diverse needs, characteristics, values, and preferences of different ethnic, gender, and age groups. Although exceptions have been reported (e.g., Hammond & Yung, 1991; Malgady, Rogler, & Costantino, 1990), culturally tailored interventions are typically not designed to be delivered in a school setting (Orlandi, 1986). Among other issues, if schools target a particular ethnic group or market the program as a prevention effort directed toward a particular health concern, they run a high risk of alienating and stigmatizing their young participants (Yung & Hammond, 1995). It appears to be much more common for schools to use "off the shelf" prevention programs (Vega, 1992), with little attention paid to ethnic and gender differences in how materials are presented, the different meanings that health information may have for different groups, and any culturally unique barriers to behavior change (Orlandi, 1986).

Acceptability

Buy in to the health-promotion program by key administrators, decision makers, service delivery and support staff, and community constituents is essential. In school settings it may be difficult to gain support for providing health education content that is especially needed for adolescents but that is sensitive or potentially controversial (e.g., AIDS prevention lessons, which typically include instruction on the use of condoms; DiClemente & Houston-Hamilton, 1989). In addition, health-promotion goals may be seen by school personnel as competitive or secondary to the school's academic mission.

Impact

There are general concerns about whether school-based programs have long-term effectiveness in preventing health problems among targeted youth. Outcome reports for substance abuse and violence prevention programs have been somewhat mixed. For example, Ellickson, Bell, and McGuigan (1993) found that initial gains of a school-based substance abuse prevention program dissipated over time. In addition, the evaluation methodology of many school-based prevention programs has been challenged for overreliance on paper-and-pencil tests; basic research design problems; and, in some cases, missing data (Guerra et al., 1994; Webster, 1993). In particular, evaluation designs for many such programs have not included collection of behavioral data from natural settings or long-term tracking of outcomes (Hammond & Yung, 1993). Thus, the lasting impact of such programs on actual rather than self-reported health behavior is often unknown (Hansen, Watson-Perczel, & Christopher, 1989; Yung & Hammond, 1994).

It is also difficult in many cases to determine the specific impact of school-based health-promotion initiatives on particular ethnic minority youth groups within a multiethnic population. Many reviews or individual reports of school-based programs either do not examine outcome differences by ethnicity or do not report on ethnicity at all (Hammond & Yung, 1993). Also, it is common practice to "lump together" less numerous ethnic minority subjects under the category of "other," so that effects on entire ethnic minority groups and their widely diverse subgroups (e.g., Southeast Asian refugee populations) are essentially unknown (Uehara, Takeuchi, & Smukler, 1994). Some studies have reported differential outcome effects according to ethnicity–race and socioeconomic status, finding, for example, that broadly targeted primary prevention programs have been less effective with African American, Hispanic, Native American, and Asian American youth than with White adolescents (Hansen et al., 1989), yet others have not reported this difference (e.g., Caplan et al., 1992; Ellickson et al., 1993). One culturally sensitive HIV–AIDS prevention program for African American adolescents found greater impact on related postintervention knowledge, beliefs, and attitudes when the intervention recipients were in an ethnically homogeneous classroom (Damond, Breuer, & Pharr, 1993). More evidence of how specific factors can contribute to varying impacts is a critical need.

Advantages and Limitations of Community-Based Health-Promotion Programs

As our review of community-based health-promotion programs demonstrates, some of the same concerns about access, acceptability, cultural relevance, and impact on ethnic minority youth can be raised for programs located in community settings that are raised for those in school settings. However, we feel that community-based programs are ideally suited to overcome many of the identified limitations inherent to interventions in school-based locations. First, neighborhood programs may be perceived to be more "consumer-friendly" by youth for whom school has not been a positive experience (i.e., those who are alienated, frequently absent, or truant from school or who have already dropped out). Also, community-based organizations may be aided in their access efforts by broader or health-specific missions, more flexible service agendas or hours of operation, a positive reputation and connections in the community, and more personalized outreach methods (Isaacs & Benjamin, 1991).

In addition, except for recent experiments with Afrocentric schools designed exclusively to serve African American boys, schools may be limited in their ability to focus on culturally unique needs and characteristics, because they typically serve children and youth of different ethnic and cultural backgrounds. In contrast, there are many community-based health and social service organizations that primarily serve one ethnic minority group and describe themselves as operating on principles of cultural competency (Isaacs & Benjamin, 1991). Such programs have demonstrated greater success with bringing in and retaining ethnic minority consumers than have mainstream organizations that make no culturally oriented outreach, staffing, linguistic, service, or policy accommodations (Sue, Fujino, Hu, Takeuchi, & Zane, 1991; Yeh, Takeuchi, & Sue, 1994).

It may also be easier for programs such as community-based health agencies to offer certain types of health-promotion programs (e.g., adolescent AIDS or pregnancy prevention) because of their health-related missions and their access to exceptionally high-risk populations, such as adolescents with sexually transmitted diseases (Mansfield, Conroy, Emans, & Woods, 1993).

Community-based programs also have some built-in limitations. For example, they do not have free access to the large, "captive" population of ethnic minority children and adolescents that schools do. Recruitment, transportation, and retention efforts can be costly both in terms of staff time and financial resources, and these expenses may be even higher where hard-to-reach dropout youth are the focus. In fact, the significant work and expense involved in bringing together groups of dropout or other high-risk ethnic minority adolescents in community-based settings for health-promotion programs is a powerful argument for early, intensive, and sustained school-based prevention programs targeted to younger age groups. Mobile units, such as vans carrying health personnel teams to community-based sites, may offer a viable alternative method for reaching out-of-school youth for health screenings or health education programs.

The greatest potential for impact on ethnic minority adolescent health behavior may be through combined school and community partnership prevention efforts. It has been suggested that many school-based programs may not have produced significant and sustained behavior change because of a lack of integration between school-based health education and skill development training and other pervasive, negative environmental influences outside of school (Pentz et al., 1989; Tobler, 1986). Because of their greater ability to tailor programs for sensitivity to ethnic and cultural factors, neighborhood norms and conditions, and life circumstances, community-based programs are well positioned to supplement school efforts, providing multiple doses of reinforcing and culturally relevant prevention messages to adolescents who also receive health-promotion services in the classroom (Isaacs, 1993; St. Pierre, Kaltreider, Mark, & Aikin, 1992).

Review of Selected Community-Based Health-Promotion Programs

Empirical evaluations of community-based health-promotion programs for all adolescents have been limited (Tolan & Guerra, 1994). Published research on outcomes of prevention efforts directed to specific ethnic minority adolescent groups are even more rare (Hammond & Yung, 1993; U.S. General Accounting Office [U.S. GAO], 1992). In this review, we focus mainly on demonstration programs with published outcome results and on health-promotion initiatives designed to influence behavior change in individuals. So that common issues can be highlighted, we have organized our discussion around these health-behavior target areas: substance abuse prevention, HIV and AIDS prevention, violence prevention, and substance abuse and violence.

Substance Abuse Prevention

A common approach to substance abuse prevention programming in community-based settings (as well as in schools) is skills-based training of ethnic minority adolescents to enhance their abilities to resolve problems, make health-enhancing decisions, cope constructively with stress, and resist peer pressure to use or abuse alcohol or other drugs. One such program targeting Native American adolescents from two western reservation sites was reported by Schinke et al. (1988). This program used a bicultural competence approach, focusing on skills that would enable Native American youth to blend adaptive values from both their native and surrounding majority cultures in support of a drug-free lifestyle. In 10 sessions, two adult Native American counselors taught participants communication skills (e.g., how to refuse alcohol or other drugs without offending friends), coping skills to deal with acculturative stress, and discrimination skills (e.g., prediction of high-risk situations). Typical of a social-skills-training method, "homework" was assigned in the form of skill tryouts in which fellow group members were to monitor and support each other's efforts at real-life skill use. Participants also received instruction and practice in ways to build social networks with friends, family, and tribal members who could support abstinence. The evaluation design included random assignment of participants to experimental and control groups and pre- and postmeasures at program entry, exit, and 6-month follow-up. At the end of treatment and at 6-month follow-up, the experimental group had significantly higher scores on self-control, ability to generate alternative suggestions to using drugs, assertiveness, and knowledge about substance use and abuse. They also held less favorable attitudes about substance use in Native American culture and self-reported less use of tobacco, smokeless tobacco, marijuana, and inhalants.

Earlier, Gilchrist, Schinke, Trimble, and Cvetkovich (1987) had reported a very similar skills enhancement program for Native American preadolescents from rural and urban reservation and nonreservation settings in the Pacific Northwest. Because the project targeted younger participants, alternative teaching methods were used, including the use of puppets to practice the target skills; the provision of educational information about alcohol and drugs through games, films, handouts, and posters; and a group-generated media project. The program was offered in both classrooms and tribal centers, and co-leaders from the university research team worked alongside trained indigenous community leaders (teachers, school counselors, or alcohol and drug treatment staff). At 6-month follow-up, the intervention group reported less use of alcohol, marijuana, and inhalants than did a randomly assigned control group. Although there were positive changes in tobacco use at posttest, they were not evident at follow-up. Additionally, no differences were found between the groups on measures of self-esteem or attitudes toward drug use.

Although the substance abuse prevention program set up by Bobo, Gilchrist, Cvetkovich, Trimble, and Schinke (1988) did not demonstrate statistically significant positive outcomes, the description of this project is especially valuable for its detailed outline of the processes involved in the cultural tailoring of a health-promotion program for Native American youth. Having determined that many of the tribal groups in the region had purchased packaged drug abuse prevention curricula but had infrequently or never used it, the project team made special efforts to select a substance abuse approach compatible with traditional Native American values, to prepare culturally sensitive teaching materials that would be appealing and relevant, and to in-volve tribal leaders in evaluating the suitability of the curriculum and the teaching–learning approach. An advisory committee consisting of social service personnel, tribal council members, and employees of Native American education programs established criteria for cultur-ally appropriate materials that emphasized the need to acknowledge the reality of substance use in Native American communities (rather than suggesting abstinence as the only appropriate behavior), the harm that substance abuse has brought to Native American people, and the non-drug-abusing lifestyles of most contemporary Native Americans. Advisory committee members further made an extensive effort to generate widespread tribal support through a series of infor-mal community workshops, some involving more than 12 hours of discussion and hands-on manipulation of materials. The program in-corporated other culturally sensitive elements, such as the use of Na-tive American artwork and role models in visual aids and room dec-orations. Native American adolescent norms against self-disclosure were also taken into account in decisions about teaching methods. In early sessions, participants practiced communication skills by writing responses to personal questions before verbalizing them, completing cartoon strips, and acting out dialogues with puppets before moving into more conventional role-plays. The reasons for the apparent failure of this seemingly well-designed program are unknown. Bobo et al. noted that they had to simplify their intended outcome measures be-cause of complaints about length and complexity by the advisory com-mittee, leading to speculation as to whether the measures used were sophisticated enough to pick up behavioral change.

DePerry (1994) described a similar approach of promoting total community involvement to support a skill development program for Native American youth, in this case, with positive outcomes reported. Funded by the Federal Center for Substance Abuse Prevention, this project served youth from three Chippewa Indian reservations in the Great Lakes region of Minnesota and Wisconsin. Its components in-cluded a kindergarten through twelfth-grade curriculum designed to be implemented by classroom teachers, training and on-site technical assistance to teachers and school staff to implement the curriculum, training of community volunteers to implement the curriculum in nonschool sites, and training of parents and extended family to sup-port the program concepts. The curricular emphasis was on improving participants' knowledge of the harmful impact of substance abuse on spiritual and cultural health. Outcome results at 1-year follow-up showed less use of alcohol and marijuana by participants than by comparison group youth, but no effects on cigarette smoking. These results were reported as preliminary outcome data in a replication guide published by the Center for Substance Abuse Prevention and did not include information on statistical significance.

Substance abuse prevention programs primarily serving African American adolescents have also been reported. Bruce and Emshoff (1992) described a project targeting African American boys ages 10 to 15 years that was offered at Boys and Girls Clubs, parks, and other recreational sites in ethnic minority neighborhoods. This intervention provided a seven-session program of drug education from a police officer, refusal skills role-play training for the boys, and companion parent-training sessions on building children's self-esteem. In comparison with pretest scores, boys improved their knowledge about drugs, the effects of substance use and abuse, and resisting peer pressure, with results approaching significance levels. Parents showed statistically significant improvement in knowing how to talk to their children about drugs. The limitations of this research included the absence of a control group and that a posttest was given only 2 weeks after the intervention.

The substance abuse prevention initiative of Gross and McCaul (1992) served an extremely high-risk group of ethnic minority adolescents whose parents were substance abusers. This intervention involved establishing social support groups in schools and community centers; youth were also exposed to a life skills curriculum to help them develop problem-solving and stress management skills. In addition, outreach workshops on addressing the special needs of children of substance abusers were offered to various community and professional groups who had contact with these and other high-risk youth. Although the target adolescent population was 75% African American, the researchers did not identify any culturally specific features of the intervention, apart from the use of popular music as a prompt for group discussion. At posttest and at 1-year follow-up, the research team did not find statistically significant improvements in depression, self-esteem, behavior problems, or drug use for the intervention group or for a no-contact comparison group of high-risk youth whose parents were not substance abusers. There were slight increases in self-esteem measures at posttest for the experimental group, but these were not maintained at 1-year follow-up. The experimental group showed a modest reduction in the numbers of youth who experimented with gateway drugs (alcohol and tobacco) during the intervening 1-year follow-up period. This project had a small sample size that was reduced by significant attrition (from 108 to 35), with possible bias toward retaining the least distressed youth. Other limitations included the use of a comparison group that was not matched on the risk factor of primary interest (parental substance abuse).

One of the few reported health-promotion programs serving Asian American youth has addressed the issue of substance abuse. The Asian Youth Substance Abuse Prevention Project (AYSAPP, 1994) was carried out by a consortium of seven community-based agencies in the San Francisco, California, area. The project primarily served at-risk Chinese, Southeast Asian, Filipino, Japanese, and Korean adolescents but also included small numbers of Native American, African American, Hispanic, and White youth. The approach was multifaceted, including components of youth skill development, drug-free recreational activities, collaboration among institutional systems to plan for service provision to high-risk Asian youth and their families, and outreach to families to help them access support services. Activities were carried out in neighborhood centers using multilingual staff. Preliminary descriptive outcome data as reported in the project's replication manual suggested promising results in several areas: decreases in self-reported drug use and other health-risk behavior, an increase in targeted social skills, an increase in community knowledge about drug abuse issues, enhanced awareness of environmental risk within the community, and activism by families and community agencies to reduce personal and environmental risk for substance abuse.

Several substance abuse prevention programs have been provided for adolescent populations that include youth of different ethnicities. One project involved a multiagency collaboration that served youth involved with the juvenile justice system (Stein et al., 1992). Participants included Hispanics (33%), African Americans (20%), Asians (2%), Native Americans (2%), and Whites (43%). The prevention approach involved affective education (individual counseling, drug and alcohol self-help groups, and skill-building groups); drug-free alternative activities, beginning with a 15-day wilderness experience; a residential program, which included academic and vocational education; and a relationship with an adult mentor. This project had initial difficulties with attrition of ethnic minority participants, and Stein et al. noted that they had paid little attention to ethnic–cultural issues in their intervention design. For example, the residential program was located in a community where there was much gang-related activity. There were constant issues with student safety, particularly for African American participants, who were frequent targets of assaults or threats. The ethnic minority adolescent retention rates improved from 40% to 80% with the hiring of additional ethnic minority counselors and greater attention paid to participant safety. However, there were no significant changes over time in outcomes related to approval for prosocial behavior, family bonding, moral rules of conduct, self-esteem, and use of alcohol or other drugs. The project also faced significant challenges related to the interagency collaborative process.

Public housing projects have also been the site for substance abuse prevention efforts for children and adolescents of different ethnic backgrounds. St. Pierre et al. (1992) looked at the behavior change effects of a substance abuse prevention program offered through Boys and Girls Clubs located in such sites. Participants were of different ethnic backgrounds, including Hispanic (14%), African American (42%), and White (45%). In addition to recreational alternatives, the intervention included a life-skills-training component and placed heavy emphasis on experiential activities and efforts to customize the curricular support materials for cultural relevance to the ethnically diverse subgroups. The effects of adding booster sessions were also studied. Participants were tracked at 24 months and retested for effects on drug-related attitudes and behavior. The project showed significant effects on lowering self-reported marijuana use and overall drug use, with marginal effects on cigarette and alcohol use, in comparison with youth at control sites. The booster sessions produced significant effects only on attitudes toward alcohol and marijuana.

We found few attempts to evaluate modifications of macrolevel influences (e.g., social policy, legal, or social value changes) in our review of health-promotion programs for ethnic minority adolescents. An exception was in a culturally sensitive intervention designed to promote tobacco control policies in northwest Native American tribes (Lichtenstein et al., 1995). The authors described the potential impact of communitywide tobacco control policies on the health of children and adolescents by decreasing exposure to secondary smoke; enhancing participation in smoking cessation programs; and establishing nonuse of tobacco as a social norm, thus reducing the likelihood that youngsters will start or keep smoking. In collaboration with two research institutions, the Northwest Portland Area Indian Health Board initiated a consultative process to facilitate adoption by 39 tribal councils of more stringent tobacco-use policies in council meeting rooms, tribal schools, and bingo halls. Participating tribes were randomly assigned to early or late intervention groups. The early intervention group received consultation over an 18-month period on establishing written smoking control policies at the local tribal level, with stated consequences for violations. Problem-solving assistance was provided to help the local tribal health committees overcome policy development and implementation barriers and to publicize tobacco-policy-related articles in tribal newsletters in order to gain community support. The consultation team demonstrated cultural sensitivity in distinguishing between traditional or ceremonial use of tobacco in tribal rituals versus addictive or recreational use. Late intervention tribes received no assistance in modifying tobacco-use policies until the intervention had been evaluated, after which they received the same consultative services as the early intervention group. Early intervention tribes were significantly more likely to have placed greater restrictions on smoking in workplaces, council meetings, and private offices. Although no progress was reported for banning smoking in bingo halls or in reducing youth access to tobacco, there were an increased number of related public awareness messages in tribal newsletters, suggesting high potential for continued policy development.

HIV and AIDS Prevention

Community-based HIV–AIDS prevention programs have often targeted high-risk African American and Hispanic adolescent males. Mansfield et al. (1993) reported on a physician-provided AIDS education and counseling intervention for young men in their late teens or early twenties with sexually transmitted diseases. Youth were randomly assigned to either a control group, where they received standard care (risk assessment, counseling on condom use, an informational pamphlet, and offer of free condoms), or to an experimental group, which received the standard care intervention plus an additional 20-min counseling session with a physician in which there was fuller discussion of AIDS risk, drug and needle use, and condom use.

At 2 months postintervention, participants in both groups reported significantly less sexual activity, fewer sexual partners, less drug use, and increase in condom use. There were no significant differences between the groups: The shorter intervention appeared to be as effective as the lengthier one.

Magura, Kang, and Shapiro (1994) have also researched change in risky sexual behavior among male adolescents. Their target population was incarcerated African American and Hispanic drug users. The prevention program was provided in eight small-group sessions facilitated by an ethnically similar male counselor. The program included information on HIV and AIDS, drug abuse, sexual behavior and reducing AIDS risk, and skill development in problem solving and help seeking. A waitlisted control group was used to gauge intervention effects. In this extremely high-risk group, more than half of the adolescents had prior arrests for such offenses as drug abuse, murder, attempted murder, robbery, rape, and assault. Intervention results were only tracked for the portion of the participants who were incarcerated while awaiting trial but who were not sentenced to prison; thus, the sample underrepresented the most serious or persistent offenders in the population. The follow-up interviews were conducted at a median of 10 months after baseline and 5 months after release from jail. At follow-up, members of the experimental group were significantly more likely to report having changed their sex-risk behavior (e.g., reduced number of sexual episodes with high-risk partners and increased acceptability and use of condoms).

AIDS prevention programs for younger participants at somewhat less risk have reported more use of interactive skill-building activities in addition to the provision of health education information. One such program, serving a predominantly Hispanic male adolescent population, integrated AIDS-prevention concepts into existing community-based after-school programs (Kipke, Boyer, & Hein, 1993). In addition to receiving information about HIV and AIDS, methods of transmission, and instruction on the use of condoms, the adolescents participated in skill-building exercises intended to help them recognize and respond to high-risk situations. The intervention was very brief (two sessions for pre- and postassessment and three 90-min intervention sessions), and the authors did not specifically report on any adaptations to make content or materials culturally relevant. Postassessment occurred 4 weeks after the intervention. In comparison with members of a waitlisted control group, experimental group members showed significant increases in knowledge and perception of risk, as well as increases in assertiveness and communication skills as assessed by videotaped role-plays.

Schinke, Gordon, and Weston (1990) tested the effectiveness of self-instruction interventions to reduce the risks for HIV and AIDS among African American and Hispanic male adolescents enrolled in an urban job-training program. Participants were randomly assigned to one of three groups. Group 1 received a self-instructional guide about AIDS and its transmission plus a social problem-solving intervention and small-group instruction in using the guide. Group 2 received only the written guide, and Group 3 received no intervention. The researchers made efforts to create written materials that were culturally appropriate and adjusted for consumer literacy level. The guide was written in comic book format, with graphics and rap music lyrics presented by a cartoon character drawn to mirror participants' age and ethnic backgrounds. Participants in the two self-instructional interventions improved more from pretest to posttest than did control participants, but there were few differences that reached levels of significance.

Thomas and Quinn (1993) evaluated the impact of an HIV-prevention program provided to African American residents of a low-income public housing complex. Although this project also served adults, the modal age of participants was 16 years. The health-promotion program included presentation of a custom-made slide show and a workshop on risk reduction, designed to be culturally sensitive to the needs of the target population. Effects were evaluated with pretests and posttests of knowledge about AIDS, including methods of reducing risk. Findings showed that, compared with control groups (who received only a smoking cessation program), the experimental groups significantly increased knowledge and use of risk-reduction behaviors. The study also examined the effects of the characteristics of whoever delivered the prevention message by setting up three experimental groups: one facilitated by an African American health care professional, another by a White health care professional, and the third by a recovered intravenous drug user who was a neighborhood resident and was considered a community leader. No statistical differences were found for outcomes among the three experimental groups.

Violence Prevention

Violence prevention represents a newer field of health-promotion activities. In fact, violence has only been widely recognized as a health
rather than a juvenile justice concern within the past decade. Thus,
there is less of a base of health-promotion literature dealing with this
issue than might be expected. Certainly there are other bodies of research information that may provide useful guidance in designing violence prevention programs, including literature on delinquency prevention and psychoeducational interventions with antisocial or
conduct-disordered children and adolescents. We do not review this
related literature here because of its extensiveness and its focus on
other target behaviors in addition to violence (but see Kazdin, 1994;
Lipsey & Wilson, 1993; Tolan & Guerra, 1994 for reviews of literature
on delinquency preventions and interventions with antisocial children
and adolescents).

There are few empirically oriented reports on outcomes of violence
prevention programs and still fewer report on programs targeting ethnic minority youth (Hammond & Yung, 1993; Wilson-Brewer & Jacklin, 1990). Exceptions appear in the studies of school-based programs
described by Gainer, Webster, and Champion (1993) and by Hammond
and Yung (1991).

The U.S. GAO (1995) report on violence prevention programs described results of a community-based gang prevention program in
California (called "Alternatives to Gang Membership") that primarily
serves a Hispanic youth population and includes school and community components. The school program targets elementary students,
with a follow-up at seventh-grade level, and covers content related to
peer pressure, drug abuse, the consequences of a criminal lifestyle,
positive self-esteem, and career exploration. The community program
involves a series of bilingual neighborhood meetings held in schools,
parks, churches, community centers, and private homes in which parents are given information to help them prevent their children from
joining gangs. Pre- and posttests are given to participants to assess
their attitudes toward joining gangs and self-reported gang membership. Some longitudinal follow-up has been done; for example, participants who were in a fifth-grade cohort were retested at ninth grade,
and more than 90% reported that they were staying out of gangs. A
cross-check of participants was made through the sheriff's department

to identify whether these participants were known as gang members. Police identification suggested that the self-reports were fairly accurate, with only 4% of the participating students identified as belonging to gangs. Information on the outcome of this program was not published as a research report, so it was difficult to fully understand the evaluation design. However, it appeared that there was no control community for comparison and no baseline data on gang activity in the area before the program was initiated.

Guerra and Slaby (1990) implemented a social skills training intervention to modify the violence-related beliefs and behavior of African American adolescents incarcerated for acts of aggression. In a controlled study using participants randomly assigned to a cognitive–behavioral intervention group, an attention control group, or a no-treatment control group, they found associated increases in social problem-solving skills, a reduction in endorsement of beliefs supporting aggression, and a decrease in aggressive behavior as rated by neutral observers for those participants receiving the preventive intervention.

Similar to initiatives related to other health concerns, there have been little evaluation data on violence prevention approaches directed toward environmental or agent-related change. In the area of violence, it makes sense to address the issue of gun control policies and programs in light of the impact of firearms on mortality and morbidity. At present, this area remains largely unexplored. Recently, however, Callahan, Rivara, and Koepsell (1994) did examine the impact of a gun buy-back program on firearms-related death and injury in a northwestern city. They found no significant changes in deaths and hospital admissions related to firearms and concluded that a much larger number of guns would have to be collected to begin to see an impact. However, Callahan et al. did find high community support for the project, even among gun owners. They also noted the participation by young people (of unspecified ethnicity) in the program, estimating that about 5% of the total group returning guns (approximately 70 young people) were under 18. They recommended that there should be future gun buy-back programs specifically designed to remove weapons possessed by minors and that such events might be better attended if offered in community centers or youth clubs during after-school or weekend hours.

Substance Abuse and Violence

Friedman and Utada (1992) compared the effects of two different types of early secondary level interventions on substance abuse and violence for ethnic minority adolescents at high risk for, or actively demonstrating, both problems. One group received an intervention using an adaptation of a popular life-skills-training (LST) model, and the other received an intervention that combined a values-clarification model with the violence prevention curriculum of Prothrow-Stith (1987). The target youth, who were all male and 75% African American, were students in day-school treatment centers who were court adjudicated for illegal offenses, primarily violence related. Most also had histories of use of gateway drugs and self-reported family and school problems. The project had mixed results, and the evaluators indicated several problems in the area of youth resistance to the program (which we discuss in later sections of this chapter). Both groups showed decreases in getting into fights or into trouble with police while drinking, increases in knowledge about smoking and drinking, and increases in negative attitudes toward marijuana use. There were also significant decreases in delinquent behavior and related legal problems and in the number and seriousness of illegal offenses committed. On the negative side, participants showed no changes in smoking behavior; experiencing trouble at home; having accidents or injuries due to drinking; or interpersonal skills, such as decision making; and self-reported drug use as well as emotional problems actually increased between pre- and posttesting. Friedman and Utada found the combined violence curriculum and values-clarification program to have been more effective than the LST in several areas, including a reduction in going to bars, more reliance on what participants' mothers told them, less money spent on drugs, and more reduction in illegal offenses committed and in the amount of illegal activity. Although not entirely successful, this program provides valuable guidance in its description of problems of engaging youth and finding culturally appropriate resource materials as well as in noting group leader variables that may affect success.

Limitations of This Review

By focusing on published outcome studies, we have covered only a small portion of the existing community-based programs to promote healthier behavior among ethnic minority adolescents. In most cases, the studies we reviewed were demonstration projects collaboratively conducted by community-based organizations and university or other research institution staff, often in conjunction with evaluation requirements of federal grants, rather than descriptive results of ongoing health-promotion efforts of neighborhood or tribal service agencies. Many neighborhood agencies may place primary importance on service delivery rather than on pilot testing or evaluation (Bernal, Bonilla, & Bellido, 1995; Isaacs & Benjamin, 1991; Orlandi, 1986; U.S. GAO, 1992). They may also lack funding support or the technical knowledge needed to design and carry out scientifically sound outcome studies (Isaacs & Benjamin, 1991; U.S. GAO, 1992; Webster, 1993). As a result, there are many community-based health-promotion programs for ethnic minority adolescents whose behavioral impact is simply not known. For example, after reviewing culturally competent community-based health and social service agencies and programs, Isaacs and Benjamin concluded that there had been few attempts to measure impact outcomes for clients served in ethnic-specific programs. Among the programs they described, there were eight culturally specific child-oriented prevention or health-promotion programs. These programs were directed to diverse health and behavior problems (substance abuse, school dropout, juvenile delinquency, and teenage pregnancy) and to diverse populations. The authors noted that the programs generally only tracked process outcomes, such as service delivery statistics and consumer satisfaction surveys. The only two that did conduct outcome evaluations were substance abuse prevention programs receiving federal funds for specific initiatives.

A similar finding emerged from a review of substance abuse prevention programs (primarily serving high-risk ethnic minority children and adolescents) conducted by the U.S. GAO (1992). On the basis of site visits to 10 programs that had been nominated as exemplary, the GAO found that only 3 of the programs had completed some type of outcome evaluation and that only 1 of the evaluations included data from a comparison group.

Outcomes related to the work of community coalitions—an increasingly popular approach to addressing particular health problems—are also noticeably absent from this review. They were not a major focus primarily because we found it difficult in these types of studies to distinguish outcomes for ethnic minority adolescents as a subset of the larger target population. In addition, as Tolan and Guerra (1994) have noted, it appears to be more typical of the literature on coalition programs to describe the process and activities of the partnership rather than the effects on specific health problems.

What Worked Well and What Did Not

We can draw some conclusions from those programs that did report outcomes. It worked well to establish health-promotion programs on-site, where adolescents were already known to gather. Three projects (Friedman & Utada, 1992; Magura et al., 1994; Stein et al., 1992) were located in residential treatment, correctional, or job-training settings. Four others linked into popular community-based educational or recreational programs in neighborhood or tribal centers (AYSAPP, 1994; DePerry, 1994; Gilchrist et al., 1987; Kipke et al., 1993; St. Pierre et al., 1992). One program recruited participants for its AIDS prevention program from among adolescents being treated at a health clinic for a sexually transmitted disease (Mansfield et al., 1993). Locating programs in such settings provided easy access to a large pool of potential participants, generally led to higher levels of attendance and retention, and reduced the need for transportation. Gross and McCaul (1992) reported that in their multisite project, attendance was best for the group of adolescents who received the intervention in school on a fixed schedule during regular hours of school operation compared with others who had a rotating schedule or met after school.

Having access to ethnic minority adolescent populations was not enough to ensure engagement, active participation, and retention of participants, however. Friedman and Utada (1992) reported that they encountered significant levels of hostility and resentment because participation in their intervention was virtually mandatory. Projects in which participation was voluntary and was encouraged by incentives of some type tended to have good attendance, high levels of youth participation in program activities, and better retention rates. Some projects gave money for participation and incorporated a bonus system for completion of all sessions (e.g., Kipke et al., 1993; Magura et al., 1994). Money may have been an especially enticing incentive for these programs, because they served older male adolescents who frequently lacked legitimate ways of earning cash. Other programs provided alternative kinds of material or activity reinforcers, such as T-shirts, prizes, food, or recreational opportunities (Bruce & Emshoff,

1992; St. Pierre et al., 1992; Stein et al., 1992). Bruce and Emshoff (1992) also found it effective to use peer group leaders as trainers for some sessions of their program. The Boys and Girls Club substance abuse prevention project (St. Pierre et al., 1992) had a formal youth leadership component where "graduates" moved into helper roles, such as assisting with club activities and providing role-model demonstrations for younger members. Projects that included parental participation also provided child care and transportation to remove attendance barriers for adults (Bruce & Emshoff, 1992; DePerry, 1994).

Using ethnically similar counselors, outreach workers, and neighborhood or tribal advisory panels to assist with such tasks as recruitment, review of curricula for cultural relevance, and prevention service delivery resulted in more successful recruitment and retention outcomes (AYSAPP, 1994; Bobo et al., 1988; Bruce & Emshoff, 1992; DePerry, 1994; Gilchrist et al., 1987; Gross & McCaul, 1992; Lichtenstein et al., 1995; Magura et al., 1994; Schinke et al., 1988; St. Pierre et al., 1992). Further evidence of the need for this practice is suggested by projects that reported attrition or poor quality of participation when there was no perceived "connection" between group leader and adolescent participants (Friedman & Utada, 1992; Stein et al., 1992). Friedman and Utada cautioned that ethnic similarity in itself was not enough to ensure that rapport would be established:

> Regardless of ... differences in the group leaders' background, it appeared that what we might call a "real desire" to work with these youth, linked with an ability to be nonjudgmental and to enjoy them for who they are, had a positive impact on the functioning of the groups. (p. 116)

The process of tailoring program content to local cultural norms and circumstances was an important one, and some projects (e.g., Bobo et al., 1988) provided an in-depth view of how this was done. St. Pierre et al. (1992) outlined a process that included having local leaders—in this case, program prevention staff in local Boys and Girls Clubs—select culturally and regionally appropriate music videos, television commercials, role-plays, and records or tapes used in specific sessions. During program implementation, there were subsequent meetings to further customize materials and activities for cultural relevance. Friedman and Utada (1992) initially had difficulties with finding culturally appropriate materials that were appealing to streetwise African American male adolescents. They addressed this by using relevant current events highlighted in local news articles to prompt discussions.

Nearly all of the projects reviewed used multimodal and interactive teaching–learning techniques, making liberal use of role-plays, group discussion, video, audio, cartoons, television, music, and newspapers. Several projects highlighted special considerations for program content and methods when working with ethnic minority adolescents: the need to be concrete and literal rather than abstract (Friedman & Utada, 1992); the need to be sensitive to the shame and stigma associated with health issues, particularly for Asian youth (AYSAPP, 1994); the need to avoid stereotypical views about the etiology or characteristics of health issues, such as myths about the biological bases for Native American problems with alcoholism (Schinke et al., 1988); and the need to adapt teaching methods for ethnic minority adolescents, particularly African American or Native American youth, who may have a culturally rooted discomfort in self-disclosure (Friedman & Utada, 1992; Schinke et al., 1988).

Several of the projects engaged in broad efforts to gain local community buy-in. This appeared to be especially needed in programs directed at Asian American and Native American adolescents (Bobo et al., 1988; DePerry, 1994; Gilchrist et al., 1987; Lichtenstein et al., 1995; Schinke et al., 1988). Alternatively, few of the programs reviewed had significant levels of parental involvement beyond securing permission for adolescents to participate. At least one program (Gross & McCaul, 1992) concluded that lack of parental involvement was a factor that negatively affected health behavior change in the African American adolescents served.

Most projects described a critical need to be flexible in program design, and nowhere was this more true than in the area of evaluation. Several authors reported having to change the evaluation design of projects because of such real-world constraints as objections by the cooperating community-based agencies to identifying a control group who would be ineligible for services (Bruce & Emshoff, 1992; Magura et al., 1994), the expense of follow-up tracking (Magura et al., 1994), or the referral source disagreeing with procedures for youth assignment (Stein et al., 1992). University-based research teams came to understand retrospectively the need for better initial communication and coordination with partner community-based sites so that the potential impact of agency policies, procedures, and values on evaluation design could be anticipated in advance and addressed proactively

(Friedman & Utada, 1992; Stein et al., 1992). Evaluators also found it helpful in some cases to make content or process adaptations in evaluation methods, such as reading questions aloud because of varying literacy levels (Bruce & Emshoff, 1992) or supplementing information provided on paper-and-pencil tests with interactive role-play skill demonstrations (Kipke et al., 1993; Schinke et al., 1988).

Conclusion and Recommendations

Community-based health-promotion programs for ethnic minority adolescents can benefit targeted youth if program designers carefully consider the impact of culture and environment on all phases of the program, from conceptualizing the prevention approach to evaluating its effects. However, cultural sensitivity in itself is not enough to guarantee positive outcomes when the preventive intervention is not lengthy or intense enough or lacks appropriate focus. Gross and McCaul (1992) speculated that the limited effectiveness of their social support and skill-building model in preventing substance abuse may have been because it was "too little, too late" for the extensive needs of children of substance-abusing parents. Certainly health-promotion programs for ethnic minority adolescents should be grounded in an understanding of the culture, needs, and characteristics of the target youth group. However, programs must also be informed by knowledge of the health problem, the theoretical frameworks guiding intervention approaches, and research-based information on what has and has not worked well in the past. Particular care should be taken to ensure the relevancy, appropriateness, appeal, and potential for effectiveness of "canned" curricula; such materials should be reviewed by focus groups who are ethnically and culturally similar to the intended audience and should be extensively pretested (Vega, 1992).

The issue of gaining adequate access to ethnic minority adolescent groups is paramount to the success of any health-promotion program, and the issue is much broader than simply locating programs in convenient settings with physical proximity to youth. Language compatibility (including the use of familiar slang expressions), program name and image, "social marketing" techniques to increase the acceptability of participation (Mrazek & Haggerty, 1994), incentives and motivational systems of retention, and removal of any barriers to entry and full participation are equally important facets of an accessible program. Another access issue is the provider's recognition of cultural style and group norms common to adolescents of different ethnic groups. This understanding is key to engaging and retaining adolescents in health-promotion programs and influencing them to adopt or maintain positive health practices. For example, it is important to take into account the tremendous impact of the peer pressure pushing youth to engage in fighting, carrying weapons, or high-risk sexual and drug-related behaviors that may be prominent in their neighborhoods, as well as the sanctions that may be directed at those who attempt to engage in health-promoting behaviors (DiClemente & Houston-Hamilton, 1989). Access also must involve examination of the health service provider's own cultural biases, particularly in cases where ethnic dissimilarity exists between the researcher and the targeted culture (Cross, Bazron, Dennis, & Isaacs, 1989).

There is a growing body of literature on the attainment of cultural competency that can be extremely helpful to those wishing to design and implement health-promotion programs for ethnic minority adolescents. This literature includes general guidelines and recommendations (Bernal et al., 1995; Cross et al., 1989; Isaacs & Benjamin, 1991); theoretical perspectives (Rogler, Malgady, Constantino, & Blumenthal, 1987; Szapocznik, 1993; Tharp, 1991); individual studies, such as the programs we have cited; program inventories and summaries (Isaacs & Benjamin, 1991; Office of Substance Abuse Prevention, 1990; Wilson-Brewer & Jacklin, 1990); model program databases (e.g., from the Office of Minority Health); and studies of clinical and research issues related to specific ethnic groups or particular health problems (DiClemente & Houston-Hamilton, 1989; Gong-Guy, Cravens, & Patterson, 1991; Hammond & Yung, 1993; Huang, 1994; Pernice, 1994).

To validate that health-promotion programs are indeed making an impact on the critical health problems they are designed to address, community-based programs should seek to evaluate their outcomes in scientifically sound studies. The ideal is for programs to include behavioral measures and long-term tracking. The federal government can offer significant help in this effort by funding well-designed longitudinal evaluation research projects. Where community-based agencies lack the personnel or technical knowledge needed to carry out this work, partnerships between the academic research and ethnic minority communities might be established. Such partnerships would capitalize on the unique expertise of both groups and begin to build the information base needed for a sustained impact on the health of ethnic minority adolescents.

REFERENCES

Asian Youth Substance Abuse Prevention Project. (1994). *Guidance manual.* Rockville, MD: Center for Substance Abuse Prevention.

Bernal, G., Bonilla, J., & Bellido, C. (1995). Ecological validity and cultural sensitivity for outcome research: Issues for the cultural adaptation and development of psychosocial treatments with Hispanics. *Journal of Abnormal Child Psychology, 23,* 67–81.

Bobo, J., Gilchrist, L., Cvetkovich, G., Trimble, J., & Schinke, S. (1988). Cross-cultural service delivery to minority communities. *Journal of Community Psychology, 16,* 263–272.

Boles, S., Casas, M., Furlong, M., Gonzalez, G., & Morrison, G. (1994). Alcohol and other drug use patterns among Mexican-American, Mexican, and Caucasian adolescents: New directions for assessment and research. *Journal of Clinical Child Psychology, 23,* 39–46.

Brooks-Gunn, J., Boyer, C., & Hein, K. (1988). Preventing HIV infection and AIDS in children and adolescents: Behavioral research and intervention strategies. *American Psychologist, 11,* 958–964.

Bruce, C., & Emshoff, J. (1992). The SUPER II Program: An early intervention program. *Journal of Community Psychology,* (OSAP Special issue), 10–21.

Callahan, C., Rivara, F., & Koepsell, T. (1994). Money for guns: Evaluation of the Seattle Gun Buy-Back Program. *Public Health Reports, 109,* 472–477.

Caplan, M., Weissberg, R., Grober, J., Sivo, P., Grady, K., & Jacoby, C. (1992). Social competence promotion with inner–city and suburban young adolescents: Effects on social adjustment and alcohol use. *Journal of Consulting and Clinical Psychology, 60,* 56–63.

Chavez, E., Edwards, R., & Oetting, E. (1989). Mexican American and White American school dropouts' drug use, health status, and involvement in violence. *Public Health Reports, 104,* 594–604.

Chavez, E., Oetting, E., & Swaim, R. (1994). Dropout and delinquency: Mexican-American and Caucasian non-Hispanic youth. *Journal of Clinical Child Psychology, 23,* 47–55.

Cross, T., Bazron, B., Dennis, K., & Isaacs, M. (1989). *Towards a culturally competent system of care.* Washington, DC: CASSP Technical Assistance Center, Center for Child Health and Mental Health Policy, Georgetown University Child Development Center.

Damond, M., Breuer, N., & Pharr, A. (1993). The evaluation of setting and a culturally specific HIV / AIDS curriculum: HIV / AIDS knowledge and behavior intent of African American adolescents. *Journal of Black Psychology, 19*, 169–189.

DePerry, R. (1994). *Parent, school, and community partnership program: Documentation/replication manual.* Bayfield, WI: First American Prevention Center.

DiClemente, R., & Houston-Hamilton, A. (1989). Health promotion strategies for prevention of human immunodeficiency virus infection among minority adolescents. *Health Education, 20*, 39–43.

Ellickson, P., Bell, R., & McGuigan, K. (1993). Preventing adolescent drug use: Long-term results of a junior high program. *American Journal of Public Health, 83*, 856–861.

Friedman, A., & Utada, A. (1992). Effects of two group interaction models on substance-using adjudicated adolescent males. *Journal of Community Psychology*, (OSAP Special issue), 106–117.

Gainer, P., Webster, D., & Champion, H. (1993). A youth violence prevention program: Description and preliminary evaluation. *Archives of Surgery, 128*, 303–308.

Gilchrist, L., Schinke, S., Trimble, J., & Cvetkovich, G. (1987). Skills enhancement to prevent substance abuse among American Indian adolescents. *International Journal of the Addictions, 22*, 869–879.

Gong-Guy, E., Cravens, R., & Patterson, T. (1991). Clinical issues in mental health service delivery to refugees. *American Psychologist, 46*, 642–648.

Gross, J., & McCaul, M. (1992). An evaluation of a psychoeducational and substance abuse risk reduction intervention for children of substance abusers. *Journal of Community Psychology*, (OSAP Special issue), 75–87.

Guerra, N., & Slaby, R. (1990). Cognitive mediators of aggression in adolescent offenders, 2: Intervention. *Developmental Psychology, 26*, 269–277.

Guerra, N., Tolan, P., & Hammond, R. (1994). Prevention and treatment of adolescent violence. In L. Eron, J. Gentry, & P. Schlegel (Eds.), *Reason to hope: A psychosocial perspective on violence and youth* (pp. 383–403). Washington, DC: American Psychological Association.

Hammond, R., & Yung, B. (1991). Preventing violence in at-risk African-American youth. *Journal of Health Care for the Poor and Underserved, 2*, 359–373.

Hammond, R., & Yung, B. (1993). Psychology's role in the public health response to assaultive violence among young African-American men. *American Psychologist, 48*, 142–154.

Hansen, D. J., Watson-Perczel, M., & Christopher, J. S. (1989). Clinical issues in social skills training with adolescents. *Clinical Psychology Review, 9*, 365–391.

Huang, L. (1994). An integrative approach to clinical assessment and intervention with Asian-American adolescents. *Journal of Clinical Child Psychology, 23*, 21–31.

Isaacs, M. (1993). Developing culturally competent strategies for adolescents of color. In A. Elster, S. Panzarine, & K. Holt (Eds.), *Adolescent health promotion* (pp. 35–54). Arlington, VA: National Center for Education in Maternal and Child Health.

Isaacs, M., & Benjamin, M. (Eds.). (1991). *Towards a culturally competent system of care: Programs which utilize culturally competent principles, II.* Washington, DC: CASSP Technical Assistance Center, Center for Child Health and Mental Health Policy, Georgetown University Child Development Center.

Kazdin, A. (1994). Interventions for aggressive and antisocial children. In L. Eron, J. Gentry, & P. Schlegel (Eds.), *Reason to hope: A psychosocial perspective on violence and youth* (pp. 341–382). Washington, DC: American Psychological Association.

Kipke, M., Boyer, C., & Hein, K. (1993). An evaluation of an AIDS risk reduction education and skills training (ARREST) program. *Journal of Adolescent Health, 14,* 533–539.

Lichtenstein, E., Galsglow, R., Lopez, K., Hall, R., McRae, S., & Meyers, B. (1995). Promoting tobacco control policies in Northwest Indian tribes. *American Journal of Public Health, 85,* 991–994.

Lipsey, M., & Wilson, D. (1993). The efficacy of psychological, education, and behavioral treatment: Confirmation from meta-analysis. *American Psychologist, 48,* 1181–1209.

Magura, S., Kang, S., & Shapiro, J. (1994). Outcomes of intensive AIDS education for male adolescent drug users in jail. *Journal of Adolescent Health, 15,* 457–463.

Malgady, R., Rogler, L. & Constantino, G. (1990). Hero/heroine modeling for Puerto Rican adolescents: A preventive mental health intervention. *Journal of Consulting and Clinical Psychology, 58,* 469–474.

Mansfield, C., Conroy, M., Emans, J., & Woods, E. (1993). A pilot study of AIDS education and counseling of high-risk adolescents in an office setting. *Journal of Adolescent Health, 14,* 115–119.

Mrazek, P., & Haggerty, R. (Eds.). (1994). *Reducing risks for mental disorders: Frontiers for preventive intervention research.* Washington, DC: National Academy Press.

Office of Substance Abuse Prevention. (1990). *Breaking new ground for American Indian and Alaska Native youth at risk: Program summaries* (OSAP Tech. Rep. No. 3; DHHS Publication No. [ADM]90-1705).

Orlandi, M. (1986). Community-based substance abuse prevention: A multicultural perspective. *Journal of School Health, 56,* 394–400.

Pentz, M., Dwyer, J., MacKinnon, D., Flay, B., Hansen, W., Wang, E., & Johnson, C. (1989). A multi-community trial for primary prevention of drug abuse: Effects on drug use prevalence. *Journal of the American Medical Association, 261,* 3529–3266.

Pernice, R. (1994). Methodological issues in research with refugees and immigrants. *Professional Psychology: Research and Practice, 25,* 207–213.

Prothrow-Stith, D. (1987). *Violence prevention curriculum for adolescents.* Newton, MA: Education Development Center.

Rogler, L., Malgady, R., Constantino, G., & Blumenthal, R. (1987). What do culturally sensitive mental health services mean? The case of Hispanics. *American Psychologist, 42,* 565–570.

Schinke, S., Botvin, G., Trimble, J., Orlandi, M., Gilchrist, L., & Locklear, V. (1988). Preventing substance abuse among American-Indian adolescents:

A bicultural competence skills approach. *Journal of Counseling Psychology,* *35,* 87–90.

Schinke, S., Gordon, A., & Weston, E. (1990). Self-instruction to prevent HIV infection among African-American and Hispanic-American adolescents. *Journal of Consulting and Clinical Psychology, 58,* 432–436.

Shafer, M. (1995). Transition and Native American youth: A follow-up study of school leavers on the Fort Apache Indian Reservation. *Journal of Rehabilitation, 61,* 60–65.

Sheley, J. (1994). Drug activity and firearms possession and use by juveniles. *Journal of Drug Issues, 24,* 363–382.

Soriano, F. (1994). U.S. Latinos. In L. Eron, J. Gentry, & P. Schlegel (Eds.), *Reason to hope: A psychosocial perspective on violence and youth* (pp. 119–132). Washington, DC: American Psychological Association.

St. Pierre, T., Kaltreider, L., Mark, M., & Aikin, K. (1992). Drug prevention in a community setting: A longitudinal study of the relative effectiveness of a three-year primary prevention program in Boys and Girls Clubs across the nation. *American Journal of Community Psychology, 20,* 673–706.

Stein, S., Garcia, F., Marler, B., Embree-Bever, J., Garrett, C., Unrein, D., Burdick, M., & Fishburn, S. (1992). A study of multiagency collaborative strategies: Did juvenile delinquents change? *Journal of Community Psychology,* (OSAP Special issue), 88–105.

Sue, S., Fujino, D., Hu, L., Takeuchi, D., & Zane, N. (1991). Community mental health services for ethnic minority groups: A test of the cultural responsiveness hypothesis. *Journal of Consulting and Clinical Psychology, 59,* 533–540.

Szapocznik, J. (1993). Family psychology and cultural diversity. *American Psychologist, 48,* 400–407.

Tharp, R. (1991). Cultural diversity and treatment of children. *Journal of Consulting and Clinical Psychology, 59,* 799–812.

Thomas, S., & Quinn, S. (1993). An evaluation of HIV education messengers in a Black low income housing complex. *Journal of Health Education, 24,* 135–140.

Tobler, N. (1986). Meta-analysis of 143 adolescent drug prevention programs: Quantitative outcome results of program participants compared to a control of comparison group. *Journal of Drug Issues, 16,* 537–567.

Tolan, P., & Guerra, N. (1994). *What works in reducing adolescent violence: An empirical review of the field.* Boulder, CO: Center for the Study and Prevention of Violence.

Uehara, E., Takeuchi, D., & Smukler, M. (1994). Effects of combining disparate groups in the analysis of ethnic differences: Variations among Asian American mental health service consumers in level of community functioning. *American Journal of Community Psychology, 22,* 83–99.

U.S. Department of Education. (1992). *Digest of education statistics, 1992.* Washington, DC: National Center for Education Statistics.

U.S. General Accounting Office. (1992). *Adolescent drug use prevention: Common features of promising community programs* (Publication No. GAO/PEMD 91-2). Washington, DC: Author.

U.S. General Accounting Office. (1995). *School safety: Promising initiation for addressing school violence* (Publication No. GAO/HEHS-95-106). Washington, DC: Author.

Vega, W. (1992). Theoretical and pragmatic implications of cultural diversity for community research. *Journal of Community Psychology, 20,* 375–390.

Webster, D. (1993). The unconvincing case for school-based conflict resolution programs for adolescents. *Health Affairs, 12,* 126–141.

Wilson-Brewer, R., & Jacklin, B. (1990). *Violence prevention strategies targeted at the general population of minority youth.* Newton, MA: Education Development Center.

Yeh, M., Takeuchi, D., & Sue, S. (1994). Asian-American children treated in the mental health system: A comparison of parallel and mainstream outpatient service centers. *Journal of Clinical Child Psychology, 23,* 5–12.

Yung, B., & Hammond, R. (1994). The positive case for school-based violence prevention programs. *Health Affairs, 13,* 170–173.

Yung, B., & Hammond, R. (1995). *PACT—Positive Adolescent Choices Training: A model for violence prevention groups with African-American youth. Program guide.* Champaign, IL : Research Press.

IV

Health Policy and Special Concerns for Minority Adolescent Populations

INTRODUCTION

Health Policy and Special Concerns for Minority Adolescent Populations

This last part of the book addresses special issues of access to health care and health policy as they relate to minority adolescents. Whereas much of the focus of Parts I through III has been on conceptualizing and understanding adolescent health behaviors and relevant clinical interventions, this part of the book provides insight into broader issues of health policy. The two chapters in this part discuss policy issues with a particular focus on the unique health concerns of minority adolescents. From a clinical perspective, it is important to understand that there are constraints within the health care system that may hinder practitioners' efforts to enhance and promote healthier lifestyles among minority adolescents. By gaining a better understanding of these constraints, practitioners may begin to establish better opportunities for minority adolescents who are especially vulnerable to health risks.

Access to health care may be particularly problematic among minority populations, and this may have profound consequences on health status. In chapter 13, Giachello and Arrom emphasize the role that poverty plays in limiting minority access to health care. These authors highlight the barriers of obtaining adequate health care across diverse ethnic groups and propose important solutions for improving access for minority adolescents in general. The chapter also provides an appropriate segue between the previous parts of the book and the final chapter on health care policy. In this last chapter, Kaplan and Friedman take a special look at pertinent issues for minority adolescents given the current status of relevant health-related policies. The authors emphasize that adolescents and children are one of the largest uninsured groups in the United States today with African Americans and Hispanics being the most prevalent among the uninsured. They offer specific case studies of policy that provide suggestions for future health initiatives that could improve the health status of such minority adolescents. In summary, this last part of the book provides an important perspective on policy issues that will have significant implications for the future health of minority adolescents.

Dawn K. Wilson

13

Health Service Access and Utilization Among Adolescent Minorities

Aida L. Giachello and Jose O. Arrom

Considerable barriers to health care access exist at a time when minority youth are most at risk for acquiring communicable and sexually transmitted diseases and for developing dependencies on tobacco, alcohol, and other drugs. Many minority youth have been exposed to adverse conditions such as injury and social violence, malnutrition, family dysfunction, alcoholism, and poverty that may lead to school failure and drop out, gang membership, adolescent pregnancy, or the tendency to run away. Those youth most affected live in extreme poverty, and experience a number of social stressors. Therefore, to understand and to improve minority youth health status and to design and implement appropriate health-promotion activities, it is critical that health care providers take into consideration adolescents' living conditions; the social, cultural, and environmental conditions that may affect their health; age; gender; national origin; levels of ed-

ucation; income and poverty; family composition; and levels of acculturation and assimilation to the mainstream society.

Many of these issues have been addressed in other chapters of this
volume; therefore, we focus on issues of access to health care as they
affect minority youth and their families; and conclude with findings
and recommendations for programs, policies, and future research. The
terms *people of color* and *minority* cover a broad spectrum of groups
and cultures who experience a series of socioeconomic and political
disadvantages. These groups traditionally have experienced segrega-
tion, prejudice, and social discrimination. Given the diversity of the
minority youth population in regard to country of origin, cultures,
value systems, socioeconomic characteristics, migration patterns, living conditions, levels of acculturation and assimilation, and the impact
of these factors on their health, caution is needed in the generalization
of their experiences across all groups. Most of the limited research
data included in this chapter refer to African Americans and Hispanics
or Latinos. Whenever data are available on any other specific minority
group, we identify them by their national origins.

Changing Demographics

The demographics of people of color portend a dramatic change in
the composition of American society. Racial and ethnic minorities as
a whole are the fastest growing group in the United States. For example, from 1980 to 1990, the African American population increased
by 13%, from 26.5 million in 1980 to approximately 30 million in 1990;
the Asian population increased 95%, from 3.7 million to 7.2 million;
Native Americans grew 28%, from 1.5 million to almost 2 million; and
Hispanics and Latinos increased 53%, from 15.7 million to 22.3 million
(U.S. Bureau of the Census, 1990). During the same period, the White
population increased only 5.6%.

Even more striking is the age composition of racial and ethnic minorities. People of color tend to be concentrated in two age groups:
They are extremely young (21 years or younger) or they are in the
prime-age workers group (22–55 years). Very few are of retirement
age. Given that the fertility of women of color is almost one third to
one half times higher than that of White women and given the size
of the cohort of minority groups moving into their reproductive years,

people of color are expected to sustain their high population growth in the near future (U.S. Bureau of the Census, 1990; National Center for Health Statistics, 1993). Their population increase relative to the overall population may provide the political base from which to address the social, economic, and health concerns of their diverse populations.

Poverty and Health

Given the young age and high fertility rate of most people of color, the economic status of minority children and youth is of critical concern. Minorities of all ages are more apt to live in poverty than non-minorities. In 1991, 32.7% of African Americans, 28.7% of Hispanics and Latinos, and 13% of Asian and Pacific Islanders, were living below poverty level compared with 9.4% of Whites (Mendoza, 1994). The percentage of minority children and adolescents living below poverty levels were even higher (Children's Defense Fund [CDF], 1990b; Mendoza, 1994). The percentage of children and youth in poverty between 1986 and 1990 was 43.6% for African Americans and 37.4% for Hispanics, compared with 14.7% for Whites (Annie E. Casey Foundation, 1992). High poverty rates for people of color are linked to a number of factors. The inability of poor minority parents to protect children's and adolescents' well-being results primarily from insufficient economic resources, often combined with a lack of knowledge and personal and social support.

Limited Research and Data on Minority Youth

There are a number of reasons for the limited health information available on minorities as a whole. Some have to do with the government data organization and classification practices and the limited public interest in minority health. Many minority groups such as Latinos and Asians are usually merged into such categories as "White," "Non-White," "Others," or "Racial and Ethnic Minorities." Racial and ethnic identifiers have been routinely omitted, at least until recently, from the major national and state data resources. At present, a number of states continue to omit key items (i.e., place of birth and language preference) from their databases, impeding analysis of their data for specific subgroups. Interstate comparison of health data remains a nearly impossible task.

As a result, there is a distinct lack of epidemiological data on minority youth for such significant indicators as mortality rates, incidence rates, morbidity, and survival rates for certain illnesses, such as cancer. In researching public health, investigators lack databases (or registries) in key areas related to chronic disease and mental health. Therefore, they often depend on utilization and mortality data, when these are available. Hospital utilization databases lack identifiers or cannot generate data on Hispanics and Latinos, Asian Americans, Native Americans, and other such groups because of nonreporting and misclassification (Kozak, 1995). An added difficulty is the small number of studies conducted on minority youth as a whole, and the even smaller number that address minority youth by national origin or by gender. When available, the data seldom provide information on cultural, national, and lifestyle differences that may affect the health of adolescents. The data do not allow for analysis of differences by levels of education and literacy, levels of acculturation and assimilation, immigration history or socioeconomic status, all of which have been shown to affect the rates and types of certain diseases as well as patient access to the health care system (Arrom, 1993; Giachello, 1994). Furthermore, little intervention research has been conducted on minority youth and even fewer clinical trials have included or focused on minority youth or young women of color, hampering effective interventions with these populations. The overall lack of data available to measure the health status of the variety of minority youth populations may lead to hypotheses and conclusions that are wholly inadequate for addressing each population's specific health needs (Ramirez, Valdez, & Carter-Pokras, 1994).

Issues of Access: Understanding the Problem

Public debates on health and welfare reform have focused on issues of cost containment, the impact on business, governance, financing, health insurance, and the appropriate role of the public and private sector in the health and human services delivery system (Valdez, Morgenstern, et al., 1993). Limited discussions have taken place about how to improve the health status and address the health needs of vulnerable populations such as adolescents and people of color in a comprehensive fashion. Such discussions are critical, however, to minimizing the social and economic consequences to the nation when these people are unable to work or contribute to society because of illness or when their untreated health problems grow more severe, eventually requiring more expensive hospital and specialty care. Health and social policies, whether related to managed care or to Medicaid reform, must embrace a broader view of these issues if the health needs of people of color are to be served well.

Access refers to the entry into the system for either preventive and maintenance health care or for the treatment of illness (Aday, Andersen, & Fleming, 1980). Minorities confront a series of problems in accessing the health and the medical system in the United States. Giachello (1994), in a recent review of the literature, summarized the barriers to health care that Latinos confront on the basis of a number of indicators: whether or not a person has a regular source of care, financial barriers, including the lack of health insurance coverage, and cultural and institutional barriers. We briefly summarize these factors below as they relate to minority youth and their families.

Regular Source of Care

The phrase "regular source of care" refers to an established and identifiable facility or medical source that an individual or a family uses on a routine basis. Having a regular source of care is a good indicator of health services utilization because it facilitates entry into the health care system, continuity of care, and better quality of care (Aday, 1984; Aday et al., 1980). According to a 1986 survey, 15% of all poor children (Whites and minorities) under age 17 lacked a regular source of pediatric care (CDF, 1987). This is twice the proportion of that of nonpoor children. Studies consistently document that minorities are less likely than majority Whites to be linked to a regular source of care, such as a family doctor or a private clinic (Andersen, Giachello, & Aday, 1986; Giachello, 1994; Robert Wood Johnson Foundation, 1983, 1987; U.S. General Accounting Office [U.S. GAO], 1992; Valdez, Morgenstern, et al., 1993). Approximately 20% of African Americans and 35% of Latinos do not have a family physician or clinic for medical care. This percentage is even higher among minority groups with low family income (Aday, Andersen, & Fleming, 1980) and among minority children and adolescents (Garcia, Saucedo-Gonzalez, & Giachello, 1985; Giachello, 1994).

Where regular sources of care are reported, it is important to note poor and uninsured minority children and adolescents tend to use public health care facilities or hospital outpatient clinics. They tend to receive less continuous care from a regular provider who knows their medical history, their family situation, and their special needs (CDF, 1987). They are also most likely to be disproportionately linked to facilities with limited medical services outside regular office hours or to those that provide emergency treatment (Andersen et al., 1986; Garcia et al., 1985; Giachello & Aponte, 1989; Giachello & Arrom, 1989). As a result, minority children and youth are most likely to be taken to hospital emergency rooms, where care is episodic. A 1986 national survey (Giachello, 1994) found that Latinos and African Americans use hospital emergency rooms to a greater extent than Whites (22%, 19%, and 18%, respectively). This may be attributable to their different health status or to their higher probability of being exposed to violence, trauma, and injury (Giachello, 1994).

Youth often find that health care facilities are not user-friendly. Frequently, to receive health services, they need to be accompanied by a parent or an adult relative. Youth and their parents are forced to complete complicated forms, and when services are provided, they tend to come from the pediatric clinic (where, in most instances, most of the other patients are children under the age of 5). Furthermore, by observation we find that providers are less trained in adolescent health and less skilled in interviewing adolescents, particularly when such sensitive issues as substance use (or abuse) and sexually transmitted diseases need to be discussed.

If there is a clinic in their neighborhood, teens may avoid it, worrying that community workers or patients may recognize them and find out the purpose of their visits. Some poor minority teens have reading and writing difficulties and, at times, cannot fully comprehend family planning literature or written instructions, which tend to be geared to the educated adult population.

Health Insurance and Financing

Lack of health insurance is frequently cited as the single greatest problem that minorities face in the health care system. The high cost of health care, particularly for acute care for complications related to such chronic conditions as juvenile diabetes and asthma, is another barrier that minorities confront in obtaining medical care (Giachello, 1994). The lack of health insurance makes it difficult for minorities to have access to a broad array of health services, especially primary care (Aguilera, 1992; Giachello, 1994; U.S. GAO, 1992). In 1989, 39% of all Latinos (7.2 million) under 65 years of age did not have health insurance, compared with 14% for Whites and 24% for African Americans. The National Council of La Raza (Aguilera, 1992) documented that in 1990, nearly one third of Latinos nationwide did not have health insurance, compared with 13% of Whites and 20% of African Americans. Aguilera also found that, since 1985, the number of uninsured increased 1.4 million among Latinos and more than 400,000 among African Americans, whereas uninsured Whites decreased by 2.7 million.

Family income, type of family structure, and parents' employment status are perhaps the most important determinants of whether children and youth have health insurance coverage and of the type of coverage they have (Cunningham & Hahn, 1994). Nearly one third of children in female-headed families did not have any insurance coverage (either public or private) for all or part of 1987, compared with nearly one fourth of children in two-parent families (Cunningham & Hahn, 1994).

A recent report issued by the U.S. GAO (1992) on Hispanic access to health care stated that 35% of Latinos (over 6 million persons) were uninsured during all or part of 1989, compared with 19% of African Americans and 12% of Whites. This report indicated that 78% of Latino family members under the age of 65 who were uninsured lived in families who had an adult worker (U.S. GAO, 1992). The report also stated that uninsured Latinos were more likely than Whites and African Americans to work in industries that were less likely to provide health insurance coverage, such as construction and agriculture. Lack of health insurance coverage varies across racial and ethnic groups, by age group, by gender, by type of occupation, and by income.

Treviño, Moyer, Valdez, and Stroup-Benham (1991), using data from the 1989 Current Population Survey, reported that the following populations were the least likely to have health insurance (percentage uninsured is shown in parentheses): Mexican Americans (43.7%), Puerto Ricans (43.6%), and African Americans (45.4%). Furthermore, Puerto Ricans were the most likely of all racial and ethnic groups to report Medicaid coverage (32.5%), followed by African Americans (23.3%), Mexican Americans (13.7%), and Cuban Americans (11.9%), and compared with the total U.S. population (8.3%).

The high percentage of African Americans and Puerto Ricans enrolled in Medicaid programs was explained by the high prevalence of female-headed households, among these poor families, which makes them more likely to be eligible for Medicaid coverage. The low prevalence of Medicaid coverage among Mexican Americans was explained by the fact that many states exclude two-parent families from the Medicaid program (regardless of whether they meet the income requirements). Differences in Medicaid eligibility criteria vary across states. Texas and Florida represent the most restrictive states, compared with the less restrictive states of New York and New Jersey (National Coalition of Hispanic Health and Human Services Organizations [known as COSSMHO], 1990; U.S. GAO, 1992).

Finally, the problem of the lack of insurance coverage is very severe among minority children and adolescents (Bloom, 1990; Giachello & Aponte, 1989). The Children's Defense Fund (1990a) found that 24.8% of African American children and 34.7% of Hispanic children did not have health insurance during 1987–1991 compared with 18.1% of White children. Some local studies have indicated that the situation may be even worse. For example, Giachello and Aponte (1989) found in Chicago that 38% of Mexican American children and adolescents were uninsured. Mexican adolescents experienced the greatest disadvantage, with over half of 18 to 19 year olds (56%) uninsured.

Even minority children and youth who have insurance coverage cannot be assured of equal access to health care, because of inequities in benefits packages, providers' discretion in deciding which health insurance programs to accept, increased service costs because of private cost-containment efforts (e.g., deductibles and copayments), requirements that parents pay additional premiums for dependents, and poor quality of care. Thus, even the presence of insurance (public or private) may not adequately provide for the needs of these populations. More than half of private health insurance plans do not cover pre- or postnatal care, both of which are critical time periods for ensuring a child's future health, as well as have limited coverage for dental care and other preventive services. Of employment-based insurance plans, only 9% cover preventive care, 15% cover eyeglasses, and 32% cover dental care. Similar inadequacies are also found in public programs (COSSMHO, 1990). Furthermore, having access to the medical care system does not guarantee good quality of care. Mc-Dermott et al. (in press) found that African Americans and Hispanics with asthma who reported a regular source of health care were undertreated for asthma, despite having more symptoms that interfere with their daily functioning. These authors also found that providers' limited knowledge of clinical guidelines for good asthma management and control were associated with the poor care received by the minority groups studied.

Structural and Institutional Barriers to the Health Care System

As mentioned earlier, the health care system in America has limited flexibility to meet the needs of populations who are poor or who may have different illnesses, cultural practices, diets, languages, or age groups. The U.S. medical care system operates as a fragmented, loosely tied network of providers and institutions (Valdez, Morgenstern, et al., 1993). The organization and delivery of health care services rarely reflect the cultural or social concerns of the communities in which the services are located.

In reference to minority youth health, we have found that there are few adolescent health clinics. The maternal–infant model in place is designed for the convenience of providers and from an adult perspective with complicated forms to be filled out and with scheduled services organized around the needs of health care providers, not the consumers. Services to teens do not include adolescents in the planning and implementation process. Therefore, users of public primary health care facilities experience long waiting times between calling for an appointment and actual visits, and long waits once they arrive at the doctor's office or clinic. This creates system stress, encourages inefficient use of available resources, and causes overcrowding. As a result, the health care "system" uses a large share of its resources for emergency services and for admissions of those with increasingly serious conditions (Valdez, Morgenstern, et al., 1993).

Poor and uninsured minority youth, who may have limited ability to speak English, face a health system that lacks bilingual and bicultural services and providers who have limited cultural understanding, sensitivity, and competency. Providers' lack of knowledge about the health beliefs of minority cultures may result in a series of stereotypes and racial attitudes that may negatively affect the provider–consumer relationship. Some stereotypes that prevail among nonminority providers are the tendency to view minorities as both uninterested in preventive health care and noncompliant (Gregory, 1978). In addition, a 1987 mail survey in Chicago found that 50% of health care providers had limited knowledge about Latino health and stated that Latinos should learn English instead of expecting bilingual services to be provided (Aponte & Giachello, 1989). Such perceptions lead to poor communications between providers and consumers and poor quality of care.

These communication barriers can be reduced or eliminated with the use of interpreters. However, few health care systems (e.g., hospitals and clinics) have such procedures in place to deal effectively with clients who do not speak English well. For example, Aponte and Giachello (1989) found in Chicago that only 40% of health care providers reported having a procedure for dealing with monolingual Spanish-speaking clients. Of those who reported a procedure, close to one third stated that it consisted of telling the client to bring his or her own interpreter, and two thirds indicated that an interpreter was available on-site. Providers serving primarily Latino clients were the least likely to report having any sort of arrangements for serving clients who spoke only Spanish.

Even when health care facilities do establish a pool of interpreters, often not enough time and resources are invested to train interpreters with the necessary skills, medical terminology, and information about health and illnesses (Putsch, 1985). Usually the responsibility for interpretation in a health or mental health facility falls to anyone who is bilingual, such as an employee, family members (e.g., children), or friends—all of whom have no training (Putsch, 1985). This may lead to inaccuracies, failure to disclose information, violations of confidentiality, and failure of the provider to develop rapport with the patient (only with the interpreter; Giachello, 1994).

The middle-class orientation of the medical care system also leads to communication problems between providers and minority youth of low socioeconomic status. For example, providers tend to use too many technical terms, which confuse further minority youth and families, and they tend to have behavioral expectations for youth that reflect their own middle-class training, background, and orientation.

Transportation and child care pose serious barriers to minorities, particularly those who live outside major cities (e.g., suburban or rural areas), where public health care facilities tend to be limited or nonexistent. Minorities have reported lengthy, time-consuming travel to reach a health care facility (Valdez, Morgenstern, et al., 1993). Others forego seeking medical care because of a facility's lack of flexible hours of services or household, job, or family responsibilities. Minority youth are not only exposed to the poor design of services but also to a lack of providers, especially physicians, who may practice in their own middle-class communities, leading to severe shortage of health care professionals in other areas (Giachello, 1994).

In summary, there are a number of institutional and cultural characteristics of the health delivery system that serve as barriers to the initial entry or the further utilization of health care services by minority youth. Many of these are related to the organization of the health care services and to the culture that prevails. These are some of the discouraging features of the health care system that lead minority youth to noncompliance or poor adherence to treatment. Such barriers have an impact on health services use as we illustrate next.

Use of Health Services

Health services utilization is the true measure of access to health care. The literature on minority use of health services has indicated that compared with majority Whites, minorities as a whole and minority youth in particular use health and medical services less (Cunningham & Hahn, 1994; Giachello, 1994; Mendoza, 1994; Treviño & Moss, 1984). For example, minorities are less likely overall to see a physician, to be hospitalized during the year, or to use preventive health services. However, differences do prevail among the various racial and ethnic groups in the pattern of health services use. African Americans and Puerto Ricans, for example, report higher levels of use. Two main explanations have been given for this: These two groups reportedly have the worst health status (measured on a number of indicators), and both groups are most likely to have health insurance (e.g., Medicaid coverage), which allows them to access the health care system more often (Giachello & Andersen, 1986).

Patterns of health service utilization also vary by gender, with women overall using the health care system more. Women in their child-bearing years reported higher use than men of general preventive services, but lower use of mental health services (Giachello, 1994).

Use of health services also varies by age group, with preventive services being used the most by infants and young children. Adolescents use health services the least. An explanation for their underuse may very well be that adolescents tend to be healthier and to experience less chronic conditions. Although this may be true for adolescents in general, it is questionable for minority youth, considering the high poverty and violence experienced by many of them. Minority adolescents may actually have stronger needs for using the health care system, yet barriers to care may prevent them from doing so. Unfortunately, the limited data on minority youth health status and their patterns of health service use do not allow for a clear understanding of the dynamics at work for health care delivery to this population.

Summary and Recommendations

In summary, minorities overall are least likely to be able to afford medical care and to have health insurance coverage. The situation has become more acute in the past decade and appears to be more severe among certain communities in the nation and among certain subgroups, such as children and adolescents and those with lower incomes. Among minority groups, Hispanics are the most likely to be uninsured. When health insurance is reported, African Americans and Puerto Ricans are the most likely to be covered by government-sponsored programs such as Medicaid. Finally, lack of health insurance appears to be associated with low linkages with a regular source of medical care and low use of health services. This contributes to the disproportionate use by uninsured people of more costly services, such as hospital emergency rooms, when symptoms of illness persist or when an illness reaches an advanced stage.

Minority youth experience poor health status and poor access to health care services. These factors, combined with their disproportionately high rate of school drop-out, academic underachievement, and low literacy rates, are critical concerns that will affect their employment, insurance coverage, and access to preventive care and health education. Minority youth lack positive self-esteem, experience few viable opportunities for a productive and successful future, and have only limited exposure to role models. Such realities promote a sense of powerlessness and hopelessness in these youth, often leaving them to accept a marginal existence, or to become involved in social violence (e.g., gang-related activities) and substance abuse.

Minority youth health must be viewed within a broader societal context. Most of the health problems of these adolescents are caused by structural conditions in society. These include a weak and deteriorating public school system, poverty, and environmental and occupational hazards, among others. Health care providers often treat the most costly symptoms and do not address the origins of the problems. Therefore, there is a need for long-term institutional and structural changes to deal effectively with the health and social problems of minority youth. Likewise, social changes must occur in U.S. society to minimize poverty and improve levels of education and incomes among these groups.

It is important to recognize that institutional racism, sexism, and classism account for many of the health and social problems of minority groups, including minority youth. Such prejudices are reflected in the type of policies that are developed and implemented in the United States, as well as in the lack of action taken on behalf of disadvantaged groups.

Reforms are also needed in the medical care and social service systems. Reforms currently proposed in Congress will not assume a compassionate and humane role toward the needy. Instead, they will increase the gap between the "haves" and the "have-nots," at a time when a move should be made toward supporting a health care system where everyone can have access regardless of their ability to pay, or their gender, age, race, or nationality. This should not only eliminate financial barriers but also remove structural, distributional, and cultural barriers in accessing and using the health care system in different settings.

Comprehensive and culturally sensitive services, as well as a high quality of medical care, can be key elements to improving the health status, access, and quality of health services for minority youth. Adolescent health service capacity must be increased in minority communities. Services should be reorganized so that they can be relevant and accessible to minority youth in their neighborhoods and schools. Institutional policy changes should be promoted that reward the delivery of primary care and increase cooperation between the education and the health systems in terms of increasing school clinics, providing comprehensive health education, and offering preventive and early intervention services aimed at minority youth. Lack of community outreach efforts and the exclusion—or limited participation—of minorities in planning and managing health care services create intended and unintended barriers to medical care.

Health-promotion interventions must be conducted through a variety of settings and channels, primarily the health care system, schools, worksites, the community, and the media (Mullen, Evans, Forster, & Gottlieb, 1995). Schools provide great opportunities to intervene with minority youth, providing a captive audience with which a series of health-promotion activities can be implemented. Most states have health-promotion components to their school codes, requiring a minimum number of hours of physical education and health education at different grade levels, as well as physical examinations and immunization compliance.

In addressing the well-being of minority youth in a comprehensive way, schools also have a critical role to play in identifying social and learning problems at an early stage and to intervene appropriately to boost poor academic performance. Non-English-speaking students are often segregated into bilingual education tracks, with deficient curriculums and teaching, when they could be placed in classes where culturally competent teaching techniques can be used. Unfortunately, children of migrant workers tend to move frequently, failing to receive a continuous education and often falling behind in their learning. Their limited literacy skills often impede their appreciation of health education and their ability to receive continuous health care.

Part of a comprehensive minority youth prevention strategy is for schools and community groups to work together to reduce violence in the street and in the home. Violence results in posttraumatic stress disorders and appears to increasingly link to alcohol and other drugs.

Implementation of a comprehensive health-promotion strategy aimed at minority youth is a major problem. In the case of schools, we have found that they have few certified bilingual health educators. In Chicago, it has been our experience that immigrant bilingual teachers have very low levels of knowledge about such issues as HIV, sexually transmitted diseases, and violence and demonstrate great discomfort in discussing these issues, let alone in teaching them. There are no health curriculums in the languages of the major immigrant minorities in the United States, whether epidemiologically relevant or specifically tailored to their needs. The often limited economic resources of school systems do not allow them to make up-to-date health education materials and resources available.

Adult education programs are critical for integrating older immigrant youth, who can learn English and catch up with the education they missed in their home countries. These programs often present major access barriers of their own, particularly for working youth, in terms of class times, enrollment dates, instructional technology, and fees. Curriculum content is often not relevant to young workers, and education on life skills, health, and legal procedures is difficult to integrate with needed basic levels of English instruction.

Health-promotion activities at the community level should be increased to target minority youth. Neighborhood organizations such as churches, park programs, and youth clubs have offered traditional bases for health promotion in many minority communities. Yet, attachment to and use of community-based organizations and facilities by minority youth is highly variable. Non-English-speaking and other minority youth also face language and cultural barriers. At the community level, there are often fewer activities for young women. In addition, gang affiliations often prevent youth from accessing youth facilities (i.e., when they are located on gang "turf").

Media campaigns and frequent news items are effective ways of increasing awareness of health issues and making people aware of health services. Minorities face major media barriers in health promotion in that few minority health educators have media skills and media campaigns are expensive to design and produce. Sponsorship is also difficult to secure, because many health messages may work against key advertisers (e.g., beer companies).

English-speaking minority children have been said to spend more time watching television than attending school. Therefore, an avenue for reaching them is through either radio or television. Unfortunately, without clear intentions, many television programs promote violence, alcohol abuse and smoking and glamorize sexuality. Immigrant non-English-speaking minorities have few media channels; it is only when such groups become a major advertising market that the media begin broadcasting to them in major cities. Cable television is a rapidly emerging venue for media influence and even provides opportunities for interactive education. However, in many small minority population areas, access is a continuing issue, both to local production and national channels, as are high cable subscription rates (Giachello & Arrom, 1989).

Finally, environmental, social, and physical health care issues must be given equal consideration in any public health care policy discussion or reform agenda when one is addressing barriers to care faced by minority groups. Reducing barriers requires strengthened organization of public health and medical care delivery. Academic institutions must recognize the importance of cultural competency issues. Their curriculums need to be modified and training efforts reoriented to include greater understanding of culturally based perspectives regarding adolescent health and illness.

REFERENCES

Aday, L. A. (1984). National profile on access to medical care: Where do we stand? *American Journal of Public Health, 74*, 1331–1339.

Aday, L. A., Andersen, R. M., & Fleming, G. V. (1980). *Health care in the U.S.: Equitable for whom?* Beverly Hills, CA: Sage.

Aguilera, E. (1992). *Hispanics and health insurance, Vol. I. Status.* Washington, DC: National Council of La Raza and Labor Council for Latin American Advancement.

Andersen, R. M., Giachello, A. L., & Aday, L. A. (1986). Access of Hispanics to health care and cuts in services: A state-of-the-art overview. *Public Health Reports, 101*, 238–252.

Annie E. Casey Foundation. (1992). *Kids count data book.* Baltimore: Author.

Aponte, R., & Giachello, A. L. M. (1989). *Health care provider's knowledge, attitudes, and practices in reference to Hispanics in Chicago: Analysis of a 1988 citywide survey.* Chicago: Hispanic Health Alliance.

Arrom, J. (1993, March). *Research and data on Latinos in the Midwest.* Paper presented at the Surgeon General Regional (Midwest) Meeting on Hispanic / Latino Health, Chicago.

Bloom, B. (1990). Health insurance and medical care: Health of our nation's children, United States, 1988. *Advance Data From Vital Health and Statistics, 188.* (DHHS Publication No. PHS 90-1250). Washington, DC: U.S. Government Printing Office.

Children's Defense Fund. (1987). *A children's defense budget: An analysis of the FY 1987 Federal budget and children.* Washington, DC: Author.

Children's Defense Fund. (1990a). *Latino youth at a crossroads.* Washington, DC: Author.

Children's Defense Fund. (1990b). *A report card, briefing book, and action primer.* Washington, DC: Author.

Cunningham, P. J., & Hahn, B. A. (1994). The changing American family: Implications for children's health insurance coverage and the use of ambulatory care services. *The Future of Children, 4*(3), 24–42.

Garcia, R., Saucedo-Gonzalez, I., & Giachello, A. L. (1985). *Access to health care and other social indicators among Hispanics in Chicago.* Chicago: Latino Institute.

Giachello, A. L .M. (1994). Issues of access and use. In C. W. Molina & M. Aguirre-Molina (Eds.), *Latino health in the US: A growing challenge* (pp. 83–111). Washington, DC: American Public Health Association.

Giachello, A. L. M., & Andersen, R. M. (1986, September). *Variations in access to medical care among Mexican Americans and Puerto Ricans in different regions of the U.S.* Paper presented at the 114th annual meeting of the American Public Health Association, Las Vegas, NV.

Giachello, A. L. M., & Aponte, R. (1989). *Health status and access issues of Hispanic children and adolescents in Chicago: Analysis of a 1984 citywide survey.* Chicago: Hispanic Health Alliance.

Giachello, A. L. M., & Arrom, J. O. (1989). *Access to health care among Hispanics, Whites, and Blacks in selected communities in Chicago's northwest side.* Chicago: Hispanic Health Alliance.

Gregory, D. (1978). Transcultural medicine: Treating Hispanic patients. *Behavioral Medicine, 5,* 22–29.

Kozak, L. M. (1995, July 6). Underreporting of race in the National Hospital Discharge Survey. *Advance Data From Health and Vital Statistics, 265.* Washington, DC: U.S. Government Printing Office.

McDermott, M., Silva, J., Rydman, R., Giachello, A. L. M., Yarzagaray, E., Peragallo, N., Barquolo, H., Arrom, J. O., & Robinson, D. (in press). *Practice variations in the treatment of asthma. Journal of Medical Systems.*

Mendoza, F. S. (1994). The health of Latino children in the United States. *The Future of Children, 4*(3), 43–72.

Mullen, P. D., Evans, D., Forster, J., & Gottlieb, N. H. (1995). Settings as an important dimension in health education / promotion policy, programs, and research. *Health Education Quarterly, 22,* 329–345.

National Center for Health Statistics. (1993, February). Advance report of final natality statistics, 1990. *Monthly Vital Statistics Report* (DHHS Publication No. DHS92-1120). Washington, DC: Author.

National Coalition of Hispanic Health and Human Services Organizations (COSSMHO). (1990). *". . . And access for all: Medicaid and Hispanics."* Washington, DC: COSSMHO.

Putsch, R. W., III. (1985). Cross-cultural communication: The special case of interpreters in health care. *Journal of the American Medical Association, 254,* 3344–3348.

Ramirez, A. G., Valdez, R. B., & Carter-Pokras, O. (1994). Cancer. In C. W. Molina & M. Aguirre-Molina (Eds.), *Latino health in the US: A growing challenge* (pp. 211–246). Washington, DC: American Public Health Association.

Robert Wood Johnson Foundation. (1983). *Update report on access to health care for the American people.* Princeton, NJ: Author.

Robert Wood Johnson Foundation. (1987). *Access to health care in the United States: Results of a 1986 survey.* Princeton, NJ: Author.

Treviño, F. M., & Moss, A. (1984). Health indicators for Hispanic, Black, and White Americans. *Vital Health Statistics* (DHHS publication PHS 84-1576). Washington, DC: U.S. Department of Health and Human Services.

Treviño, F. M., Moyer, M. E., Valdez, R. B., & Stroup-Benham, C. A. (1991). Health insurance coverage and utilization of health services by Mexican-Americans, mainland Puerto Ricans, and Cuban Americans. *Journal of the American Medical Association, 265,* 233–237.

U.S. Bureau of the Census. (1990). *P.L. 194 for 1980 and 1990.* Washington, DC: U.S. Government Printing Office.

U.S. General Accounting Office. (1992, January). *Hispanic access to health care: Significant gaps exist.* Washington, DC: Author.

Valdez, R. B., Morgenstern, H., Brown, E. R., Wyn, R., Wang, C., & Cumberland, W. (1993). Insuring Latinos against the costs of illness. *Journal of the American Medical Association, 269,* 889–894.

Health Care and Health Policy for Adolescents

Robert M. Kaplan and Lawrence Friedman

The purpose of this chapter is to provide an overview of health policy issues relevant to adolescents from underrepresented groups. The term *public policy* is often misunderstood. A policy is a plan of action, often selected from several competing alternatives, that is meant to guide and define future directions. The term *policy* is often used in the limited sense of legislative actions. However, policy is made at different levels, including governments, organizations, and communities. It would not be possible to review all issues in health policy in the confines of a single chapter. Therefore, we focus on some specific policy issues that are relevant to minority adolescents.

Before proceeding, we must clarify our use of the term *adolescent*. In public policies, the use of this term has been inconsistent. Some federal and state programs cover individuals beginning at age 11 years, whereas others do not initiate coverage until age 16 years. Some other definitions even include people up until age 24. Certainly, the medical and developmental issues for 11- and 24-year-olds are remarkably different. For this chapter, we follow the American Medical Association (AMA) interval of 11 to 21 years of age to define an adolescent (AMA, 1992).

This chapter addresses several issues. First, we give an overview of adolescent health. Next, we review the conceptualization and measurement of health status relevant to adolescents. Third, we consider medical care policy guidelines for adolescents. We then evaluate the funding of health care for adolescents. The remainder of the chapter touches on other policy issues. We offer two specific policy case studies, one a medical policy and the other a legal policy. The policies include adolescent hepatitis B vaccination and the case of cigarette advertising. These examples are not intended to be comprehensive. Instead, our purpose is to introduce several different examples of policies that may affect adolescent health in minority communities.

Is Public Funding for Adolescent Medical Care Necessary?

One of the major public policy questions concerns whether it is necessary to invest public resources in health services for adolescents. The reason this is an issue is that adolescents tend to be healthy, at least in terms of traditional biomedical indicators. Other age groups are more likely to be at risk for serious illness and death. Figure 1 shows the deaths per 100,000 persons in the population as a function of age in 5-year intervals. In 1987 there were approximately 872 deaths for each 100,000 people in the population. For those in early adolescence, there were approximately 27 deaths per 100,000 persons. In other words, mortality rates for those in early to midadolescence were remarkably low. Furthermore, morbidity associated with serious chronic illness was also very low during this phase of life.

Although there are some adolescents who have chronic illnesses, the great majority of medical visits for this age group are for acute, self-limiting illnesses. The three most common reasons for office-based physician visits are general examinations, acne, and sore throats (U.S. Department of Health and Human Services, 1988). It might be argued that providing extensive services for adolescents diverts resources

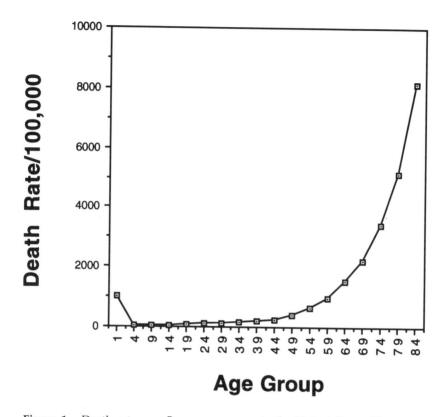

Figure 1. Death rates per 5-year age group in the United States. The initial data point is for children under the age of 1. The points on the x-axis represent the remaining intervals. For example, the Point 9 represents interval ages 5–9 (U. S. Department of Commerce, 1991). Data are adapted from the U.S. Congress Office of Technology Assessment and are in the public domain.

away from groups that are more likely to benefit from acute medical intervention.

The arguments presented above may be compelling from the perspective of the traditional biomedical model. The traditional model focuses on disease and emphasizes mortality as the principal outcome. Under an alternative outcomes model, the objectives of health care are twofold. First, health care and health policy should increase life expectancy. Second, the health care system should improve the quality of life during the years that people are alive. Traditional biomedical indicators and diagnoses are important because they may be related to mortality or to quality of life. We prefer the term *health-related quality of life* to refer to the impact of health conditions on function. Thus, health-related quality of life may be independent of quality of life relevant to work setting, housing, air pollution, or similar factors.

The appropriate conceptualization of health outcomes requires consideration of quality of life in addition to life duration. Furthermore, models must consider future as well as current health. Many adolescent health problems do not affect near-term mortality. However, good health care for adolescents might prevent mortality from HIV, accidents, or other chronic illnesses at some point in the future. Thus, an adequate conceptualization of adolescent health must consider future as well as current outcomes. For example, it is valuable to invest in smoking prevention programs that will reduce the burden of adult lung disease. Likewise, prevention of teen pregnancy may prevent problems throughout the life cycle. A conceptual model of health outcome must recognize that near-term benefits may be few but long-term benefits may be great (Kaplan, 1993).

Health services for adolescents are different from those for adults for several reasons. First, services for adolescents may be more psychosocial than biomedical in nature. In other words, the purpose of the services may not necessarily be to diagnose and treat an acute or chronic disease. Instead, services might offer support and guidance during developmental phases as teenagers struggle to separate from parents and establish their own set of behaviors and health beliefs. In the next section, we consider what services are appropriate for adolescents.

Practice Policy: Guidelines for Adolescent Preventive Services

In 1992, the AMA released a set of Guidelines for Adolescent Preventive Services (GAPS). The GAPS report represents a major change in the recommendations for physicians' treatment of adolescents and offers a framework for the organization and delivery of preventive services. Table 1 summarizes the services and the stages of adolescence at which services are recommended. In addition to traditional medical services, the guidelines recommend guidance services on parenting, safety, diet and fitness, and lifestyle. Screening measures are expanded to include substance use, sexually transmitted diseases (STDs), and

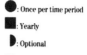

Key and Notations:

● : Once per time period

■ : Yearly

◗ : Optional

HR : High Risk Category

1. Recommendation developed by the National Heart, Lung, and Blood Institute Second Task Force on Blood Pressure in Children.

2. Recommendation developed by the National Cholesterol Education Program: Report of the Expert Panel on Blood Cholesterol Levels in Children and Adolescents, 1991.

3. Recommendation developed by the Advisory Committee for Immunization Practices.

* Screening should be performed if the adolescent is currently sexually active.

** Screening should be performed if the adolescent female is sexually active or 18 years of age or older.

HR-1: Test should be performed if there is a family history of cardiovascular disease prior to age 55 or parental history of high cholesterol. Physician may choose to perform test if family history is unknown or if adolescent has multiple risk factors for future cardiovascular disease.

HR-2: Syphilis test should be performed on and HIV test offered to adolescents who are at high risk for infection. This includes having had more than one sexual partner in last six months, having exchanged sex for drugs, being a male who has engaged in sex with other males, having used intravenous drugs (HIV), having had other STDs, having lived in an area endemic for infection, and having had a sexual partner who is at risk for infection.

HR-3: Test should be performed on adolescents who have been exposed to active TB, have lived in a homeless shelter, have been incarcerated, have lived in an area endemic for TB, or currently work in a health care setting.

HR-4: Vaccination should be provided to adolescents who have had only one previous MMR.

HR-5: Vaccination should be given 10 years following previous dT booster.

HR-6: Hepatitis B virus vaccination (HBV) should be given to susceptible adolescents at high risk for infection (see HR-2).

	Stage of Adolescence		
	Early (11-14 yrs.)	Middle (15-17 yrs)	Late (18-21 yrs)
Health Guidance			
Parenting	●	●	◗
Adolescent Development	■	■	■
Safety Practices	■	■	■
Diet and Fitness	■	■	■
Healthy Lifestyles (sexual behavior, smoking, alcohol and drug use)	■	■	■
Screening			
Hypertension[1]	■	■	■
Hyperlipidemia[2]	HR-1		●
Eating Disorders	■	■	■
Obesity	■	■	■
Tobacco Use	■	■	■
Alcohol & Drug Use	■	■	■
Sexual Behavior	■	■	■
Sexually Transmissible Diseases (STDs)			
Gonorrhea	■ *	■ *	■ *
Chlamydia	■ *	■ *	■ *
Genital Warts	■ *	■ *	■ *
Syphilis	HR-2	HR-2	HR-2
HIV Infection	HR-2	HR-2	HR-2
Cervical Cancer	■ *	■ *	■ **
Depression/Suicide Risk	■	■	■
Physical, Sexual or Emotional Abuse	■	■	■
Learning Problems	■	■	■
Tuberculosis	HR-3	HR-3	HR-3
Immunizations[3]			
Measles, Mumps, & Rubella	HR-4	HR-4	HR-4
Diphtheria & Tetanus		HR-5	
Hepatitis B	HR-6	HR-6	HR-6

Source: Guidelines for Adolescent Preventive services, American Medical Association, copyright 1992.

learning problems. The GAPS recommendations differ from traditional medical care in several ways. For example, traditional approaches to screening emphasize the diagnosis and treatment of defined diseases. The GAPS approach emphasizes health promotion and disease prevention. The GAPS approach recommends at least two parental guidance consultations, whereas the traditional approach leaves consultations with parents to the discretion of the physician.

A major component of adolescent health service is preventive in nature. Certain problems, such as growth abnormalities, can be detected through other regular examinations. Yet many of the services could be directed toward preventing future problems. For example, tobacco use, drug use, and dietary and sexual habits are likely to be established during adolescent years, and services that deal directly with these problems may help prevent morbidity and mortality in the near- or long-term. Other programs for adolescents might include AIDS education and prevention of teen pregnancy. There has been evidence that such prevention programs are well received and that they can affect behavior changes.

An example of an intervention with potential benefit for minority adolescents was recently reported in the *Journal of the American Medical Association* (DiClemente & Wingood, 1995). African American women are at particularly high risk for HIV disease. In fact Centers for Disease Control and Prevention (CDC) data from 1994 indicated that African American women were 16 times more likely to be infected with the HIV virus than White non-Hispanic women (CDC, 1995). To reduce this trend, it has been suggested, a condom should be used during each episode of sexual intercourse. Yet some researchers (e.g., Ickovics & Rodin, 1992) have suggested that compliance with condom use is significantly lower among African American adolescents than in most other groups. In one clinical trial (DiClemente & Wingood, 1995), 127 sexually active young African American women were randomly assigned to a social skills intervention or to a control group that was given a single session of information about HIV. The social skills intervention used five sessions to develop ethnic and gender pride and to provide instruction on HIV risk reduction, self-control, assertiveness, and communication skills. Follow-up data showed that participants in the intervention group used condoms more often, had greater sexual self-control and communication, and exhibited better sexual assertiveness. Furthermore, women in the social skills intervention group achieved greater use of condoms by their partners than did those in the control group. Overall, the study suggested that programs sensitive to culture and gender can achieve significant behavior change among members of high-risk groups.

One of the difficulties in establishing a health care policy for adolescents is that supportive and preventive services may not be covered under reimbursement schedules for traditional health care policies. For example, it is often difficult for providers to get reimbursed for counseling visits; depending on the program, counseling adolescents on issues relevant to sexuality may or may not be a reimbursable expense. It is actually easier for providers to be reimbursed for treatment than for prevention of an STD or pregnancy. Thus, it may be unlikely that interventions such as those we have described will be widely used. In health care, physicians are given primary responsibility for patient care. Yet, most patient encounters last less than 10 min, and in this short time, it is difficult to provide instruction for safety, prevention of alcohol, STDs, unwanted pregnancies, and drug-related problems. Furthermore, resources are rarely available to support nonphysicians in disseminating this information.

Although managed care plans may be interested in health promotion and disease prevention, their commitment to prevention services for teenagers is not universal. Therefore, it is likely that the responsibility for the health of a teenager will not be taken on by the provider until he or she becomes ill or is an adult.

Public Policy Relevant to Funding Health Services

This part of the chapter concerns policies relevant to the funding of health care services for adolescents. Although the exact numbers are uncertain, nearly all observers agree that a substantial proportion of Americans are uninsured. The number 37 million is cited most frequently whereas other estimates range between 32 and 43 million (Chollet, Folley, & Mages, 1990; Nelson & Short, 1990; Short 1990; Short, Monheit, & Beauregard, 1989). Although somewhat out of date, the 1987 National Medical Expenditure Survey (Short, 1990; Short et al., 1989) remains the most complete data set on insurance coverage. The survey found that 47.8 million Americans did not have health insurance during some part of calendar year 1987. On any particular day during that year, between 34 and 36 million people were uninsured, whereas 24.5 million were uninsured throughout the entire year.

Those who are uninsured are not a random sample from the general population. The only group that is immune is elderly people, because virtually all Americans older than 65 years are covered under Medicare (Lee & Estes, 1990). Those in the age range from 19 to 25 years are most likely to be uninsured (23.3% according to the NMES), and the second most likely group to be excluded are children and adolescents under 18 years of age. In 1988, 17% of children and adolescents had no health insurance from either public or private sources (Bloom, 1990).

Members of different racial and ethnic groups have very different rates of health care coverage. The NMES suggested that 18.6% of non-Hispanic Whites were uninsured for all or part of 1987. This stands in contrast to 29.8% of uninsured Black respondents and 41.4% of uninsured Hispanic respondents. Hispanics, the least likely to be insured, also represent the most rapidly growing demographic group in the United States (see chap. 13, in this volume).

What is more, problems with health insurance are not limited to those who do not have insurance. Many individuals who have private health insurance are underinsured. Being underinsured is defined as being at risk for financial difficulty because of large out-of-pocket expenditures in the event of a catastrophic illness. Recent evidence has suggested that, in addition to the 40 million Americans who have no health insurance, another 29 million privately insured people do not have enough insurance (Short & Banthin, 1995). Among privately insured individuals, African Americans and Hispanics are significantly more likely to be underinsured than White non-Hispanics, and individuals less than 19 years of age are more likely to be underinsured than adults (Short & Banthin, 1995). In addition, even some adequately insured teenagers may not access services because of confidentiality concerns. Fear that a provider may inform parents or that parents will receive insurance notification about a visit to receive birth control services may deter some teens from seeking preventive health services.

Medicaid

Very low-income individuals in the United States may qualify for a Medicaid program. Originally, Medicaid was designed to help low-income women and children and those with certain defined disabilities. However, Medicaid covers families with dependent children and thus may also include coverage for some men. In contrast to Medicare, which is a federal program, Medicaid is jointly funded by states and the federal government and administered by the states. However, because of the federal involvement, all programs must meet national standards for eligibility. States are allowed to define their own eligibility thresholds. The national average for Medicaid eligibility is set at less than 50% of the federal poverty level, which is about $13,000 per year. This means that a family of three with a yearly income of $7,500 may be too rich to be considered eligible for Medicaid support in many states. As a result, the majority of low-income people are not eligible. In a 1987 survey (which remains the best data source), 47.5% of individuals or families with incomes below the poverty level were reportedly uninsured. The situation was not much better for people between the poverty line and 125% of poverty (between about $11,000 and $13,750 in 1990 dollars). Among this group, about 45% had no source of health insurance (Short, 1990).

Medicaid decides on eligibility by category. For example, Congressional action in the 1980s required Medicaid coverage for pregnant women with incomes below 133% of the federal poverty level (states could also elect to use 185%). Governors of 49 states have asked Congress to cease requesting special coverage because states simply do not have the money to expand services. Current policies sometimes seem counterproductive. For example, all states now provide Medicaid coverage for pregnant women, yet a nonpregnant low-income woman without children does not fit any category to receive coverage. Thus, for many low-income women, the only way to obtain health insurance is to become pregnant. Furthermore, states are required to provide Medicaid for low-income families that receive financial support for dependent children born after September 30, 1993. Thus, a family may get coverage for young children but may be denied services for adolescents. For some low-income adolescents, incarceration in a correctional facility or participation in a federally funded program such as the Job Corps provides a first opportunity for comprehensive health care.

Medicaid and Adolescents

The Medicaid program actually has opportunities to exclude adolescents. Federal policies require states to provide Medicaid for all pregnant women and for children under the age of 6 if family income is below 133% of the federal poverty level. New rules, enacted in 1988 and 1989, permitted states to provide Medicaid funding up to 100% of the poverty level for children older than 6 years if they were born after September 30, 1983. By 2002, this will include all children under the age of 19 from families with incomes up to the federal poverty level. For now, though, adolescents born before September 30, 1983 are not covered in many states. In other words, adolescents as of the time of this writing are not covered under Medicaid. States have the option of covering pregnant women and infants up to 1 year of age if women's incomes are 185% of the federal poverty level or below. Rich states typically offer this program but poor states do not.

The Medicaid programs must provide mandatory coverage for the aged, blind, disabled families receiving aid to families with dependent children, and pregnant women with children under 6 years of age. The programs have the option of covering medically needy children and adolescents up to age 18 years. The difficulty is that the states often cannot afford this coverage. California, for example, has traditionally had one of the most generous Medicaid programs (Medicaid is called *MediCal* in California). The MediCal program tripled in cost between 1988 and 1995. By 1993, an estimated 5 million people—one in six California citizens—received MediCal. Currently, the cost of the MediCal program is about 25% of the state general fund. The costs of the program grew over $800 million in 1992 alone (Kaplan, 1993).

In recent years, the Medicaid program has been severely strained. In 1995, Medicaid is expected to serve about 36 million people. This is up from about 22 million served in 1988. The Medicaid program is particularly relevant to adolescents from minority populations. Increasingly, Medicaid is the safety net for low-income persons. However, the program covers only 58% of poor Americans. About half of all people enrolled in Medicaid are children or adolescents. An estimated one in four children or adolescents in the United States are currently covered by Medicaid. However, twice this many may be in need of coverage (Kaiser Commission on the Future of Medicaid, 1995).

In the coming years, it is almost certain that Medicaid will face serious problems. The Clinton administration proposed that the growth in the expected costs of Medicaid be reduced by $55 billion over 7 years. However, recent budgets passed in the U.S. House of Representatives and Senate have called for cutting Medicaid spending growth by $182 billion during the same period. This would represent nearly a 19% reduction in projected expenses (Newachek, Hughes, et al., 1995).

The Congressional proposal for cutting Medicaid spending gives states more discretion in making cuts. The group most likely to be adversely affected by cuts is minority youth, because Medicaid is the primary source of health care funding for low-income children. Data show that this category of children continues to grow at a fast pace: The number of children living below the poverty line grew by over 2 million between 1988 and 1992 (Newachek, Hughes, & Cistneras, 1995). Such growth in the face of proposed Congressional cuts is of major concern, because the burden of illness disproportionately falls on poor children and adolescents from underrepresented groups who have low family incomes. Clinical studies (e.g., Newachek, Hughes, & Cistneras, 1995) have shown that these children and adolescents are more likely to have vision and hearing problems, dental problems, speech defects, sickle cell disease, anemia, skin problems, high blood pressure, and hyperactivity.

To keep Medicaid costs down, the only alternatives are for providers to refuse service to individuals in the optional groups (i.e., adolescents) or to refuse coverage for some services. Most states have been reluctant to deny services to those who gain eligibility for the program. In other words, once enrolled in the Medicaid programs, individuals receive the full range of services. However, some of these services, such as antibiotic treatments for the common cold, may provide little benefit. Furthermore, for obvious reasons, it is difficult to justify denying services to blind and disabled people. Thus, when cuts are necessary, healthy adolescents from low-income families are a convenient target.

To qualify for Medicaid, a family with dependent children must have a low enough income to be medically needy. The definition of *medically needy* varies by state. For example, in 1992, Tennessee defined a family as medically needy if a family of three people were subsisting on less than $250 per month ($3,000 per year), whereas California defined the medically needy as those making $934 per month ($11,208 per year). In Tennessee, then, a family of three making $4,000 per year is too wealthy to receive full Medicaid benefits. If they have additional resources, they have to "spend down" in order to be eligible for the program. For example, if the family made $350 per month and they had $200 of medical bills, they would have to pay the first $100 out of pocket before they would be eligible to have Medicaid cover the additional expenses. Differentials across states have made migration to more accommodating states attractive. California Governor Pete Wilson has argued in public political speeches that many low-income families have moved to California because its benefits are so much more attractive.

A common misunderstanding is that most Medicaid costs are attributed to low-income families. In fact, the increase in Medicaid costs are primarily attributable to growth in services for aged and disabled people. Figure 2 shows the increases in the costs of the Medicaid program between 1975 and 1991 for three groups: aged people, disabled people, and children. As Medicaid has assumed more responsibility for older people and those with disabilities, a smaller portion of the total Medicaid budget has been made available for children and adolescents. Efforts to balance the federal budget by early in the 21st century almost certainly mean that Medicaid will encounter major cuts. It might be argued that expenditures on healthy adolescents take resources away from those who are truly medically needy. Federal Medicaid policy requires that some services be offered to all recipients, but other services are optional, and whole categories of service might therefore be eliminated. Optional services include in-patient psychiatric care for those under 21 years of age or nursing home care for those under 21 years of age. Services offered by practitioners who are not MDs (psychologists, social workers, optometrists, and so on) are also in the optional category. Furthermore, nonbasic services for pregnant women are optional, including needs assessment, case management, and nutritional counseling. As Medicaid costs have escalated from providing services for older and disabled people, programs have had difficulty limiting costs. As budgets have tightened, most programs have looked closely at eliminating optional categories or at redefining eligibility.

It is clear that current Medicaid policy has failed. In particular, it has failed adolescents, because they are among the most likely to be ignored under budgetary pressure. Some think that costs are avoided

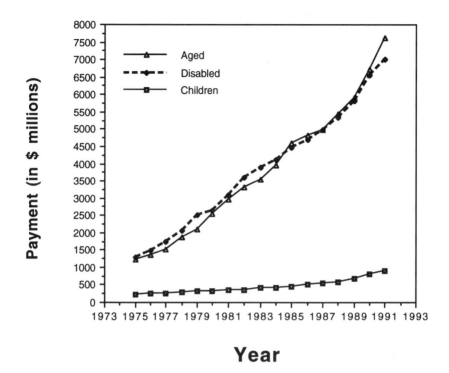

Figure 2. Medicaid payments by beneficiary group, 1975–1991 (U.S. Department of Commerce, 1991). Data are from the Congressional Research Service and are in the public domain.

by denying services to low-income adolescents and their families. However, this will result in costs being shifted rather than saved. We address these cost-shifting issues in the next part of the chapter.

Cost Shifting

Some members of U.S. society feel that we should not care about the uninsured. They believe that the uninsured are typically poor people who do not take care of themselves and that their failure to plan should not be our problem. However, it is not necessarily true that people without insurance do not get care. In fact, they do get health care by going to emergency rooms, and they are often unable to pay for these services. When a patient is unable to pay, the hospital still has to reimburse its nurses, support its pathology labs, and so forth;

someone also has to pay for the surgeons and for the other physicians (Eddy, 1994).

It is also not necessarily true that patients who are uninsured get free care. In fact, the costs are just shifted. When an uninsured patient comes to the hospital and cannot pay, his or her charges are shifted to insured patients through increased costs of care. When the insured patients get charged, insurance rates go up. As a result of this series of shifts, charges in fancy suburban clinics, where most patients are insured, may be lower than they are in inner-city hospitals, where a high percentage of patients are uninsured. The reason is that the people who are able to pay in inner-city hospitals are subsidizing a larger number of patients who are uninsured. A corollary is that insurance rates should be higher in areas of the country where there are high rates of people who are medically uninsured. In fact, this seems to be true. For example, in cities such as Los Angeles and Miami, many people have no medical insurance. As a result charges to businesses for health insurance are higher than in such cities as Minneapolis and Seattle, where the percentages of people without insurance are lower (Kaplan, 1993).

In summary, cost shifting resulting from caring for uninsured patients suggests that costs are not avoided but, instead, are just charged to someone else. Uninsured people obtain services in a costly way because they are often more seriously ill at entry to the system, and they are cared for inefficiently through emergency rooms. Examination of alternative health care systems in the United States illustrates possible solutions to these problems. In Hawaii, for example, providing universal coverage has actually decreased health care costs (Lewin & Sybinsky, 1993). In Oregon, an innovative experiment has greatly expanded the availability of Medicaid services by excluding payment for ineffective services. In this case, savings from denial of payment for ineffective services were used to increase the number of people covered under the program, which resulted in increased access to care for adolescent minorities. Furthermore, it opened the door for the inclusion of psychological and substance abuse services for adolescents (Kaplan, 1993).

Case Examples

In the preceding sections, we have focused on reviewing medical policies. However, public policy relevant to adolescent health goes far beyond funding for health services. The remainder of this chapter is therefore devoted to consideration of policy case studies. Our first example concerns a medical practice policy and the second a legislative and legal policy. Both examples involve attempts to improve the health status of minority adolescents, but each addresses the problem from a different perspective.

Medical Case Example: Hepatitis B Immunization

Public financing choices, such as Medicaid, are among the most difficult and complex policies. Another level of policy involves recommendations for clinical care. With the right endorsements, clinical guidelines can become the standard of care and can be used as the basis of practice in managed care or for guidelines for reimbursing providers. When composed properly, the guidelines are based on the best available scientific and clinical data. However, there are often disagreements about what constitutes the best standard of care. One such debate concerns the prevention of hepatitis B in adolescents.

Deaths from childhood illnesses have decreased remarkably during the twentieth century. To a large extent, decline in childhood illness can be attributed to successful public health immunization campaigns. To many traditional biomedical practitioners, vaccines are the core of the prevention program. Today, infants receive between 13 and 15 immunizations for such diseases as polio, diphtheria, pertussis, tetanus, influenza, measles, mumps, and rubella. All of these diseases affect young children, and there is significant justification for policies that require vaccination of young children. Furthermore, those who have not been vaccinated during childhood may be afflicted with these diseases during adulthood.

Vaccinating newborns is a desirable policy for several reasons. First, it protects children from these diseases early in life. Second, early childhood is a time during which most children are exposed to the health care system. Parents are highly motivated and programs, including Medicaid, require coverage for young children. Immunizations for adolescents are more difficult. Adolescents may be unwilling to get injections, and significant numbers of adolescents are not covered by standard health insurance policies. Until recently, few immunization programs required the first inoculation during adolescence. However, several issues were raised by the development of a vaccine for hepatitis B.

Hepatitis B virus is a serious illness that can cause death in about 5% of cases. Only about 10% of infections occur in infants and young children, but the risk increases sharply during adolescent years. Furthermore, minority youth are at a significantly higher risk than are nonminority youth. Hepatitis B is spread through exposure to bodily fluids, including blood and semen. A vaccine against hepatitis B virus became available in the mid-1980s, and so the disease can be significantly reduced by vaccinating sexually active people. Thus, it has been recommended that adolescents be inoculated against hepatitis B prior to their initiation of sexual activity.

The dilemma is that many adolescents do not see their doctors on a regular basis during early or midadolescent years. Even when visits occur, they are often brief and do not include discussions about prevention issues. Visits are particularly rare for minority adolescents. As a result, many adolescents initiate sexual activity without the protection of the vaccine for hepatitis. The CDC recommended that the vaccine be given at birth in order to provide adequate protection (Cassidy & Mahoney, 1995). Shortly thereafter, the American Academy of Pediatrics and the American Academy of Family Physicians concurred, suggesting that all newborns be given three injections of the vaccine. The rationale for inoculating newborns rather than adolescents was that teenagers are difficult to immunize and that children should be vaccinated for as much as possible whenever they are available. In one analysis, Margolis et al. (1995) suggested that the 5% lifetime risk of hepatitis B virus could be reduced by 68% with infant inoculation programs.

The hepatitis B vaccine policy was recently examined by Ganiats, Bowersox, and Ralph (1993), who challenged the notion of early inoculation on a variety of grounds. There is no question that hepatitis B is a serious public health problem: An estimated 300 million people in the world are now believed to be infected (Lawrence & Goldstein, 1995). The disease is contagious, and those infected have a 5%–10% chance of developing chronic hepatitis. People with chronic hepatitis have 100 times the risk of developing liver cancer (DiBisceglie, 1989). Yet, even though hepatitis B is largely preventable and disproportionately affects minority communities, public health officials have not launched major campaigns for vaccination programs (Francis, 1995).

Despite the seriousness of hepatitis B, the lifetime risk of acquiring it is only about 5% (Immunization Practices Advisory Committee, 1991), and up to 70% of the cases occur in high-risk populations (Alter et al., 1990; Lawrence & Goldstein, 1995). Furthermore, the disease is very rare among children under the age of 10. Although there are no known risks of initiating the immunization after age 10, there has been evidence that providing too many inoculations to young children may suppress their immune reaction. In other words, adding an additional vaccine to an infant's already crowded schedule may render the vaccine less useful during a child's lifetime (Ganiats et al., 1993).

A third argument for delaying immunization is that the vaccine may lose its effectiveness over the course of time. Studies have shown that the immunization is about 90% effective in the short term and loses potency over time (Immunization Practices Advisory Committee, 1991). In fact, by 10 years following immunization, there is little evidence of its effectiveness. Therefore, for the vaccine to be useful at the time adolescents who are inoculated in infancy begin gaining exposure to hepatitis B, boosters may be needed.

Perhaps the most important issues in developing the strategy for the prevention of hepatitis B are based in behavior. There is concern that vaccination programs will be unacceptable to adolescents, parents, and physicians. The adolescent may be concerned about getting a shot, whereas, for parents, the vaccination program may symbolically represent preparation for the initiation of sexual activity. Ganiats et al. (1993) have offered several policy suggestions for implementing vaccination programs for adolescents. Vaccination programs for younger children have been successful because vaccination records are often required for enrollment in kindergarten. Similarly, documentation of hepatitis B vaccine might be used as a requirement for getting a driver's license or for enrollment in the ninth grade. Another alternative would be to base the immunization program in schools. The CDC is currently sponsoring several school-based demonstration projects in various cities. One recent study found that, if parents were supportive of the vaccines, they could positively influence acceptance of the vaccine by their teenage children (Rosenthal, Kottenhahn, Biro, & Succop, 1995). In British Columbia, the vaccine was offered to all sixth-grade students in one community. Analysis of the program showed that, among over 43,000 students, 95% participated. Adverse reactions to the vaccine were rare, and the program did not result in increased absenteeism or physician visits. Among students who received the series of injections, 98% showed active antibodies to the hepatitis B surface antigen (Dobson, Scheifele, & Bell, 1995). School-based programs may be less expensive and more acceptable to students, and there is growing evidence that such programs can be successfully implemented in middle schools (Cassidy & Mahoney, 1995). The program could be tied to administration of tetanus and rubella booster shots, which would increase compliance and reduce costs. However, analysis is still unavailable to suggest which grade level will have the greatest compliance. Reimbursement is also an issue because, under capitated payment systems, providers must pay for the new vaccines. Not all insurance companies have built payment for hepatitis B vaccine into their fee structures. When new vaccines for other illnesses are developed (for example a vaccine for chicken pox), providers are often required to absorb the cost. Thus, separation of vaccination from traditional office visits may be of value. For a variety of reasons, school-based programs may be most advisable, because current approaches are more likely to leave minority adolescents unprotected even though they are at highest risk.

Health policy goes beyond rules for reimbursing or providing clinical care. Many public policies are designed to promote population health status but have little to do with health care providers. In the following sections, we offer an example of efforts to control tobacco use.

Legislative and Legal Policy Example: Tobacco Advertising

Although few adolescents die of chronic diseases, the risks for many diseases of adulthood begin during the second decade of life. Tobacco use is an important example. Cigarette smoking remains the greatest single cause of preventable death in contemporary U.S. society. The health consequences of smoking cigarettes has been documented in literally thousands of studies (e.g., Kaplan, Orleans, Perkins, & Pierce, 1995). Although there has been some decline in cigarette use in the United States, the worldwide trend is in the opposite direction.

It has been estimated that there will be 10 million tobacco-related deaths in the world by the Year 2010 (Peto, Lopez, Boreham, Thun, & Heath, 1992). In the United States, tobacco use has been estimated to be responsible for 434,000 adult deaths each year (McGinnis & Foege, 1993). By comparison, motor vehicle crashes and illicit drug use are relatively minor problems. Tobacco use causes 20 times as many deaths as other drug use and 16 times as many deaths as motor vehicle crashes. Despite societal concern about homicide, tobacco use causes 15 deaths for every 1 death by murder. Tobacco use most directly affects health outcomes for pregnant women. It has been estimated that 17%–26% of low-birth-weight deliveries are associated with maternal tobacco use and that 5%–6% of prenatal deaths can be traced to smoking by the mother (U.S. Surgeon General, 1989).

Tobacco regulation. Recently, the Society of Behavioral Medicine issued a policy statement directed toward the regulation and control of tobacco products (Kaplan et al., 1995). Similarly, the Society of Adolescent Medicine, the American Psychological Association, the American Lung Association, the American Heart Association, and the American Cancer Society have all argued for policies that would require greater regulation of tobacco products. Regulation of tobacco products is supported by a variety of different arguments. Perhaps the most important argument is that cigarettes are not considered to be drugs, and so, cigarettes and other tobacco products are not regulated by the Federal Food and Drug Administration (FDA). The FDA has broad authority to regulate drugs. Other pharmaceuticals must be shown to be safe and efficacious, and there are strict limits on the distribution and marketing of these controlled substances. Under the Food, Drug, and Cosmetic Act, the FDA must certify that drugs are safe. The evidence that cigarettes are unsafe is overwhelming. Indeed, scientific evidence suggests that tobacco is the most dangerous product on the consumer market (U.S. Department of Health and Human Services, 1988, 1989, 1990). There is extensive evidence that cigarettes are addicting and that they function much like pharmaceutical agents (Kaplan et al., 1995). Yet cigarettes and other tobacco products clearly do not meet the safety and efficacy requirements required of other drugs. If tobacco was to be classified as a drug, and cigarettes needed to withstand the same safety requirements as other drugs, then they almost certainly would be eliminated from the market. The evidence for the addictive nature of tobacco products has been reviewed elsewhere (Kaplan et al., 1995). In this chapter, we consider the more difficult problem of the regulation of tobacco advertising.

Tobacco regulation for adolescents and youth. The regulation of tobacco advertising is particularly important for adolescent health because virtually all smokers initiate the habit during youth. Estimates have suggested that approximately 3,000 adolescents start smoking each day (Pierce, 1991). The number of adults age 20 years or older who begin smoking has declined in recent years (L. L. Lee, Gilpin, & Pierce, 1993). Today, it is extremely rare that the tobacco habit is initiated during adulthood. More than 90% of all smokers started when they were teenagers, and many initiated the habit before the age of 16 (Gilpin, Lee, Evans, & Pierce, 1994).

Public statements by both the tobacco industry and public policy makers emphasize that cigarettes should not be marketed to youth. Thus, most states have a legal age for cigarette purchases, and these policies have been in effect throughout the twentieth century. Nevertheless, studies repeatedly demonstrate that adolescents can easily obtain cigarettes in supermarkets, from vending machines, and in other locations (U.S. Department of Health and Human Services, 1990). The tobacco industry needs to recruit new smokers to replace the 3,000 smokers who die or quit every day. Because few people start smoking during adulthood, these new smokers must be recruited almost exclusively from people in their adolescent years. An industry policy of advertising to minors would be unacceptable on moral and ethical grounds. The tobacco industry denies such a policy, and their intent must be inferred from other evidence.

Several studies have documented the role of advertising in attracting adolescents who are below the legal age to purchase cigarettes (DiFranza & Brown, 1992; DiFranza et al., 1991; Fischer, Schwartz, Richards, Goldstein, & Rojas, 1991). Other evidence supports the argument that tobacco advertising is targeted at minors. For example, a major survey of tobacco use in California demonstrated that adolescents are significantly more likely to report having a favorite cigarette advertisement than people in other age groups (Pierce et al., 1991). The R. J. Reynolds Company spent over $100 million on the Joe Camel campaign in the 1990. The Joe Camel ad was featured on billboards and was commonly displayed in media that are most available to youths. A large study in California demonstrated that the Joe Camel character was particularly attractive to children and adolescents and less recognized by adults (Pierce et al., 1991). The study involved telephone interviews with 24,296 adults and 5,040 adolescents contacted by using a random-digit-dialing method. Respondents were asked if they smoked cigarettes and, if so, what brand they smoked. In addition, they were asked what brand they had seen advertised on billboards. Both adults and adolescents identified Marlboro as the most advertised brand of cigarettes. The Camel brand, however, was noted by 28.5% of the adolescents in contrast to 13.7% of the adults. Furthermore, the 12- and 13-year-old respondents identified Camel as the most advertised brand. Among adolescents smoking cigarettes, Camel was the most preferred cigarette by 12- and 13-year-olds. With advancing age, fewer adolescents chose Camel as their preferred brand (Pierce et al., 1991). Other studies have confirmed that younger children have been attracted by the Joe Camel campaign. A study by DiFranza et al. (1991) suggested that Joe Camel was recognized more often than Mickey Mouse by 6-year-olds. Even an industry study designed to refute these findings confirmed that Joe Camel was recognized by two thirds of those 6 years of age (Catanoso, 1993).

It is impossible to prove that the tobacco industry systematically targets youth in their advertising. However, several lines of evidence converge to suggest that marketing efforts do, indeed, focus on adolescents. For example, there is circumstantial evidence indicating that tobacco use in adolescents follows intense investments in tobacco advertising. One of the most interesting analyses concerns the Virginia Slims campaign, which attempted to increase cigarette use among young women. The campaign, created by the Philip Morris Company, targeted younger women by using such phrases as "You have come a long way, baby." In an attempt to study the influence of the campaign, Pierce, Lee, and Gilpin (1994) used data from the National Health Interview Study for the years 1970, 1978, 1979, 1980, 1987, and 1988. Each of these surveys asked if the respondents had ever smoked cigarettes. Among those who had smoked at least 100 cigarettes in their lifetime, respondents were asked how old they were when they started smoking cigarettes fairly regularly. The respondents were between the ages of 20 and 50 at the times the surveys were conducted. By using data from more than 100,000 people, it was possible for researchers to estimate the year that respondents began smoking cigarettes. Figure 3 shows the smoking initiation rates among 16-year-old females between the calendar years of 1944 and 1988. As the figure suggests, smoking initiation among teenage females peaked around 1967. This is precisely the year that the Virginia Slims campaign was conducted. In other words, the data provide circumstantial evidence that the campaign directed toward young females successfully initiated this target audience as cigarette smokers.

Supporting a total ban. The First Amendment to the U.S. Constitution guarantees freedom of speech. However, not all speech is protected. In the case of *Virginia State Board of Pharmacy v. Virginia Citizens Consumer Council* (1976), the Supreme Court noted that some advertising comes under the category of commercial speech. *Commercial speech* was defined as "expression related solely to the economic interests of the speaker and its audience." Defining cigarette advertising

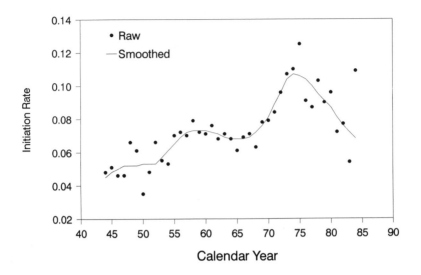

Figure 3.   Smoothed (line) and raw (points) smoking initiation rates among 16-year-old girls, 1940–1984. (From Gilpin et al., 1994 permission required). From "Smoking Initiation by Adolescent Girls, 1944 Through 1988: An Association With Targeted Advertising," by J. P. Pierce, L. Lee, & E. A. Gilpin, 1994, *Journal of the American Medical Association, 271*, pp. 610–611. Reprinted with permission.

as commercial speech allowed the Supreme Court to uphold a ban on advertising in the electronic media (Gostin & Brandt, 1993). However, the court later changed its position to allow commercial speech limited protection under the First Amendment. This gave legislatures greater leeway in the regulation of advertising for dangerous products such as cigarettes (Ile & Kroll, 1990).

There are several reasons why a total ban on tobacco advertising may benefit society. There would be a substantial public health benefit resulting from an advertising ban and significant implications with regard to taxpayer expenses. Furthermore, the evidence is compelling that tobacco advertising is directed toward individuals younger than the legal age for consent. Therefore, we believe, a total ban on tobacco advertising would be in the interest of adolescents and all members of society (Kaplan et al., 1995).

Summary and Conclusions

Adolescent medicine is a broad field. Most effort has been devoted to clinical diagnosis and treatment, with the intended goals being to improve health outcomes. However, the goal of improving adolescent health status can be achieved in several ways. In this chapter, we have discussed a selected set of policy interventions to improve the health status of adolescents. These range from structural change of reimbursement under a state Medicaid program to efforts for reducing the use of tobacco among youth.

Policy proposals can take different forms and can be developed by different groups. The examples reviewed in this chapter include federal and state policy (Medicaid), policies of health care practitioners (with regard to hepatitis B vaccine), and statutory regulation (tobacco advertising). To be truly effective, public policy should have a strong empirical base. We therefore encourage more research that will provide the justification for future policy approaches to the problems of minority adolescents.

REFERENCES

Alter, M. J., Hadler, S. C., Judson, F. N., Mares, A., Alexander, W. J., Hu, P. Y., Miller, J. K., Moyer, L. A., Fields, H. A., & Bradley, D. W. (1990). Risk factors for acute non-A, non-B hepatitis in the United States and association with hepatitis C virus infection. *Journal of the American Medical Association, 264,* 2231–2235.

American Medical Association. (1992). *Guidelines for adolescent preventive services.* Chicago: Author.

Bloom, B. (1990). Health insurance and medical care: Health of our nation's children: United States, 1988. Hyattsville, MD: National Center for Health Statistics.

Cassidy, W. M., & Mahoney, R. J. (1995). A hepatitis B vaccination program targeting adolescents. *Journal of Adolescent Health, 17,* 244–247.

Catanoso, J. (1993, April 14). Old Joe's influence inflated, study says. *Greensboro News and Record,* p. A6.

Centers for Disease Control and Prevention. (1995). Update: AIDS among women: United States, 1994. *Morbidity and Mortality Weekly Report, 10*(44), 81–84.

Chollet, D., Folley, J., & Mages, C. (1990). *Uninsured in the United States: The non-elderly population without health insurance, 1988.* Washington, DC: Employee Benefit Research Institute.

DiBisceglie, A. M. (1989). Hepatocellular carcinoma: Molecular biology of its growth and relationship to hepatitis B virus infection. *Medical Clinics of North America, 73,* 985–997.

DiClemente, R. J., & Wingood, G. M. (1995). A randomized controlled trial of an HIV sexual risk-reduction intervention for young African-American women. *Journal of the American Medical Association, 274,* 1271–1276.

DiFranza, J. R., & Brown, L. J. (1992). The Tobacco Institute's "It's the Law" campaign: Has it halted illegal sales of tobacco to children? *American Journal of Public Health, 82,* 1271–1273.

DiFranza, J. R., Richards, J. W., Paulman, P. M., Wolf-Gillespie, N., Fletcher, C., Jaffe, R. D., & Murray, D. (1991). RJR Nabisco's cartoon camel promotes Camel cigarettes to children. *Journal of the American Medical Association, 266,* 3149–3153.

Dobson, S., Scheifele, D., & Bell, A. (1995). Assessment of a universal, school-based hepatitis B vaccination program. *Journal of the American Medical Association, 274,* 1209–1213.

Eddy, D. M. (1994). Clinical decision making: From theory to practice. Rationing resources while improving quality. How to get more for less. *Journal of the American Medical Association, 272,* 817–824.

Fischer, P. M., Schwartz, M. P., Richards, J. W., Jr., Goldstein, A. O., & Rojas, T. H. (1991). Brand logo recognition by children aged 3 to 6 years. Mickey Mouse and old Joe the camel. *Journal of the American Medical Association, 266,* 3145–3148.

Francis, D. P. (1995). The public's health unprotected: Reversing a decade of underutilization of hepatitis B vaccine [Editorial comment]. *Journal of the American Medical Association, 274,* 1242–1243.

Ganiats, T. G., Bowersox, M. T., & Ralph, L. P. (1993). Universal neonatal hepatitis B immunization: Are we jumping on the bandwagon too early? *Journal of Family Practice, 36,* 147–149.

Gilpin, E. A., Lee, L., Evans, N., & Pierce, J. P. (1994). Smoking initiation rates in adults and minors: United States, 1944–1988. *American Journal of Epidemiology, 140,* 535–543.

Gostin, L. O., & Brandt, A. M. (1993). Criteria for evaluating a ban on the advertisement of cigarettes. Balancing public health benefits with constitutional burdens. *Journal of the American Medical Association, 269,* 904–909.

Ickovics, J. R., & Rodin, J. (1992). Women and AIDS in the United States: Epidemiology, natural history, and mediating mechanisms. *Health Psychology, 11,* 1–16.

Ile, M. L., & Kroll, L. A. (1990). From the Office of the General Counsel: Tobacco advertising and the first amendment. *Journal of the American Medical Association, 264,* 1593–1594.

Immunization Practices Advisory Committee. (1991). Hepatitis B virus: A comprehensive strategy for eliminating transmission in the United States through universal childhood vaccination. *Morbidity and Mortality Weekly Report, 40,* 1–8.

Kaiser Commission on the Future of Medicaid. (1995, April). *Health needs and Medicaid financing: State facts.* Washington, DC: Author.

Kaplan, R. M. (1993). *Hippocratic predicament: Affordability, access, and accountability in health care.* San Diego, CA: Academic Press.

Kaplan, R. M., Orleans, C. T., Perkins, K. A., & Pierce, J. P. (1995). Marshaling the evidence for greater regulation and control of tobacco products: A call for action. *Annals of Behavioral Medicine, 17,* 3–14.

Lawrence, M. H., & Goldstein, M. A. (1995). Hepatitis B immunization in adolescents. *Journal of Adolescent Health, 17,* 234–243.

Lee, L. L., Gilpin, E. A., & Pierce, J. P. (1993). Changes in the patterns of initiation of cigarette smoking in the United States: 1950, 1965, and 1980. *Cancer Epidemiology Biomarkers and Prevention, 2,* 593–597.

Lee, P. R., & Estes, C. L. (1990). *The nation's health* (3rd ed.). Boston, MA: Jones and Bartlett.

Lewin, J. C., & Sybinsky, P. A . (1993). Hawaii's employer mandate and its contribution to universal access. *Journal of the American Medical Association, 269,* 2538–2543.

Margolis, H. S., Coleman, P. J., Brown, R. E., Mast, E. E., Sheingold, S. H., & Arevalo, J. A. (1995). Prevention of hepatitis B virus transmission by immunization: An economic analysis of current recommendations. *Journal of the American Medical Association, 274,* 1201–1208.

McGinnis, J. M., & Foege, W. H. (1993). Actual causes of death in the United States. *Journal of the American Medical Association, 270,* 2207–2212.

Nelson, C., & Short, K. (1990). *Health insurance coverage, 1986–1988* (Current Population Reports, Household Economic Studies Series No. 17). Washington, DC: U.S. Department of the Census.

Newachek, P. W., Hughes, D. C., & Cisternas, M. (1995). Children and health insurance: An overview of recent trends. *Health Affairs, 14,* 244–254.

Newachek, P. W., Hughes, D. C., English, A., Fox, H. B., Perrin, J., & Halfon, N. (1995). The effect on children of curtailing Medicaid spending. *Journal of the American Medical Association, 274,* 1468–1471.

Peto, R., Lopez, A. D., Boreham, J., Thun, M., & Heath, C., Jr. (1992). Mortality from tobacco in developed countries: Indirect estimation from national vital statistics. *Lancet, 339,* 1268–1278.

Pierce, J. P. (1991). Progress and problems in international public health efforts to reduce tobacco useage. *Annual Review of Public Health, 12,* 383–400.

Pierce, J. P., Gilpin, E., Burns, D. M., Whalen, E., Rosbrook, B., Shopland, D., & Johnson, M. (1991). Does tobacco advertising target young people to start smoking? Evidence from California. *Journal of the American Medical Association, 266,* 3154–3158.

Pierce, J. P., Lee, L., & Gilpin, E. A. (1994). Smoking initiation by adolescent girls, 1944 through 1988. An association with targeted advertising. *Journal of the American Medical Association, 271,* 608–611.

Rosenthal, S. L., Kottenhahn, R. K., Biro, F. M., & Succop, P. A. (1995). Hepatitis B vaccine acceptance among adolescents and their parents. *Journal of Adolescent Health, 17,* 248–254.

Short, P. F. (1990). *National medical expenditure survey: Estimates of the uninsured population, Calendar Year 1987: Data Summary 2.* Rockville, MD: National Center for Health Services Research and Health Care Technology Assessment.

Short, P. F., & Banthin, J. S. (1995). New estimates of the uninsured younger than 65 years. *Journal of the American Medical Association, 274,* 1302–1306.

Short, P. F., Monheit, A., & Beauregard, K. (1989). *National medical expenditure survey: A profile of uninsured Americans. Research findings 1.* Rockville, MD: National Center for Health Services Research and Health Care Technology Assessment.

U.S. Department of Health and Human Services. (1988). The health consequences of smoking: Nicotine addiction. Washington, DC: U.S. Government Printing Office.

U.S. Department of Health and Human Services. (1990). *The health benefits of smoking cessation.* Washington, DC: U.S. Government Printing Office.

U.S. Surgeon General. (1989). *Reducing the health consequences of smoking: Twenty-five years of progress.* Rockville, MD: U.S. Department of Health and Human Services and Centers for Disease Control and Prevention.

Virginia State Board of Pharmacy v. Virginia Citizens Consumer Council., 425 U.S. 748, 762 (1976).

Conclusion

This volume has highlighted the special needs and cultural issues that are relevant to understanding health behaviors in minority adolescent populations. Part I of the book provided a conceptual framework for understanding the complex developmental, biological, and sociocultural issues affecting minority youth. Clearly, pubertal maturation has a strong impact on both the emotional and the behavioral development of adolescents and may be particularly instrumental in understanding why minority adolescents engage in high-risk behaviors at such young ages. The psychological, social, and cultural aspects of understanding minority youth were also a focus of this part. The authors have emphasized that scientists and clinicians need to consider a life-course perspective in designing and implementing health-promotion efforts across diverse ethnic groups of adolescents.

Part II outlined the health-compromising and health-promoting behaviors that need to be targeted with effective intervention strategies for minority adolescents. Behaviors related to drug abuse and violence, sexually transmitted diseases, physical activity, diet, and female health issues, as well as health-risk behaviors specific to the development of chronic illness, were all examined. In each chapter of this part, authors emphasized the need for further research across various ethnic groups, particularly with such understudied groups as Asians and Native Americans. Furthermore, these chapters suggested that health-promotion efforts should incorporate a more comprehensive approach in addressing the overlap across health behaviors.

The third part of the book provided an innovative and culturally sensitive review of relevant intervention approaches that are effective in promoting healthy habits among minority adolescents. In particular, chapters in this part suggested that such factors as individual differences in self-efficacy, family, school, and community involvement are all at the heart of establishing integrated and thoughtful intervention strategies. Specifically, the research presented indicates a need to maintain insight into the diverse and unique needs of different ethnic groups. Finally, Part IV of the book addressed the special problems of access and health policy for minority adolescents. Clearly, minority adolescents are at a disadvantage with respect to both of these issues. From a public health perspective, health care access and policies are needed that support the establishment of more healthful behaviors among minority youth.

This book has provided a comprehensive view of minority adolescent health, ranging from basic theoretical issues and clinical interventions to the broader issues of policy. The innovative and culturally appropriate interventions that authors have proposed should assist clinicians and health care providers in improving the quality of life and longevity of culturally diverse groups of adolescents.

Dawn K. Wilson

Author Index

Subject Index

Adolescence, as period of transition, 6

Adolescent (term), 321–322

Adult education programs, 317

Adulthood, transition into, 15–17

Advertising
and adolescent dietary behavior, 141
by tobacco industry (policy case study), 338–342

African American females
body image among adolescent, 143–144
body size of, 145
perceived self-efficacy in adolescent, 162
physical activity in, 111, 114
program promoting, 118–119
pregnancy in adolescent, 158
risky behaviors by adolescent, 190
STD incidence in adolescent, 158, 159
substance use by adolescent, 159, 160
weight-loss program for adolescent, 134

African Americans. *See also* African American females
cardiovascular disease and diabetes in
and modifiable health behaviors, 178–179
and prevalence of risky health behaviors, 185–186, 188–190
caregiving responsibilities of adolescent, 9–10
children, African American
cognitive flexibility in, 14
in poverty, 39
cholesterol levels in, 178
demographics of adolescent, 36

developmental differences in, 8
dietary interventions with, 133, 139–140, 142
school-based programs, 136–137
social support, 135
diet of, 121, 131
diversity among, 33
drug abuse by young
prevalence, 56–57
risk status, 58
generalizability of research on, to other racial/ethnic groups, 30
health care coverage rate for, 328
HIV-prevention programs
community-based program, 283
self-instruction program, 97–99
homicide risk for young, 59
Life Skills Training as drug abuse prevention approach with, 72–73
and Medicaid, 310
multisystemic therapy with, 230–242
client preferences for counselor characteristics in, 232–233
and cultural competence, 237–238
effectiveness of, 230–231
and lack of client cooperation, 236
and minority family structure, 234
misinterpretation of client behavior by therapist in, 231–232
outcome studies, 239–242
and social isolation, 235
and socioecological pressures, 235

About the Editors

Dawn K. Wilson is Assistant Professor of Internal Medicine in the Division of Clinical Pharmacology and Hypertension at the Medical College of Virginia/Virginia Commonwealth University. She received her PhD in social psychology from Vanderbilt University in 1988 and completed a 1-year postdoctoral fellowship on alcohol prevention in the School of Public Health, University of California, Berkeley. She also has been a Fellow at the American Heart Association Seminar on Epidemiology and Prevention of Cardiovascular Diseases in Lake Tahoe, California. In 1992, she received a 5-year Young Investigator Award from the National Institutes of Health's Heart, Lung, and Blood Institute for hypertension prevention in minority adolescents. Dr. Wilson has also served on the Executive Committee boards for both Division 38 (Health Psychology) of the American Psychological Association (APA) and the Society of Behavioral Medicine. She is currently an associate editor for *Mind/Body Medicine*. She has authored numerous scholarly papers and book chapters on health promotion, hypertension prevention, and adolescent health psychology.

James R. Rodrigue is Associate Professor of Clinical and Health Psychology and Director of Child Clinical and Pediatric Psychology Training at the University of Florida Health Science Center. He is also an Affiliate Associate Professor in the Department of Pediatrics and Director of the Family Therapy Clinic in the Department of Clinical and Health Psychology at the University of Florida. Dr. Rodrigue received his PhD in clinical psychology from Memphis State University in 1989 and was a predoctoral intern at the University of Florida Health Science Center. He has authored over 50 articles and chapters on clinical child, pediatric, and health psychology. Professional service activities have included Member-at-Large for the Society of Pediatric Psychology, Chair of the Division 38 (Health Psychology) Committee on Children and Health, member of the APA's Division 12 (Clinical Psychology) Task Force on Diversity in Clinical Psychology, member of the Division 12 Task Force on Innovative Models of Service Delivery in

Clinical Child Psychology, and regional trainer for the HIV Office for Psychology Education Program of APA.

Wendell C. Taylor is Assistant Professor of Behavioral Sciences at the University of Texas–Houston Health Science Center, School of Public Health. He is also Adjunct Assistant Professor in the College of Education Graduate Studies at the University of Houston and Adjunct Assistant Professor in the Communications Department at Texas Southern University. He received his AB from Grinnell College, his MS in psychology from Eastern Washington University, his PhD in social psychology from Arizona State University, and his MPH from the University of Texas–Houston Science Center, School of Public Health, and has also completed a 2-year postdoctoral fellowship in Health Promotion and Health Education at the Center for Health Promotion Research and Development, University of Texas. Dr. Taylor has received outstanding faculty awards and is the principal investigator for research grants from the National Heart, Lung, and Blood Institute, National Cancer Institute, and American Heart Association. His research interests include health promotion in adolescents, health behaviors in underserved communities, and cancer prevention. Taylor has authored and coauthored numerous book chapters and scholarly articles.